T0309163

Brain Tumors: Therapeutics and Management

Brain Tumors: Therapeutics and Management

Editor: Michael Jones

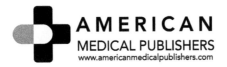

AMERICAN
MEDICAL PUBLISHERS
www.americanmedicalpublishers.com

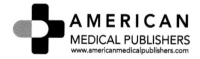

Cataloging-in-publication Data

Brain tumors : therapeutics and management / edited by Michael Jones.
    p. cm.
Includes bibliographical references and index.
ISBN 978-1-63927-944-9
1. Brain--Tumors. 2. Brain--Tumors--Treatment.
3. Brain--Tumors--Diagnosis. I. Jones, Michael.
RD663 .B73 2023
616.994 810 59--dc23

American Medical Publishers,
41 Flatbush Avenue,
1st Floor, New York,
NY 11217, USA

ISBN 978-1-63927-944-9 (Hardback)

This book contains information obtained from authentic and highly regarded sources. Copyright for all individual chapters remain with the respective authors as indicated. All chapters are published with permission under the Creative Commons Attribution License or equivalent. A wide variety of references are listed. Permission and sources are indicated; for detailed attributions, please refer to the permissions page and list of contributors. Reasonable efforts have been made to publish reliable data and information, but the authors, editors and publisher cannot assume any responsibility for the validity of all materials or the consequences of their use.

Trademark Notice: Registered trademark of products or corporate names are used only for explanation and identification without intent to infringe.

Contents

Preface

A brain tumor develops when the cells of brain start growing abnormally within the brain. These brain tumors may be malignant or benign. Primary brain tumors begin within the brain whereas secondary tumors usually spread from cancers outside the brain and are known as brain metastasis tumors. Symptoms of all types of brain tumors vary depending on the size of the tumor, rate of growth of tumor and part of the brain affected. Headaches, seizures, eyesight problems, vomiting, and mental abnormalities are some of the symptoms of brain tumor. Other signs and symptoms include trouble walking, speaking, numbness, or loss of consciousness. Surgery, radiation therapy, and chemotherapy are all options for treating brain tumors. This book includes some of the vital pieces of research works being conducted worldwide with respect to brain tumors. It aims to shed light on some of the unexplored aspects of the brain tumors and their management. Those in search of information to further their knowledge will be greatly assisted by this book.

Significant researches are present in this book. Intensive efforts have been employed by authors to make this book an outstanding discourse. This book contains the enlightening chapters which have been written on the basis of significant researches done by the experts.

Finally, I would also like to thank all the members involved in this book for being a team and meeting all the deadlines for the submission of their respective works. I would also like to thank my friends and family for being supportive in my efforts.

Editor

Systems Biology of Glioblastoma Multiforme

Caroline Agha, Hannah C. Machemehl and
Hassan M. Fathallah-Shaykh

1. Introduction

Gliomas encompass approximately 80% of primary brain malignancies [1]. The five-year survival rate is dependent on the subtype of glioma. According to the Central Brain Tumor Registry there are about 13,000 deaths and 18,000 new cases per year of primary brain cancer in the United States and the overall average annual age-adjusted incidence rate for 2006-2010 for primary brain and CNS tumors was 21.03 per 100,000 [2]. In this chapter, our main focus is glioblastoma (GBM), which is by far the most common and the most malignant of all primary brain tumor [2]. Often described as the most lethal or the most devastating brain tumors, gliomas continue to carry a very poor prognosis at all levels, quantity and quality of life. GBM almost exclusively recurs despite meticulous conventional therapies, including surgical resection, radiation, and chemotherapy and bevacizumab. Despite all advances, the survival rates continue to be low, with a median survival of approximately 15 months in patients with malignant gliomas [3].

The multiple hit theory of cancer speculates that the origin and progression of GBM is the product of complex series of molecular processes like activation of oncogenes and alterations in tumor suppression genes. However, the complexity of the molecular interactions in malignant gliomas imposes a great challenge that indeed has crucial implications on treatment. This cannot be achieved without a meticulous understanding of this multifaceted process and its molecular mechanism, and therefore dictates dissection at systems level. The Cancer Genome Atlas Research Network has sequenced the genome of GBM and deduced that the apparatus of tumor growth and recurrence is the result of complex epigenetic mechanisms and gene interactions [4]. The twenty first century has been referred to as the genomic millennium, thus in an era where genes dictate remedy a comprehensive understanding of the systems biology of gliomas may be a key to the cure. Our goal in this chapter is to touch on the complexity of the molecular networks of GBM by presenting on an overview without delving into details. We will focus on how molecules and pathways are dysregulated in GBM rather than presenting detailed graphs of networks as the latter are readily easily found. To illustrate the clinical relevance of a systems approach to molecular networks, we dissect the case of the use of rapamycin in a GBM clinical trial and discuss the pathogenesis of its adverse effect in causing activation of AKT, an oncogene.

2. Classes of GBM

Malignant gliomas develop as part of a multistep process comprising chronological and collective genetic modifications resulting from core and environmental dynamics. Cowden, Turcot, Li-Fraumeni, neurofibromatosis type 1 and type 2, tuberous sclerosis, and familial schwannomatosis are among the predisposing syndromes for glioblastoma occurrence [15]. From a molecular perspective, malignant gliomas are greatly heterogeneous tumors [14]. In a nutshell, 4 transcriptional subclasses of GBM have been proposed: *classical, mesenchymal, proneural*, and *neural* [1]. The classical type glioblastoma typically exhibits chromosome 7 amplifications, chromosome 10 deletions, *EGFR* amplification, *EGFR* mutations (point and vIII mutations), and *Ink4a/ARF* locus deletion. The mesenchymal subclass shows a high frequency of *NF1* mutation/deletion and high expression of *CHI3L1, MET*, and genes involved in tumor necrosis factor and nuclear factor–κB pathways. Proneural type glioblastoma is characterized by changes of *PDGFRA* and mutations in *IDH1* and *TP53*; these are features common to lower-grade gliomas and secondary GBM. A characteristic feature of the neural subclass of GBM is the expression of neuronal markers.

3. Gliomagenesis

The multiple hit theory of cancer stipulates sequential molecular events leading to GBM. The following is a summary of current ideas. One of the first steps in tumoregenesis is loss of cell cycle control. The cell cycle checkpoint that has been of most interest is the G1-S phase. This important checkpoint is mainly controlled by p16INK4a/cyclin-dependent kinase (CDK)-4/RB (retinoblastoma) 1 pathway, which involves p16, CDK-4, cyclin D1, and RB1[16]. The CDK/cyclin D1 complex phosphorylates RB1 therefore releasing the E2F transcription factor, which in turn activates the genes, involved in the G1/S transition [17]. Subsequent steps in gliomagenesis include the overexpression of growth factors and their receptors. A diverse array of growth factors such as epidermal growth factor receptor (EGFR), platelet-derived growth factor (PDGF), basic fibroblast growth factor (bFGF, FGF-2), transforming growth factor (TGF)-alpha, and insulin-like growth factor (IGF)-1 are overly expressed in glioblastoma [18, 19]. Malignant gliomas are highly vascular tumors; the angiogenic molecule that has been most widely implicated in GBM is vascular endothelial growth factor (VEGF), an endothelial cell mitogenic [20].

Another key event contributing to gliomagenesis is the abolishment of apoptosis, or programmed cell death. Malignant glioma cells, not only divide uncontrollably, but also intentionally lose the ability to undergo apoptosis. *p53*, a key molecule involved in apoptosis, is often mutated during gliomagenesis [21]. An important process contributing to gliomagenesis is genetic instability, which refers to the property that random mutations are introduced in dividing cancer cells because of the loss of check points and the molecular machinery that ensures that the genome is copied faithfully during mitosis [22]. A clinical correlation to genetic instability is the Turcot syndrome [23].

4. Signaling pathways

A large number of signaling pathways exchange information to generate a large molecular network that controls the phenotypes of GBM. A detailed discussion is beyond the scope of this chapter. In this section, we will discuss how the RTK/PI3K/Akt, mTOR, Ras/MEK/MAPK, p53, ATM/Chk2, Rb, and stat3 pathways are affected to GBM. Additional pathways will be briefly discussed in the section on crosstalk.

4.1. RTK/PI3K/Akt pathway

This pathway regulates a range of cellular processes such as proliferation, growth, apoptosis, and cytoskeletal rearrangement. It involves receptor tyrosine kinases (RTKs), like EGFR, PDGFR, and VEGFR, as well as tumor suppressor protein phosphatase (PTEN), and protein kinases PI3K, AKT. Irregular activation of RTK/PI3K/AKT is commonly seen in malignant gliomas [24].

4.1.1. Receptor tyrosine kinases

RTKs relay extracellular signals to activation of intracellular networks through PI3K and AKT. *EGFR* gene amplification is the most widespread alteration present in GBM [25]. The most common is EGFR vIII, which relays ligand independent accumulative growth signals [26, 27]. Some studies have previously shown a correlation between aberrance of EGFR and aggressiveness of tumor and therefore shorter survival [28, 29]. Unfortunately, EGFR inhibitors such as Gefinitib and Erlotinib have not produced promising results in clinical trials of patients with GBM [30, 31]. Overexpression of PDGFR (especially PDGFR-α) and PDGF have been documented in astrocytic tumors irrespective of the grade [32], [33]. *PDGFRA* amplification and *IDH1* mutation are a characteristic of the proneural subtype of GBM implying a possible association of the proneural subtype and secondary GBM [4]. Anti-PDGFR therapy such as imatinib has not been promising either [34].

4.1.2. PI3K–PTEN-AKT signaling

AKT, a serine/threonine kinase that acts to regulate cell growth, proliferation, and apoptosis, is activated in about 80% of human GBMs [35]. PI3K belongs to the family of lipid kinases.

PI3K enzymes produce phosphatidylinositol-3,4,5-trisphosphate (PIP3), a lipid secondary messenger, which is found to be at high levels in cancer cells [36, 37]. Binding of PI3Ks to RTKs results in activation of AKT through PiP3 and PDK1 [38]. Dissecting the PI3K complex, it is composed of a catalytically active protein, p110α, encoded by *PIK3CA*, and a regulatory protein, p85α, encoded by *PIK3R1*. In primary GBM, *PIK3CA* mutations and amplification are seen in about 5% to 13% of cases [39]. Furthermore, *PIK3R1* mutations have been reported in about 10 % in GBM patients [4].

PTEN (phosphatase and tensin homologue, located on chromosome 10) is a tumor suppressor gene. PTEN mutations are associated with several types of cancer including GBM. Loss of heterozygosity of chromosome 10, which causes deletions or mutations of PTEN, is a common event in GBMs. PTEN negatively regulates the PI3K/AKT/PKB pathway by blocking AKT signaling via the reduction of intracellular levels of PIP3. Furthermore, lower PTEN activity induces activation of the RTKs/PI3K/AKT pathway. This is due to the negative inhibition accomplished by PTEN antagonizing PIK3 [40]. GBMs typically harbor diminished expression of PTEN through homozygous deletion or mutations of PTEN, which contributes the activation of the RTKs/PI3K/Akt pathway [4, 41, 42]. Mesenchymal and classical types of GBM exhibit loss of PTEN (www.cbtrus.org). It is noteworthy that GBM cells expressing EGFRvIII with an intact PTEN appear to have a higher response rate to EGFR inhibitors [35, 43].

4.2. mTOR

Signaling through mTOR is mediated by two independent complexes, mTORC1 and mTORC2. mTORC2 is activated by growth factors and ribosomes and in turn activates AKT among other kinases via phosphorylation [44]. mTORC1 controls cellular metabolism, biosynthesis, stress, and by several growth factors such as EGF and its receptor, EGFR [45]. In settings promoting cell growth, mTORC1 phosphorylates substrates to stimulate anabolic processes such as ribosome biogenesis, translation, and synthesis of lipids and nucleotides and to abolish catabolic processes such as autophagy [45]. Likewise, mTORC2 promotes cancer growth by stimulating glucose uptake via activation of AKT and activating serum/glucocorticoid regulated kinase (SGK), which contributes to proliferation and survival [46]. Inhibitors of mTOR, like rapamycin, sirolimus, temsirolimus, everolimus have not shown efficacy in GBM [47, 48]. In fact, inhibitors of mTOR lead to elevated expression and activity of growth factor receptors, which increases PI3K activity and RAS signaling. Below we discuss the effects of rapamycin on the mTOR pathway in detail.

4.3. Ras/MAPK pathway

The 3 components of the human Ras genes (Rat Sarcoma) are transmuting oncogenes and include: H-Ras, N-Ras, and K-Ras. Ras is a member of the G protein family, which basically means that it is activated by binding to guanosine triphosphate (GTP), and deactivated by binding to guanosine diphosphate (GDP) [49]. Ras serves to activate serine tyrosine kinases (STK) including Raf, MAPK (ERK1 and ERK2), PI3K, among other proteins that influence cell proliferation, differentiation, and survival [50]. Although the mutual activation of Ras and AKT in neural progenitors contributes to gliomagenesis in mouse models [51], Ras mutations are uncommon in human GBM [4]. Activated Raf phosphorylates and activates MAPK kinase (MAPKK), also called MEK, which in turn phosphorylates and activates MAPK [52, 53][54], which then moves to the nucleus to induce other transcription factors including Elk1, c-myc, Ets, STAT (signal transducers and activators of transcription), and PPARγ (peroxisome proliferator-activated receptor γ), which induce cell cycle progression and anti-apoptosis genes [50, 55].

NF-1, a tumor suppressor gene encoding neurofibromin, negatively regulates Ras and influences adenylate cyclase- and AKT-mTOR-mediated pathways [56]. NF-1 mutation and homozygous deletions are detected in 18% of GBM [4]. Mesenchymal type GBM appears to respond to concomitant chemo-radiation therapy and happens to commonly have inactivation of the NF-1 (37%), p53 (32%), and PTEN genes [57].

4.4. The p53 pathway

The *p53* gene, labeled as the "guardian of the genome", is located at chromosome 17q13.1 and encodes a protein that takes action against miscellaneous cellular stresses to regulate the corresponding genes that provoke programmed cell death or apoptosis, cell differentiation, senescence, DNA repair, and neovascularization [58]. The p53 pathway is the most frequently mutated pathway in human cancer and is essentially disrupted in roughly 80% of high-grade gliomas. p53, activated in response to DNA damage, induces transcription of genes such as p21Waf1/Cip1 that arrest the cell cycle progression at the G1 phase [59].

An important regulator of the p53 pathway is MDM2, an E3 ubiquitin ligase that negatively modulates p53 through transcriptional inhibition by direct binding as well as by degradation through its E3 ligase activity [60] [61]. On the other hand, the transcription of the MDM2 gene is induced by wild-type p53 [62]. This creates an autoregulatory feedback loop which controls the function of both the expression of MDM2 and the activity of p53. Another regulator of the p53 pathway is the tumor suppressor protein ARF (p14ARF), which controls p53 transcriptional activities by binding to MDM2 and consequently hindering its E3 ubiquitin ligase activity [63, 64]; conversely p14ARF expression is negatively regulated by p53 [59]. Both low grade and high grade gliomas exhibit inactivation or mutation of p14ARF [65]; homozygous deletion of p16INK4a/p14ARF/p15INK4b locus is one of the common mutations in GBMs [66]. Remarkably, mouse models revealed that co-deletion of ARF and INK4a increased accordingly with tumor progression from low- to high-grade gliomas [67]. This suggests that ARF and INK4a mutations are important steps in gliomagenesis.

4.5. ATM/Chk2 pathway

Disruption of the ATM/Chk2 pathway increases the speed of growth and development of glioma [68]; it also contributes to resistance to radiation therapy by helping the malignant cell activate a group of sensor kinases including ATM, ATR, and DNA-dependent protein kinase [69]. The latter phosphorylates multiple downstream mediators such as checkpoint kinases Chk1 and Chk2 that lead to cell-cycle checkpoint initiation and/or apoptosis [70]. Chk2, encoded at chromosome 22q12.1, acts as a tumor suppressor as it regulates p53-dependent apoptosis [71]. Chk2 mutations have in general been rarely reported; however single copy loss of the chromosomal region containing Chk2 has been reported in gliomas [4].

4.6. Rb pathway

The retinoblastoma gene, Rb, is implicated in progression from low grade to higher grade astrocytoma [72], and it is inactivated in GBM [73]. The Rb pathway suppresses cell cycle entry and progression and curbs the p53 pathway by binding and inhibiting transcription factors of the E2F family. Of note, Rb controls progression from G1 to S-phase of the cell cycle [16]. Rb is regulated by the complex of cyclin-dependent kinases (CDKs); in the G1 phase, Rb is normally inactivated by Cyclin D/CDK4/CDK6- induced phosphorylation, causing its release from E2F and consequent cell cycle progression into the S phase. CDKN2B, a CDK inhibitor, which is commonly inactivated in GBM, forms a complex with CDK4 or CDK6, thus preventing the activation of CDKs. The outcome of this inhibition is prevention of cell growth. In addition to the inactivation of CDKN2B, amplification of CDK4 and CDK6 is also common in GBM, demonstrating that both CDK4 and CDK6 have a fundamental function in gliomagenesis and progression [74]. The CDKN2A (p16INK4a) protein binds to CDK4 and inhibits the CDK4/cyclin D1 complex, consequently inhibiting cell cycle transition from G1 to S phase [73]. This implies that any alteration of Rb, CDK4, or CDKN2A causes aberrant dysregulation of the G1-S phase transition. Complete loss of Rb, homozygous deletion or mutation of CDKN2A, CDK4 amplification, CDKN2B (p15INK4b) homozygous deletion, CDKN2C (p18INK4c) homozygous deletion, CCND2 (cyclin D2) amplification, and CDK6 amplification are observed in almost 80% of GBM [75-77].

4.7. STAT3

STAT (Signal transducers and activators of transcription) complexes are a family of cytoplasmic proteins that have SH2 (Src Homology-2) domains functioning as transcription factors that control cellular responses to cytokines and growth factors by signal transduction from the plasma membrane to the nucleus [78]. Target genes are then transcribed and contribute to proliferation, invasion, and apoptosis. STAT3 is an example of the STAT family proteins; it is rendered active by EGF and is overexpressed in GBM [79]. STAT3 also plays a role in the development of neural stem cells and astrocytes [80]. Targeting STAT3 may influence glioma cell motility, resistance to temozolomide, as well as clinical outcome [81-83].

5. Crosstalk

A distinguished characteristic of signaling networks in GBM is the presence of crosstalk, or communication between subnetworks, which interact to promote gliomagenesis and all the phenotypes of GBM. For example, there is evidence of mutual cross talk between cells inactivation of either Ras/Raf/MAPK or PI3K/AKT/mTOR triggering activation of the other [39]. Other examples are the interactions between Ras and stem cell factor (SCF)/c-kit signaling, mTOR, and MAP kinase pathways and the interactions between PI3Kand STAT3 pathways and NF-κB, nuclear factor kappa-light-chain-enhancer of activated B cells, in gliomas [84] [85]. In this section, we examine selected networks that play a role in glioma stem cells (GSC) and cell motility.

5.1. GSC

GSC have the particular ability to auto-renew and initiate gliomagenesis, express neural stem cell markers, and differentiate into multiple phenotypes such as neuronal, astrocytic, and oligodendroglial. Sonic hedgehog homolog (SHH) and Notch are overly expressed in GSC and therefore aberrantly regulate neural progenitor cells [86]. SHH is an important mitogen for medulloblastoma precursor cells. The SHH pathway also contributes to glioma formation as it is activated in GSCs. The SHH pathway is also closely related to the cell cycle as it inactivates Rb and causes over-expression of cell cycle regulators such as N-myc. PDGF signaling in neural stem cells is required for oligodendrogenesis, and amplification of this signal causes an abnormal proliferation of neural stem cells and the formation of large glioma-like lesions [87].

Notch (Notch1-4 in mammals) is a family of transmembrane receptors that control intercellular signaling [88]. They are transmembrane proteins that bind to notch and reveal the receptor to proteolytic activation. Notch is cleaved by presenilin 1 which generates a Notch1 intracellular domain (NICD), a nuclear transcriptional activator. Notch activation induces expression of downstream target genes, such as p53, and promotes neural stem cell growth [89]. BMPs are growth factors that act through binding to cell-surface receptor kinases (BMPRs); the effectors of BMPRs are the Smad proteins, which play a major role in bone and cartilage formation. The overall activity of BMPs is regulation of transcription. BMP ligands exhaust the GSC population by inducing the differentiation of GSCs into astroglial and neuron-like cells. Treating GSCs with BMPs *in vivo* delays tumor growth and diminishes tumor invasion [90].

miRNA is a small non-coding RNA that post-transcriptionally downregulates gene expression. Several studies have identified aberrant miRNA (microRNA-21, miR-326, microRNA-34a) expression in gliomas, and linked some of them to GSC maintenance and growth [91, 92]. Finally, Tumor Necrosis Factor alpha-Induced Protein (TNFAIP) 3 regulates both the NF-κB pathway as well as GSC self-renewal, growth, and apoptotic resistance [93].

5.2. Brain invasion and motility

Brain invasion is a hallmark of gliomas. Tumor cell migration requires highly coordinated steps of dissociation of existing cellular adhesions, remodeling of the actin cytoskeleton to project lamellipodium extensions, formation of new adhesions, and tail detachment along with proteolytic processing and secretion of extracellular matrix proteins along the trajectory. This complex phenotype requires crosstalk between networks that control the extracellular matrix, growth factors, cdc42, GTPases, actin polymerization, PAK, src, cadherins, PIP3, integrins, and myosin (see [96] for details).

Furthermore, some GBM exhibit enhanced motility at 5% ambient oxygen, which is higher than the typical 0.3-1% concentrations observed in cancer hypoxia. This result supports an increased propensity for invasion. The phenotype of increased motility in low ambient oxygen conditions is mediated by phosphorylation of src, which in turn phosphorylates NWASP, Neural Wiskott-Aldrich Syndrome Protein (see [97] for details).

6. Effects of rapamycin on AKT

In the preceding section we have highlighted the complexity of the molecular interactions in GBM and the large number of subnetworks that communicate to generate the phenotypes. Because rapamycin inhibits the mTOR complex, it was considered a hopeful prospect for pharmaceutical therapy. However, in a clinical trial using rapamycin in the treatment of PTEN-deficient GBM, researchers encountered a paradoxical increase in AKT signaling, which was unexpected and undesirable as the latter promotes oncogenic processes [98]. The exact mechanisms for this finding are not yet known. Although many scientists postulate about a simple loss of negative feedback, there may be more than what meets the eye. To illustrate this point, we will delineate a well-characterized pathway in GBM molecular biology and discuss how intersecting activation and inhibitory pathways can lead to paradoxical downstream effects.

As reviewed in Howell et al. and Huang and Manning, mTORC1 acts ultimately as a negative regulator of AKT through various mechanisms [99-101]. First, mTORC1 directly phosphory-lates IRS (insulin receptor substrate), which is thought to hinder the scaffolding ability of PI3K to activate AKT. Additionally, mTORC1 acts through its downstream effector S6K1 (S6 kinase 1), which also phosphorylates IRS at specific serine residues and reduces downstream AKT activation [102-105]. Zhang et al. in 2003 and 2007 showed that mTORC1 activation leads to repression of PDGFR A and B transcription, which inhibits PDGF signaling to AKT and blocks proper transmission of signals from other growth factors [106, 107]. AKT also acts as an activator of mTORC1; but this interaction is irrelevant to our discussion of mTORC1 inhibitors because direct inhibitors of mTORC1 are not influenced by AKT.

Since mTORC1 inhibits AKT (Figure 1, t = 0), bringing down mTORC1 via rapamycin (Figure 1, t = 1) would subsequently lead to an increase in AKT (Figure 1, t = 2).

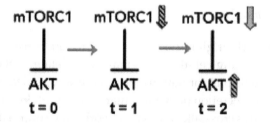

Figure 1. Cartoon depicting the negative effects of mTORC1 on AKT activation and its response to perturbations. Blocked arrows indicate repression/deactivation. The arrow pointing down indicates repression of mTORC1 activity at time = 1. The arrow pointing up indicates the response of the network by increasing the activity of AKT at time = 2.

At first sight this explanation is logical, but when we look deeper into the networks we discover additional factors to this relationship that can provide alternate explanations for the clinical trial's findings. The simple diagram of Figure 1a does not appear to be the appropriate explanation.

Subsequent studies have found that at low concentrations, rapamycin treatment leads to an increase in AKT activity; however, at high, super-physiological concentrations rapamycin causes a decrease in AKT activity [108]. Interestingly, at high concentrations of rapamycin, both mTORC1 and mTORC2 are inhibited. Hence, we need to consider the effects of mTORC2 on AKT. In fact, mTORC2 phosphorylates AKT on S473 (serine 473), which activates AKT at the plasma membrane [112]. The observation, that inhibiting both mTORC1 and mTORC2 caused a decrease in AKT activity, indicates that mTORC1 is a weak inhibitor of AKT as compared to mTORC2 as an activator (see Figure 2 for details).

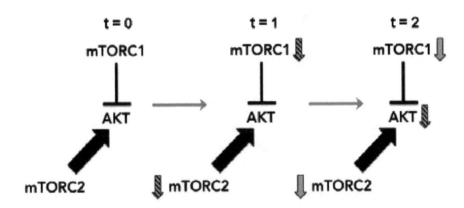

Figure 2. Cartoon depicting relative effects of mTORC1 and mTORC2 on AKT and the response of the network to high concentrations of rapamycin. Blocked and regular arrows indicate repression/deactivation and activation, respectively. The thickness of the arrows reflects the level of repression or activation. If mTORC2 is a stronger activator of AKT than mTORC1 is a repressor (time = 0), treating the cells with high concentrations of rapamycin, which inhibits both mTORC1 and mTORC2 (time = 1), causes a decrease in AKT activity (time = 2).

If we delve deeper into these pathways, we learn of a negative loop between AKT, TSC2 (tuberous sclerosis complex 2), and mTORC2 (See Figure 3) [101]. AKT directly inhibits the activity of the TSC2 complex by phosphorylating TSC2 [109-111]. Furthermore, Huang and Manning provide evidence for the subsequent arm of the loop where the TSC2 complex activates mTORC2 in a manner independent of mTORC1 [100]. These relationships together comprise the negative loop illustrated in Figure 3.

We assume that the physiological levels of rapamycin used in the clinical trial inhibit the activity of mTORC1 without any effects on mTORC2; let us now study the reaction of the network in the presence of the AKT/TSC2/mTORC2 negative loop (see Figure 4). Theoretically, if mTORC1 levels go down (Figure 4a), AKT activity should initially increase (Figure 4b). However, higher AKT activity would lead to augmented inhibition of the TSC2 complex (Figure 4c). The lower levels of TSC2 complex would then reduce the activation of mTORC2 (Figure 4c), which in turn feeds back to influence AKT. The ultimate result on AKT depends on the dynamics and the strengths of the connections the negative loop. At this stage, two possibilities arise as follows.

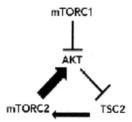

Figure 3. Cartoon depicting negative loop between AKT, mTORC2 and the TSC2 complex. Blocked and regular arrows indicate repression/deactivation and activation, respectively.

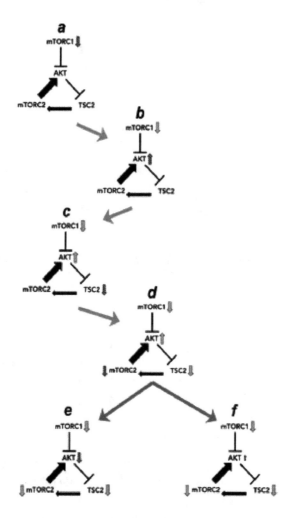

Figure 4. Cartoon depicting the reaction of the network to rapamycin in the presence of the negative loop. Blocked and regular arrows indicate repression/deactivation and activation, respectively. Arrows pointing up or down indicate perturbations causing increased or decreased activity, respectively.

Possibility A: If both AKT's inhibitory effect on TSC2 and TSC2's activation effect on mTORC2 are strong, then an increase in AKT will lead to a significant decrease in mTORC2. Because the latter is a stronger activator than mTORC1 is a repressor (Figure 3), this causes an ultimate *decrease* in AKT activity (Figure 4e).

Possibility B: The negative loop would cause a decrease in mTORC2 activity in any case. This could attenuate but may not reverse the increase in AKT (Figure 4f).

This exercise highlights the profound effects of the presence of a negative loop in the simple network. The results of the clinical trial where rapamycin leads to an increase in AKT activity would be consistent with the explanation of possibility B. However, possibility A cannot be excluded, since other regulatory loops likely influence this pathway as well. In creating treatments and therapeutic strategies in GBM, it is imperative to gain a complete picture of the complexity of intersecting pathways since inhibition can lead to paradoxical, sometimes detrimental results.

7. Conclusion

The molecular networks of GBM include a large number of molecules and interactions, as well as multiple subnetworks and crosstalk. These large networks appear to have the ability to not only bypass therapeutic blockade, but to react to therapeutic modalities by activation of oncogenic subnetworks. We are not surprised that little progress has been made against these deadly and intelligent tumors. Success requires a clear understanding of these large networks as well as predictions of their dynamical (time-dependent) behavior in response to perturbations (*ie.* therapeutic interventions). Fortunately, recent advancements in genomics and mathematical biology bring us closer to attaining these goals.

Author details

Caroline Agha, Hannah C. Machemehl and Hassan M. Fathallah-Shaykh*

*Address all correspondence to: hfathall@uab.edu

The University of Alabama at Birmingham, Department of Neurology, USA

References

[1] Phillips, H.S., et al., *Molecular subclasses of high-grade glioma predict prognosis, delineate a pattern of disease progression, and resemble stages in neurogenesis.* Cancer Cell, 2006. 9(3): p. 157-73.

[2]   Ostrom, Q.T., et al., *CBTRUS statistical report: Primary brain and central nervous system tumors diagnosed in the United States in 2006-2010.* Neuro Oncol, 2013. 15 Suppl 2: p. ii1-56.

[3]   Stupp, R., et al., *Radiotherapy plus concomitant and adjuvant temozolomide for glioblastoma.* N Engl J Med, 2005. 352(10): p. 987-96.

[4]   Cancer Genome Atlas Research, N., *Comprehensive genomic characterization defines human glioblastoma genes and core pathways.* Nature, 2008. 455(7216): p. 1061-8.

[5]   Temple, S., *The development of neural stem cells.* Nature, 2001. 414(6859): p. 112-7.

[6]   Kriegstein, A. and A. Alvarez-Buylla, *The glial nature of embryonic and adult neural stem cells.* Annu Rev Neurosci, 2009. 32: p. 149-84.

[7]   Richardson, P.M., *Ciliary neurotrophic factor: a review.* Pharmacol Ther, 1994. 63(2): p. 187-98.

[8]   Kornblum, H.I., et al., *Multiple trophic actions of heparin-binding epidermal growth factor (HB-EGF) in the central nervous system.* Eur J Neurosci, 1999. 11(9): p. 3236-46.

[9]   Powell, E.M., et al., *Mechanisms of astrocyte-directed neurite guidance.* Cell Tissue Res, 1997. 290(2): p. 385-93.

[10] van den Pol, A.N. and D.D. Spencer, *Differential neurite growth on astrocyte substrates: interspecies facilitation in green fluorescent protein-transfected rat and human neurons.* Neuroscience, 2000. 95(2): p. 603-16.

[11] Komuro, H. and P. Rakic, *Distinct modes of neuronal migration in different domains of developing cerebellar cortex.* J Neurosci, 1998. 18(4): p. 1478-90.

[12] Bacci, A., et al., *The role of glial cells in synaptic function.* Philos Trans R Soc Lond B Biol Sci, 1999. 354(1381): p. 403-9.

[13] Rasheed, B.K., et al., *Molecular pathogenesis of malignant gliomas.* Curr Opin Oncol, 1999. 11(3): p. 162-7.

[14] Theeler, B.J., et al., *Moving toward molecular classification of diffuse gliomas in adults.* Neurology, 2012. 79(18): p. 1917-26.

[15] Hottinger, A.F. and Y. Khakoo, *Update on the management of familial central nervous system tumor syndromes.* Curr Neurol Neurosci Rep, 2007. 7(3): p. 200-7.

[16] Serrano, M., G.J. Hannon, and D. Beach, *A new regulatory motif in cell-cycle control causing specific inhibition of cyclin D/CDK4.* Nature, 1993. 366(6456): p. 704-7.

[17] Sherr, C.J. and J.M. Roberts, *CDK inhibitors: positive and negative regulators of G1-phase progression.* Genes Dev, 1999. 13(12): p. 1501-12.

[18] Wong, A.J., et al., *Increased expression of the epidermal growth factor receptor gene in malignant gliomas is invariably associated with gene amplification.* Proc Natl Acad Sci U S A, 1987. 84(19): p. 6899-903.

[19] Westermark, B., C.H. Heldin, and M. Nister, *Platelet-derived growth factor in human glioma.* Glia, 1995. 15(3): p. 257-63.

[20] Louis, D.N., *Molecular pathology of malignant gliomas.* Annu Rev Pathol, 2006. 1: p. 97-117.

[21] Gomez-Manzano, C., et al., *Characterization of p53 and p21 functional interactions in glioma cells en route to apoptosis.* J Natl Cancer Inst, 1997. 89(14): p. 1036-44.

[22] Leung, S.Y., et al., *Chromosomal instability and p53 inactivation are required for genesis of glioblastoma but not for colorectal cancer in patients with germline mismatch repair gene mutation.* Oncogene, 2000. 19(35): p. 4079-83.

[23] Hamilton, S.R., et al., *The molecular basis of Turcot's syndrome.* N Engl J Med, 1995. 332(13): p. 839-47.

[24] Ekstrand, A.J., et al., *Amplified and rearranged epidermal growth factor receptor genes in human glioblastomas reveal deletions of sequences encoding portions of the N- and/or C-terminal tails.* Proc Natl Acad Sci U S A, 1992. 89(10): p. 4309-13.

[25] Ohgaki, H., et al., *Genetic pathways to glioblastoma: a population-based study.* Cancer Res, 2004. 64(19): p. 6892-9.

[26] Yamazaki, H., et al., *Amplification of the structurally and functionally altered epidermal growth factor receptor gene (c-erbB) in human brain tumors.* Mol Cell Biol, 1988. 8(4): p. 1816-20.

[27] Biernat, W., et al., *Predominant expression of mutant EGFR (EGFRvIII) is rare in primary glioblastomas.* Brain Pathol, 2004. 14(2): p. 131-6.

[28] Barker, F.G., 2nd, et al., *EGFR overexpression and radiation response in glioblastoma multiforme.* Int J Radiat Oncol Biol Phys, 2001. 51(2): p. 410-8.

[29] Shinojima, N., et al., *Prognostic value of epidermal growth factor receptor in patients with glioblastoma multiforme.* Cancer Res, 2003. 63(20): p. 6962-70.

[30] Haas-Kogan, D.A., et al., *Epidermal growth factor receptor, protein kinase B/Akt, and glioma response to erlotinib.* J Natl Cancer Inst, 2005. 97(12): p. 880-7.

[31] van den Bent, M.J., et al., *Randomized phase II trial of erlotinib versus temozolomide or carmustine in recurrent glioblastoma: EORTC brain tumor group study 26034.* J Clin Oncol, 2009. 27(8): p. 1268-74.

[32] Guha, A., et al., *Expression of PDGF and PDGF receptors in human astrocytoma operation specimens supports the existence of an autocrine loop.* Int J Cancer, 1995. 60(2): p. 168-73.

[33] Lokker, N.A., et al., *Platelet-derived growth factor (PDGF) autocrine signaling regulates survival and mitogenic pathways in glioblastoma cells: evidence that the novel PDGF-C and*

PDGF-D ligands may play a role in the development of brain tumors. Cancer Res, 2002. 62(13): p. 3729-35.

[34] Reardon, D.A., et al., *Multicentre phase II studies evaluating imatinib plus hydroxyurea in patients with progressive glioblastoma.* Br J Cancer, 2009. 101(12): p. 1995-2004.

[35] Haas-Kogan, D., et al., *Protein kinase B (PKB/Akt) activity is elevated in glioblastoma cells due to mutation of the tumor suppressor PTEN/MMAC.* Curr Biol, 1998. 8(21): p. 1195-8.

[36] Zhao, J., et al., *Signal transduction and metabolic flux of beta-thujaplicin and monoterpene biosynthesis in elicited Cupressus lusitanica cell cultures.* Metab Eng, 2006. 8(1): p. 14-29.

[37] Lemmon, M.A., *Membrane recognition by phospholipid-binding domains.* Nat Rev Mol Cell Biol, 2008. 9(2): p. 99-111.

[38] Vivanco, I. and C.L. Sawyers, *The phosphatidylinositol 3-Kinase AKT pathway in human cancer.* Nat Rev Cancer, 2002. 2(7): p. 489-501.

[39] Kita, D., et al., *PIK3CA alterations in primary (de novo) and secondary glioblastomas.* Acta Neuropathol, 2007. 113(3): p. 295-302.

[40] Furnari, F.B., et al., *Malignant astrocytic glioma: genetics, biology, and paths to treatment.* Genes Dev, 2007. 21(21): p. 2683-710.

[41] Li, J., et al., *PTEN, a putative protein tyrosine phosphatase gene mutated in human brain, breast, and prostate cancer.* Science, 1997. 275(5308): p. 1943-7.

[42] Tohma, Y., et al., *PTEN (MMAC1) mutations are frequent in primary glioblastomas (de novo) but not in secondary glioblastomas.* J Neuropathol Exp Neurol, 1998. 57(7): p. 684-9.

[43] Mellinghoff, I.K., et al., *Molecular determinants of the response of glioblastomas to EGFR kinase inhibitors.* N Engl J Med, 2005. 353(19): p. 2012-24.

[44] Zinzalla, V., et al., *Activation of mTORC2 by association with the ribosome.* Cell, 2011. 144(5): p. 757-68.

[45] Laplante, M. and D.M. Sabatini, *mTOR signaling in growth control and disease.* Cell, 2012. 149(2): p. 274-93.

[46] Zoncu, R., A. Efeyan, and D.M. Sabatini, *mTOR: from growth signal integration to cancer, diabetes and ageing.* Nat Rev Mol Cell Biol, 2011. 12(1): p. 21-35.

[47] Chang, S.M., et al., *Phase II study of CCI-779 in patients with recurrent glioblastoma multiforme.* Invest New Drugs, 2005. 23(4): p. 357-61.

[48] Galanis, E., et al., *Phase II trial of temsirolimus (CCI-779) in recurrent glioblastoma multiforme: a North Central Cancer Treatment Group Study.* J Clin Oncol, 2005. 23(23): p. 5294-304.

[49] Hurley, J.B., et al., *Homologies between signal transducing G proteins and ras gene prod-ucts.* Science, 1984. 226(4676): p. 860-2.

[50] Nakada, M., et al., *Aberrant signaling pathways in glioma.* Cancers (Basel), 2011. 3(3): p. 3242-78.

[51] Holland, E.C., et al., *Combined activation of Ras and Akt in neural progenitors induces glioblastoma formation in mice.* Nat Genet, 2000. 25(1): p. 55-7.

[52] Moodie, S.A., et al., *Complexes of Ras.GTP with Raf-1 and mitogen-activated protein kin-ase kinase.* Science, 1993. 260(5114): p. 1658-61.

[53] Thomas, S.M., et al., *Ras is essential for nerve growth factor- and phorbol ester-induced ty-rosine phosphorylation of MAP kinases.* Cell, 1992. 68(6): p. 1031-40.

[54] Krakstad, C. and M. Chekenya, *Survival signalling and apoptosis resistance in glioblasto-mas: opportunities for targeted therapeutics.* Mol Cancer, 2010. 9: p. 135.

[55] Kapoor, G.S. and D.M. O'Rourke, *Receptor tyrosine kinase signaling in gliomagenesis: pathobiology and therapeutic approaches.* Cancer Biol Ther, 2003. 2(4): p. 330-42.

[56] Gottfried, O.N., D.H. Viskochil, and W.T. Couldwell, *Neurofibromatosis Type 1 and tu-morigenesis: molecular mechanisms and therapeutic implications.* Neurosurg Focus, 2010. 28(1): p. E8.

[57] Verhaak, R.G., et al., *Integrated genomic analysis identifies clinically relevant subtypes of glioblastoma characterized by abnormalities in PDGFRA, IDH1, EGFR, and NF1.* Cancer Cell, 2010. 17(1): p. 98-110.

[58] Bogler, O., et al., *The p53 gene and its role in human brain tumors.* Glia, 1995. 15(3): p. 308-27.

[59] Stott, F.J., et al., *The alternative product from the human CDKN2A locus, p14(ARF), partic-ipates in a regulatory feedback loop with p53 and MDM2.* EMBO J, 1998. 17(17): p. 5001-14.

[60] Haupt, Y., et al., *Mdm2 promotes the rapid degradation of p53.* Nature, 1997. 387(6630): p. 296-9.

[61] Kubbutat, M.H., S.N. Jones, and K.H. Vousden, *Regulation of p53 stability by Mdm2.* Nature, 1997. 387(6630): p. 299-303.

[62] Zauberman, A., et al., *A functional p53-responsive intronic promoter is contained within the human mdm2 gene.* Nucleic Acids Res, 1995. 23(14): p. 2584-92.

[63] Kamijo, T., et al., *Functional and physical interactions of the ARF tumor suppressor with p53 and Mdm2.* Proc Natl Acad Sci U S A, 1998. 95(14): p. 8292-7.

[64] Zhang, Y., Y. Xiong, and W.G. Yarbrough, *ARF promotes MDM2 degradation and stabil-izes p53: ARF-INK4a locus deletion impairs both the Rb and p53 tumor suppression path-ways.* Cell, 1998. 92(6): p. 725-34.

[65] Nakamura, M., et al., *p14ARF deletion and methylation in genetic pathways to glioblastomas*. Brain Pathol, 2001. 11(2): p. 159-68.

[66] Solomon, D.A., et al., *Conspirators in a capital crime: co-deletion of p18INK4c and p16INK4a/p14ARF/p15INK4b in glioblastoma multiforme*. Cancer Res, 2008. 68(21): p. 8657-60.

[67] Labuhn, M., et al., *Quantitative real-time PCR does not show selective targeting of p14(ARF) but concomitant inactivation of both p16(INK4A) and p14(ARF) in 105 human primary gliomas*. Oncogene, 2001. 20(9): p. 1103-9.

[68] Squatrito, M., et al., *Loss of ATM/Chk2/p53 pathway components accelerates tumor development and contributes to radiation resistance in gliomas*. Cancer Cell, 2010. 18(6): p. 619-29.

[69] Durocher, D. and S.P. Jackson, *DNA-PK, ATM and ATR as sensors of DNA damage: variations on a theme?* Curr Opin Cell Biol, 2001. 13(2): p. 225-31.

[70] Stracker, T.H., T. Usui, and J.H. Petrini, *Taking the time to make important decisions: the checkpoint effector kinases Chk1 and Chk2 and the DNA damage response*. DNA Repair (Amst), 2009. 8(9): p. 1047-54.

[71] Hirao, A., et al., *Chk2 is a tumor suppressor that regulates apoptosis in both an ataxia telangiectasia mutated (ATM)-dependent and an ATM-independent manner*. Mol Cell Biol, 2002. 22(18): p. 6521-32.

[72] Henson, J.W., et al., *The retinoblastoma gene is involved in malignant progression of astrocytomas*. Ann Neurol, 1994. 36(5): p. 714-21.

[73] Biernat, W., et al., *Alterations of cell cycle regulatory genes in primary (de novo) and secondary glioblastomas*. Acta Neuropathol, 1997. 94(4): p. 303-9.

[74] Lam, P.Y., et al., *Expression of p19INK4d, CDK4, CDK6 in glioblastoma multiforme*. Br J Neurosurg, 2000. 14(1): p. 28-32.

[75] Schmidt, E.E., et al., *CDKN2 (p16/MTS1) gene deletion or CDK4 amplification occurs in the majority of glioblastomas*. Cancer Res, 1994. 54(24): p. 6321-4.

[76] Hayashi, Y., et al., *Association of EGFR gene amplification and CDKN2 (p16/MTS1) gene deletion in glioblastoma multiforme*. Brain Pathol, 1997. 7(3): p. 871-5.

[77] Hegi, M.E., et al., *Hemizygous or homozygous deletion of the chromosomal region containing the p16INK4a gene is associated with amplification of the EGF receptor gene in glioblastomas*. Int J Cancer, 1997. 73(1): p. 57-63.

[78] Abal, M., et al., *Molecular pathology of endometrial carcinoma: transcriptional signature in endometrioid tumors*. Histol Histopathol, 2006. 21(2): p. 197-204.

[79] Rahaman, S.O., et al., *Inhibition of constitutively active Stat3 suppresses proliferation and induces apoptosis in glioblastoma multiforme cells*. Oncogene, 2002. 21(55): p. 8404-13.

[80] Rajan, P. and R.D. McKay, *Multiple routes to astrocytic differentiation in the CNS.* J Neurosci, 1998. 18(10): p. 3620-9.

[81] Lin, G.S., et al., *STAT3 serine 727 phosphorylation influences clinical outcome in glioblastoma.* Int J Clin Exp Pathol, 2014. 7(6): p. 3141-9.

[82] Ashizawa, T., et al., *Effect of the STAT3 inhibitor STX-0119 on the proliferation of a temozolomide-resistant glioblastoma cell line.* Int J Oncol, 2014. 45(1): p. 411-8.

[83] Liang, Q., et al., *Inhibition of STAT3 reduces astrocytoma cell invasion and constitutive activation of STAT3 predicts poor prognosis in human astrocytoma.* PLoS ONE, 2013. 8(12): p. e84723.

[84] Smith, D., et al., *NF-kappaB controls growth of glioblastomas/astrocytomas.* Mol Cell Biochem, 2008. 307(1-2): p. 141-7.

[85] Romashkova, J.A. and S.S. Makarov, *NF-kappaB is a target of AKT in anti-apoptotic PDGF signalling.* Nature, 1999. 401(6748): p. 86-90.

[86] Sanai, N., A. Alvarez-Buylla, and M.S. Berger, *Neural stem cells and the origin of gliomas.* N Engl J Med, 2005. 353(8): p. 811-22.

[87] Jackson, E.L., et al., *PDGFR alpha-positive B cells are neural stem cells in the adult SVZ that form glioma-like growths in response to increased PDGF signaling.* Neuron, 2006. 51(2): p. 187-99.

[88] Artavanis-Tsakonas, S., M.D. Rand, and R.J. Lake, *Notch signaling: cell fate control and signal integration in development.* Science, 1999. 284(5415): p. 770-6.

[89] Androutsellis-Theotokis, A., et al., *Notch signalling regulates stem cell numbers in vitro and in vivo.* Nature, 2006. 442(7104): p. 823-6.

[90] Lee, J., et al., *Epigenetic-mediated dysfunction of the bone morphogenetic protein pathway inhibits differentiation of glioblastoma-initiating cells.* Cancer Cell, 2008. 13(1): p. 69-80.

[91] Kefas, B., et al., *The neuronal microRNA miR-326 acts in a feedback loop with notch and has therapeutic potential against brain tumors.* J Neurosci, 2009. 29(48): p. 15161-8.

[92] Guessous, F., et al., *microRNA-34a is tumor suppressive in brain tumors and glioma stem cells.* Cell Cycle, 2010. 9(6): p. 1031-6.

[93] Hjelmeland, A.B., et al., *Targeting A20 decreases glioma stem cell survival and tumor growth.* PLoS Biol, 2010. 8(2): p. e1000319.

[94] Chuang, Y.Y., et al., *Role of synaptojanin 2 in glioma cell migration and invasion.* Cancer Res, 2004. 64(22): p. 8271-5.

[95] Salhia, B., et al., *Inhibition of Rho-kinase affects astrocytoma morphology, motility, and invasion through activation of Rac1.* Cancer Res, 2005. 65(19): p. 8792-800.

[96]   Tang, Z., L.M. Araysi, and H.M. Fathallah-Shaykh, *c-Src and neural Wiskott-Aldrich syndrome protein (N-WASP) promote low oxygen-induced accelerated brain invasion by gliomas.* PLoS ONE, 2013. 8(9): p. e75436.

[97]   Fathallah-Shaykh, H.M., *Logical networks inferred from highly specific discovery of transcriptionally regulated genes predict protein states in cultured gliomas.* Biochem Biophys Res Comm, 2005. 336: p. 1278-1284.

[98]   Carracedo, A., et al., *Inhibition of mTORC1 leads to MAPK pathway activation through a PI3K-dependent feedback loop in human cancer.* J Clin Invest, 2008. 118(9): p. 3065-74.

[99]   Howell, J.J. and B.D. Manning, *mTOR couples cellular nutrient sensing to organismal metabolic homeostasis.* Trends Endocrinol Metab, 2011. 22(3): p. 94-102.

[100] Huang, J. and B.D. Manning, *A complex interplay between Akt, TSC2 and the two mTOR complexes.* Biochem Soc Trans, 2009. 37(Pt 1): p. 217-22.

[101] Carracedo, A. and P.P. Pandolfi, *The PTEN-PI3K pathway: of feedbacks and cross-talks.* Oncogene, 2008. 27(41): p. 5527-41.

[102] Shah, O.J. and T. Hunter, *Turnover of the active fraction of IRS1 involves raptor-mTOR- and S6K1-dependent serine phosphorylation in cell culture models of tuberous sclerosis.* Mol Cell Biol, 2006. 26(17): p. 6425-34.

[103] Harrington, L.S., G.M. Findlay, and R.F. Lamb, *Restraining PI3K: mTOR signalling goes back to the membrane.* Trends Biochem Sci, 2005. 30(1): p. 35-42.

[104] Tremblay, F., et al., *Identification of IRS-1 Ser-1101 as a target of S6K1 in nutrient- and obesity-induced insulin resistance.* Proc Natl Acad Sci U S A, 2007. 104(35): p. 14056-61.

[105] Manning, B.D., *Balancing Akt with S6K: implications for both metabolic diseases and tumorigenesis.* J Cell Biol, 2004. 167(3): p. 399-403.

[106] Zhang, H., et al., *PDGFRs are critical for PI3K/Akt activation and negatively regulated by mTOR.* J Clin Invest, 2007. 117(3): p. 730-8.

[107] Zhang, H., et al., *Loss of Tsc1/Tsc2 activates mTOR and disrupts PI3K-Akt signaling through downregulation of PDGFR.* J Clin Invest, 2003. 112(8): p. 1223-33.

[108] Costanzo, M., et al., *The genetic landscape of a cell.* Science, 2010. 327: p. 425-431.

[109] Potter, C.J., L.G. Pedraza, and T. Xu, *Akt regulates growth by directly phosphorylating Tsc2.* Nat Cell Biol, 2002. 4(9): p. 658-65.

[110] Inoki, K., et al., *TSC2 is phosphorylated and inhibited by Akt and suppresses mTOR signalling.* Nat Cell Biol, 2002. 4(9): p. 648-57.

[111] Dan, H.C., et al., *Phosphatidylinositol 3-kinase/Akt pathway regulates tuberous sclerosis tumor suppressor complex by phosphorylation of tuberin.* J Biol Chem, 2002. 277(38): p. 35364-70.

2

Radiation-Induced Brain Injury After Radiotherapy for Brain Tumor

Zhihua Yang, Shoumin Bai, Beibei Gu, Shuling Peng, Wang Liao and Jun Liu

1. Introduction

Radiation therapy is used widely for the treatment of diffuse primary and metastatic brain tumors [1]. Especially for nasopharyngeal carcinoma (NPC), the most common type of cancer in southern China, radiation therapy is the first-choice treatment and sometimes the only effective management of the disease. As many as 200,000 patients receive partial large-field or whole-brain irradiation every year, and the population of long-term cancer survivors keeps on growing. During treatment, however, some healthy brain tissues are also exposed to the radiation inevitably, and consequently many patients may experience neurological symptoms associated with damage to these healthy tissues after radiotherapy. Some of these symptoms may even last for months or years. This is known as acute and chronic radiation-induced brain injury (RIBI), also known as radiation encephalopathy (RE). Approximately 100,000 primary and metastatic brain tumor patients each year in the US survive long enough (>6 months) to experience RIBI [2]. For example, the incidence of RIBI for patients with NPC in Guangdong province is up to 3 per 100,000, to our knowledge, 40 times higher than the world average and is the most common one among head and neck tumor. RIBI includes a series of clinical manifestations, such as focal neurological deficits, secondary epilepsy, mental and behavioural disorders, elevated intracranial pressure, and the progressive deterioration of the hippocampal-associated learning and memory functions [3],which can be especially devastating to patients and caregivers.

The American Cancer Society center (ACS) stresses that in order to maximize the quality of life for tumor patients after radiotherapy, the future research should focus on preventing and curing complications of cancer therapy. RIBI, a common and devastating complication of radiotherapy for brain tumor, is now emerging as a major health problem in the treatment of brain tumor.

2. Pathogenesis

Based on the time between onset of clinical expression and radiation therapy administration, RIBI has been classified into acute, early delayed, and late delayed injury, which was first reported by Sheline [4]. Acute brain injury occurs during and/or in days to weeks after irradiation. Early delayed brain injury occurs 6–12 weeks post-irradiation [5], while some other researchers consider this time course is 1-6 months [6]. Although both of these early injuries can result in severe reactions, they rarely occur and normally resolve spontaneously or reversible after short-term treatment. In contrast, late delayed brain injury, usually developing 6 months post-irradiation, which is most significantly higher than that of acute and early delayed RIBI, have been viewed as irreversible and progressive continuously due to the pathogenesis [7].

The knowledge of the mechanisms underlying the RIBI following irradiation is the basis for improving the therapies and prophylaxes, but it is not wholly clear.

The most direct affecting risk of RIBI is the radiation doses, fractionation schemes, and adjuvant treatments. [8, 9] Liu Y and Xiao S et al. found that single-dose irradiation at 10Gy failed to induce any significant effects in young male rats whereas an exposure at 20 to 40Gy induced acute brain injury at both cognitive and pathologic levels. [10] Zhou H. and Liu Z. et al. reported that fractionated irradiation of 20 to 40Gy could also induce acute brain injury in young rats which indicated the role of fractionation schemes. [11] Furthermore, Ruben JD et al. not only demonstrated the risk of radiation dose and fraction size, but the subsequent administration of chemotherapy as well. [9]

In general, ionizing radiation can cause RIBI by either direct or indirect way and it is likely that the successful unraveling of this puzzle will not come true without the basic study of subtle molecular, cellular, or microanatomic changes in the brain. Hereon, we will discuss the pathogenesis of RIBI from oxidative stress, nonspecific inflammation, blood brain barrier(BBB) disruption as well as apoptosis and inhibition of neurogenesis which act alone or accompanied.

2.1. Oxidative stress

It is reported that in the unilaterally irradiated animals, irradiated hemispheres showed similarly significant changes in oxygenation compared to unirradiated controls. [12]

Due to radiation therapy, the microglia is activated and immune cells begin to infiltrate the brain. These cells then produce reactive oxygen species (ROS) whose production and detoxification are normal physiological processes. Nevertheless, an imbalance between ROS production and ROS removal may lead to oxidative stress [13, 14].Several components of ROS can cause damage to cardinal cellular components, such as lipids, proteins, and DNA, initiating subsequent cell death via necrosis or apoptosis [15]. Thus, ROS can be contributed to neuronal toxicity and implicated in both acute injury and chronic neuropathological conditions [16].

Many related molecules have been reported. Jun showed hydrogen peroxide (H_2O_2)-induced oxidative stress and apoptosis in HT22 cells accompany by up-regulated expression of p-ERK 1/2, p-JNK, and p-P38 [13]. What is more, the effectiveness of edaravone(a new agent of ROSscavenger), peroxisome proliferator-activated receptor (PPAR) gamma agonists, and antioxidants/antioxidant enzymes in preventing or mitigating the severity of RIBI also provided an evidence of the oxidative stress. [13, 17]

2.2. Nonspecific inflammation

Irradiation can caused an acute endothelial cell apoptosis which lead to BBB breakdown, chronic hypoxia and peritumoral tissue edema. [18] Meanwhile, nonspecific inflammation cascades which further promote the microenvironmental changes, radiation necrosis, and neurogenesis inhibition was activated [19].

Radiation could induce astrocytes proliferation and secrete a great quantity of pro-inflammatory mediators after irradiation, which may aid the infiltration of leukocytes into the brain via blood-brain barrier (BBB) breakdown [20, 21]. Microglias could also be activated by quantity of irradiation through rapid proliferation, as well as increased production of ROS and other cytokines which are involved in mediating neuroinflammation [22].

Plenty of experiments have found up-regulation of pro-inflammatory transcription factors after irradiation which constituted the evidence of nonspecific inflammation cascades in the process of RIBI. Moore, A. H. suggest that radiation-induced changes in vascular permeability are dependent on cyclooxygenase 2 (COX2), one of two isoforms of the obligate enzyme in prostanoid synthesis and the principal target of non-steroid anti-inflammatory drugs activity. [23] Lee et al. found mRNA and protein of pro-inflammatory mediators including tumour necrosis factor-alpha (TNF-alpha), interleukin-1beta (IL-1beta), and monocyte chemoattrac-tant protein-1 (MCP-1) activated significantly in regions isolated from irradiated in rat brain. [24] TNF-alpha is thought to be able to up-regulate other pro-inflammatory cytokines and increase BBB permeability, increase leukocyte adhesion, activate astrocytes, and induce endothelial apoptosis. And the further research demonstrated that anti-inflammation factor (TNF-alpha) successfully inhibited radiation-induced effects in the local as well as abscopal region in the brain. [12] Peroxisome proliferator-activated receptor (PPAR) gamma is ligand-activated transcription factor that belong to the steroid/thyroid hormone nuclear receptor superfamily. And the effectiveness of PPAR-gamma agonists is also a strong demonstration of nonspecific inflammation. [25]

What is more, radiation could induce the loss of oligodendrocyte type-2 astrocyte (O-2A) progenitor cell, the most radiosensitive type of glial cell, which leads to transient demyelina-tion soon after irradiation. Since all the brain gliocytes including oligodendrocyte, astrocytes and microglia would participate in the radioactive damage process in different ways and RIBI is predominated by white matter necrosis and demyelination, the pathological mechanism is well known as Gliocyte Hypothesis. However, there is conflicting conclusion that the targeted anti-inflammatory agent has no effect on gliocytes, but can still ameliorate RIBI [26]. Consequently, pathological mechanism of RIBI cannot be explained so simply by the Gliocyte Hypothesis despite the large amount of evidence supporting this hypothesis.

Due to the synergistic effect of oxidative stress and nonspecific inflammation after irradiation, endothelial cell nuclear, blood vessel density, and blood vessel length are vulnerable to have a reduction. The vascular damage can result in brain ischemia and even white matter necrosis. [7]. All of this elicited the Vascular Hypothesis. Paradoxically, radiation-induced necrosis has also been reported in the absence of vascular changes [27]. In addition, the PPARγ agonist, pioglitazone, and the ACE inhibitor, ramipril, which are believed to prevent RIBI in the rat do not reverse the reduction in vascular density and length that occurs after fWBI [28, 29].

Therefore, RIBI cannot be completely explained by any single cell or tissue despite a host of evidence supporting these hypotheses. It is supposed to occur and develop due to active interactions between the multiple cells. These participating cells are considered to play a synergistic rather than initial role in the radiation brain injury [30].

2.3. Blood Brain Barrier(BBB) disruption

A number of data from laboratory animals has demonstrated acute BBB disruption which was initiated by apoptosis of endothelial cells and mediated by the ASMase pathway after irradiation [18]. As a result, change of BBB permeability has been thought to be the most sensitive and reliable index for detection of early RIBI. [31] Breakdown of the BBB may also enhance the effectiveness of chemotherapeutic agents, with the unintended consequence of contributing to injury of the peritumoral tissue. Liu Y. and Xiao S. et al. found that a single-dose exposure at 20 to 40 Gy induced acute brain injury at cognitive is more or less accompanied with increased brain water content and deteriorated BBB function, though mild histopathologic alternations were only noticed in the 40-Gy-irradiated rats at 20 days. [10] Zhou H. and Liu Z. et al. reported disrupted BBB permeability was detected after fractionated irradiation of 20 to 40Gy in young rats and thus proved that the change in BBB permeability could be one of the most sensitive and reliable indices of fractionated-radiation-induced acute RIBI. [11] Besides, increased astrogliosis in the hippocampus could be detected at 4 weeks' postirradiation for 40-Gy group.

2.4. Apoptosis and neurogenesis inhibition

The pathogenesis of RIBI may also relate to the process of neuronal apoptosis and inhibition of neurogenesis.

Even gray matter contains neuronal cell bodies which is quite oxygen-dependent, neurons have been considered radioresistant since they could no longer divide. However, it is reported that apoptosis occurs in the young adult rat brain after ionizing irradiation and recent studies also demonstrated that there exists direct radiation-induced damage to hippocampal neurons with associated cognitive decline. The hippocampus consists of the DG, CA3, and CA1 regions. Irradiating the hippocampus resulted in an increase in apoptosis in the subgranular zone of the DG which are capable of both self-renewal and generating neurons, astrocytes, and oligodendrocytes [32, 33]. And blocking neurogenesis which was associated with alterations of microenvironment including disruption of the microvascular angiogenesis and increase in the number and activation status of microglia within the neurogenic zone can contribute to the deleterious side effects of radiation treatment. [14]

Neurogenesis is also related to inflammation for the reason that anti-inflammatory drug was proved to be capable of restoring and augments neurogenesis after cranial irradiation. [19]However, these changes could also be observed in the absence of demyelination, blood vessel density alternation and inflammatory cellular infiltration by a doses of ≤2 Gy that fail to produce these changes [34].

3. Clinical characteristics of RIBI

3.1. Latency

The latency of RIBI exists a long time span. Chandler reported the time interval between the end of radiotherapy to the onset of RIBI was 1 month to 16 years [35]. JY Qin et al. documented the latency of RIBI was 3 months to 38 months, median time of which was 21.7 months [36]. We collected data of 130 NPC cases who suffered RIBI post radiotherapy, the latency of them underwent a large time span from 0 to 32 years, the mean time was about 6 years [37].

Therefore, being focus on the mechanism research to get early differentiation, diagnosis, explore therapeutic strategies of late delayed RIBI become more and more urgent.

3.2. Clinical features and classification

Acute effects occur during and/or shortly after the radiation exposure and are characterized by symptoms of fatigue, dizziness, and signs of increased intracranial pressure. The acute effects are considered to be secondary to edema and disruption of the BBB. Early delayed effects of post-irradiation and usually show reversible symptoms generalized weakness and somnolence, partly resulting from a transient demyelination. It is, however, the late delayed effects that may lead to severe irreversible neurological consequences.

According to the site of involvement and corresponding clinical manifestations, the subtypes of RIBI were divided into cerebellum type, brain stem and cranial type, cerebellum type and mixed type.

3.2.1. Cerebral hemisphere type

Focal delivery of one large radiation fraction during radiotherapy can lead to focal injury of the brain adjacent to the irradiated lesion [38].Clinically, patients present with focal neurological deficits, which are often accompanied by focal increased intracranial pressure.

The most common and serious delayed complication of cerebral radiotherapy is cognitive dysfunction. Take NPC for example, since inferior temporal lobes inevitably expose to the radiation, the prominent and earliest seen symptom of RIBI is distinctive cognitive impair-ment. Recently, Hsiao demonstrated that nasopharyngeal cancer patients treated with intensity-modulated radiotherapy (IMRT) had a worse cognitive outcome if >10% of their temporal lobe volume received a total fractionated dose of >60 Gy than patients who received < 60 Gy [39]. The feature of cognitive impairment is different from those with Alzheimer's disease, it is characterized by decreased verbal memory, spatial memory, attention, novel problem-solving ability, and even executive function. Patients usually accompanied with negative emotions including depression, anxiety as well as somatization. Mental disorders such as stupor state, hallucinations and delusions could also be observed as the injury progresses [20].

It should be noted that significant cognitive impairment can be seen in the absence of radio-graphic or clinical evidence of demyelination or white matter necrosis after irradiation [40]. Therefore, conducting cognitive evaluations shortly post-irradiation at regular intervals is becoming more and more important. Once cognitive decline is detected, no matter whether there is imaging findings of brain lesions, prophylactic treatment should be given to the patients immediately. The mini-mental status examination (MMSE), a test to assess global cognitive function, is relatively insensitive to radiation-induced cognitive impairment [39, 41]. As the cognitive domains that are most affected by brain irradiation is distinct from the common causes of dementia such as Alzheimer's disease and vascular dementia, current Radiation Therapy Oncology Group (RTOG) study has established a series of tests that focuses on the cognitive domains affected by brain irradiation, such as Dutch adult reading test for assessing intelligence, vline bisection test for perception, visual verbal learning test for memory and stroop color word test for executive function [42]. The Montreal cognitive assessment (MoCA) is used to assess different cognitive domains including attention and concentration, executive functions, memory, language, visuoconstructional skills, conceptual thinking, calculations, and orientation. Sensitivity and specificity of MoCA application in radiation-induced cognitive impairment has not been reported.

Another most common injury after radiotherapy is unilateral or/and bilateral temporal lobe edema which might elevate intracranial pressure. If the pathogenesis develops persistently, the area of edema could expand to the parietal lobes and then cause rapidly deteriorating clinical course. Signs of increased intracranial pressure such as headache, nausea and vomiting would get worse progressively. Severe cerebral edema could result in compression of cerebral peduncle and cerebral hernia, which would lead to hemiplegia and even to death. Once that occurs, surgical treatment will be needed. Moreover, cerebral edema could at last get lique-factive necrosis with formation of cystic spaces. Figure.1

3.2.2. Brain stem and cranial type

It has been reported that each pair of cranial nerve could get involved in injury after irradiation in NPC patients [43]. Due to the irradiation fields mainly cover the lower part of brain stem, the last four cranial nerves, glossopharyngeal nerve, vagus nerve, accessory nerve and hypoglossal nerve, were commonly affected and leading to corresponding clinical manifesta-tions, such as atrophy of tongue muscle, dysphagia, dysphonia and dysdipsia. Severe bulbar

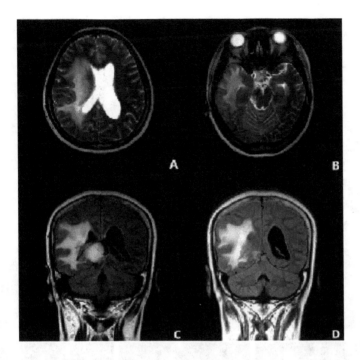

Figure 1. Cerebral edema and atrophy of a 39-year-old female cerebral hemangioma patient. 8 years after the treatment of gamma knife. Lumps-like abnormal signal was shown in the right-basolateral region, heterogeneous high signal was shown on T2W, surrounded by low signal, a large fingerlike high signal of the white matter around lesions on T2W. Cerebral gyrus of the frontal and parietal lobe narrow and cerebral sulcus widen which is the sign of cerebral atrophy. A.T2WI B. T2WI C.FLARE D.FLARE

palsy may significantly decrease the life quality of patients and sometime is fatal caused by subsequent lung infection and/or malnutrition [43]. And the frequency of upper cranial nerve injury increased greatly if the patients have to conduct re-radiotherapy.

Some other common involved cranial nerve is cochleovestibular nerve caused by not only direct effect of irradiation to the nerve but also the indirect effect of the inner ear damage after radiotherapy such as secretory otitis media or even intractable suppurative otitis media. The prime symptoms of disorders of the cochleovestibular nerve are vertigo, tinnitus and pain. Irreversible hearing loss caused by nerve deafness, conduction deafness and mixed deafness will happen in the end [43].

Radiation-induced optic neuropathy (RION) is a rare but usually devastating side effect of radiotherapy for NPC. The most frequent clinical symptoms of RION typically present with sudden, painless, irreversible vision loss in one or both eyes after radiotherapy, and occur most commonly from 3 months to more than 9 years after radiotherapy. Liu et al. reported RION in NPC patients [44]. Ophthalmologic examinations showed flake bleeding in the retina, optic nerve atrophy and cotton-wool spots. T1-weighted enhanced MRI images showed enhancement of the optic nerve and optic chiasm in six cases.

One more severe clinical manifestation is syncope. Damage to descending sympathetic nerve fibers, which anatomically run along the brain stem, may result in hazardous syncope as well

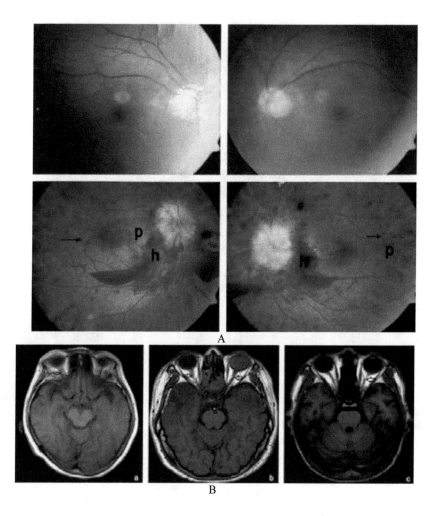

Figure 2. A. Fundus examination in radiation-induced optic neuropathy: ocular fundus showing flame-shaped and dot hemorrhage (bottom row, h, arrow) and cotton-wool spots (top row, bottom row, p). B. Axial MRI of three patients showing: (a, b) tortuous optic nerve with blurring of edges, and (b) optic nerve atrophy; (b, c) T1-weighted enhanced MRI showing enhancement of the optic nerves and optic chiasm.

as Horner syndrome. Crossed hemiplegia might also occur when pyramidal tract is involved simultaneously [43].

3.2.3. Cerebellum type

It is the least common type of RIBI. Damage to cerebellum results in edema of cerebellar hemisphere and leads to symptoms such as vertigo, stumbling, ataxia and other discomfort. The injury to cerebellum has the same prognosis as that in cerebral hemisphere and eventually develop into the tonsillar hernia.

3.2.4. Mixed type

It is a combination of two or more subtypes mentioned above.

4. Value of neuroimaging in RIBI diagnosis

Neuroimaging, including computed tomography (CT), magnetic resonance imaging (MRI) especially neurological functional imaging technology, provide valuable information in early diagnosis and differential diagnosis of RIBI. In this paragraph, we will provide a variety of neuroimaging information to readers. Including not only traditional CT/MRI imaging, but also proton magnetic resonance spectroscopy (MRS) and iffusion tensor imaging (DTI).

4.1. Computed Tomography (CT)

CT foundings of focal radiation brain edema and necrosis are generally low density, while the affected white matter is usually symmetric and exhibit no enhancement or irregular peripheral enhancement with contrast material. The brain lesions would range from small foci near the frontal or occipital horns to a confluent band extending from the ventricles to the corticomedullary junction. Figure.3

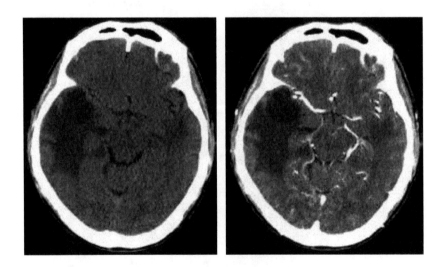

Figure 3. CT founding of a 59-year-old male patient with NPC after radiotherapy for over 10 years. A. cystic liquefactive necrosis of the right temporal lobe with edema around lesions. B. no enhancement.

4.2. Magnetic resonance Imaging (MRI)

MRI is definitely more valuable for the diagnosis of RIBI than CT. The appeerence of finger like edema and focal necrosis which shows low signal intensity on T1WI and high signal on T2WI are typical feature of MR imaging in patients with RIBI. Ringlike or irregular enhancement in the bilateral temporal lobes are also frequently seen on T1WI enhanced MR imaging while haemorrhage with heterogeneous signals is relative rare. (Figure.4)These findings on conventional MRI technology are not specific and insufficient to distinguish RIBI from tumor recurrence or other diseases. Thus various new technologies of MRI are employed to make up for this shortcoming.

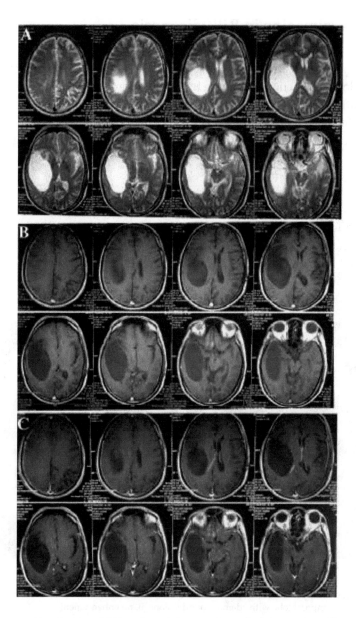

Figure 4. Radiation necrosis and edema. MRI performed 8 years after radiotherapy of one 54-years-old male patient with NPC. Necrosis of right-temporal and right-parietal lobe shows low signal intensity on T1WI and high signal on T2WI with enhanced boundary. Edema of the left-temporal lobe shows finger like low signal intensity on T1WI and high signal on T2WI with non-enhanced boundary. A. T2WI; B. T1WI; C.T1WI+C

4.3. Proton magnetic Resonance Spectroscopy (MRS)

MRS is used to display metabolite changes in normal appearing white matter after fWBI in the brain. Brain metabolites are quantified including choline(Cho), creatine(Cr), glutamate(Glu), glutamine(Gln), N-acetyl-aspartate (NAA) and lactate. It is reported that NAA, Cr and Cho change regularly from the center of the visible lesions. In the liquefaction and necrosis foci,

NAA, Cr and Cho are nearly absent. In the visible lesions, the levels of NAA increase slightly, while the contents of Cr and Cho decreased obviously. Certain extent away from the visible lesions, the contents of NAA decrease and the levels of Cr and Cho increase. Farther away from the lesions, the levels of the three substances gradually become normal. Consequently the ratios of NAA/Cr and Cho/Cr alter from periphery to the lesion, decrease from a value above 1 to one less than 1. A ratio of NAA/Cr and Cho/Cr less than 1 may be highly indicative of nerve and cell structure damage in the brain tissue [45, 46]. In view of this, MRS is supposed to indentify a larger area of abnormal metabolism in RIBI than visible lesion in MRI, which makes it possible to detect RIBI in early stage.

4.4. Diffusion Tensor Imaging (DTI)

DTI is a novel way to assess tissue microstructure by measuring the diffusion of water molecules in three-dimensional (3D) space. It is often applied to distinguish demyelination from axonal injury within white matter bundle. In a DTI study of childhood survivors after fWBI for acute lymphoblastic leukemia, fractional anisotropy (FA) decreases significantly in the frontal and parietal lobes related to declines in intelligence quotient [47]. In another study of adult survivors post fWBI for acute leukemia, FA values reduced obviously in normal appearing cerebral white matter of the temporal lobe, hippocampus, and thalamus [48]. DTI is thought to be a promising technique to detect early changes in white matter integrity before image evidence of radiation-induced demyelination or necrosis. However, the application of DTI to RIBI is just in its infancy. Figure.5

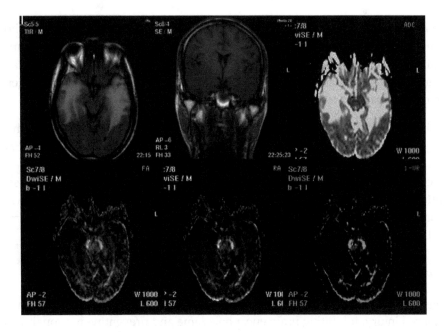

Figure 5. Delayed RIBI of bilateral temporal. Edema is obvious. Isotropic map shows high signal in the lesion area which is wider than FLAIR. Anisotropic map shows low signal in the bilateral temporal lobe and white matter fiber of the normal temporal lobe shows high signal and blurred.

5. Treatment strategies

Up to now, there has been no proven effective treatment to reverse or terminate the pathogenesis brain irradiation injury, which could be particularly devastating to patients and caregivers since the exact mechanisms of RIBI is unclear. Potential therapeutic strategies to prevent RIBI will be discussed in this part.

5.1. Glucocorticoids

Glucocorticoids play a vital role in the comprehensive therapy for RIBI. A large number of experimental and clinical studies have confirmed its polyvalent efficacy of narrowing lesions, relieving symptoms as well as improving their prognosis by counteracting the radiation-induced vascular endothelial damage and inflammatory cascade [49]. Dispute still remains over the opportunity, dose and course of glucocorticoid therapy. Many a researchers recommend maintenance therapy with regular dose for more than 3 months while some others affirm the effect of early large dosage of corticosteroids for shorter periods [49]. Some patients may be weaned off after a period of symptomatic exacerbation while in some cases symptoms can return after steroid cessation and lead to necessitating long-term steroid use. Unfortunately, the prolonged systemic administration will result in immunosupression, psychiatric distrubances, myopathy and sequelae of endocrinologic compromise such as hypertension, diabetes mellitus, osteoporosis, weight changes and thickening of facial subcutis [49].

5.2. Antiplatelets and anticoagulation

Radiation induced vascular endothelial injury may lead to subsequent mural thrombosis, thus antiplatelets may play a crucial part in preventing the RIBI. Currently exsisted antiplatelet drugs mainly include cyclooxygenase(COX) inhibitors and adenosine diphosphate (ADP) receptor antagonists. Phosphodiesterase inhibitors, a new type of antiplatelet agents, have been proved to be protective for intravascular thrombosis after radiation [2].

Another kind of drug to control thrombosis is anticoagulation drugs. It's reported that the use of heparin and warfarin lead to partial recovery of function in five of eight patients with cerebral radiation necrosis when they were proved to be unresponsive to steroid therapy [50]. One case concerning a patient experienced a recurrence of symptoms following discontinuation of anticoagulation therapy and was reversed again by resuming anticoagulation treatment [50] demonstrated the limited success of anticoagulation drug. However, this treatment need to be validated in larger trials before clinical application.

5.3. Reactive Oxygen Species (ROS) scavengers

Edaravone, a new agent of ROS scavenger, has been verified effective in reducing the vascular endothelial cell injury, inhibiting brain encephaledema and preventing neuronal cell necrosis [51]. Our clinical trails on 42 NPC patients suffered RIBI has demonstrated that efficiency (50.0%) and total efficiency (88.9%) in the edaravone administration group were significantly higher than that in the contrast group (14.3% and 42.9%). After a 4-week treatment, the lesion volume on MRI was smaller than before in edaravone group, and the scores of 6 domains, 19 aspects and the overall quality of life in edaravone group were significantly higher than those in non-edaravone group [52]. However, ROS scavengers have received not so much attention because they are likely to protect brain tumors to the same extent as they protect normal brain [2]. Another antioxidant and radioprotective drug is vitamin E. The administration of Vitamin E significantly reduced the severity of radiation-induced brain damages and increased the activity of superoxide dismutase and catalase enzymes in the brain. [53]

5.4. Refactoring microcirculation

The butyl-phthalide, a neotype of drugs reforming the microcirculation, has multiple effects of increasing the perfusion in the ischemia area, protecting the mitochondria from hypoxic injury, and also reducing neuronal apoptosis. Human urinary kallidinogenase for injection, another new agent of this type, may be instrumental in vasodilation of brain blood vessels, increasing haemoglobin in the cerebral blood flow, and also improving glucose metabolism in ischemic brain tissues [54].

5.5. Reconstructing the nerve function

Radiation injury could destroy the nerve structure and then lead to loss of neuron function. Therefore neural plasticity is thought to play a vital role in the comprehensive treatment for RIBI. As our data from animals and humans shows that gangliosides is helpful in promoting the recovery of nerve function in lesioned brain, spinal cord and also peripheral nerve. A host of in vivo and in vitro studies also demonstrated that neurotrophic factors are neuroprotective in radiation-induced nouropathy. Curative effect has been proved in patients with temporal lobe injury after two-month injection with mouse nerve growth factor, both MR imaging and cognitive function of them were improved significantly [55].

5.6. Renin–Angiotensin System(RAS) inhibitors

The RAS has been viewed as a classical systemic hormonal system. Recently several intra-organ RAS including a brain RAS have been identified. The brain RAS is involved in modulation of the BBB, stress, memory, and cognition. Both angiotensin-converting enzyme inhibitors (ACEI) and angiotensin receptor blockers (ARB) have been proved effective in treating experimental radiation nephropathy and pneumopathy [56, 57]. As for their effect on encephalopathy, studies of Jenrow et al. (2010) show that administration of the ACEI, ramipril has modest protection against WBI-induced decreases in neurogenesis, but did not modulate radiation-induced neuroinflammation while other report has different conclusion with a different timing of chronic administration of theramipril and/or the response after single or fractionated doses on rodent [58, 59]. Whether all of the drug mentioned above can be useful for the patient of RIBI remains to be further elucidated.

5.7. Symptomatic treatment

Dehydration medicine such as mannitol and albumin should be given to patients with high cranial pressure. Antiepileptic drugs (AED) should be chosen according to the forms of epilepsy seizures. Serotonin (5-HT) reuptake inhibitors and psychological therapies might be preferred when anxiety and depression are the cardinal symptoms.

It should be mentioned that there has been no known preventive medications for radiation-induced cognitive impairment in humans, although several pharmacologic agents have been assessed for symptomatic management [2]. The Wake Forest Community Clinical Oncology Program Research Base completed a phase II study using 10mg/day of a cholinesterase inhibitor namely donepezil, which showed significant improvement in energy level, mood, and cognitive function in radiation-induced brain injury survivors [60]. Memantine, an NMDA receptor antagonist being able to block ischemia-induced NMDA excitation, was proven to be effective in vascular dementia. Thus it is supposed to be conducive to radiation-induced cognitive impairment if radiation-induced ischemia occurs after fWBI. Other potential pharmacological mediators based on preclinical researches suggesting that anti-inflammatory agents could prevent or ameliorate radiation-induced cognitive function. As for anti-inflammatory peroxisome proliferator-activated PPARγ agonists, researchers have found some evidence that they maight prevent/ameliorate radiation-induced cognitive impairment when given for only a few weeks after fWBI on rodent [61].

5.8. Surgical management

Surgical resection can be considered when the patient's necrosis are symptomatic and have no take a turn for the better after medical treatments. For example, when suffering from large area-cerebral edema, and the condition progressively exacerbated active medications although has been given, patients should also be recommended to surgically remove the focal brain lesions in time when the location is in a region that is surgically accessible. During this process, the surgeon should avoid incurring additional significant neurologic morbidity. [85]

5.9. Neural Stem Cells(NSCs) therapies

In addition to drug therapeutics, there has been increased interest in the use of various NSCs therapies. Pioneering researchers directly inject NSCs into rodent brains after WBI and found it partially restores cognitive function [62, 63]. Interestingly, these NSCs not only differentiate into neurons, but also oligodendrocytes, astrocytes and endothelial cells that can alter the hippocampal microenvironment [63]. However, the use of exercise or NSCs transplantation to prevent/ameliorate RIBI in humans will require considerably more research before it can be translated to the clinic.

5.10. Organ-sparing approach

To date, one of the strategies to prevent RIBI in the clinic involves organ-sparing approach which is based on neuroanatomical target theory. Technology has evolved to potentially allow for selective avoidance of the regions of adult neurogenesis, including the hippocampus and neural stem cell niche in the periventricular regions. With the help of advanced radiation techniques, such as 3D conformal image guidance [64], inverse-planned intensity modulated radiotherapy (IMRT) [65] and proton beam radiotherapy [66], it is expected to reduce the occurrence of RIBI by limiting the dose to critical organs and possibly increasing locoregional tumor control. [67]

5.11. Anti-VEGF antibody

As is mentioned above, the necrosis is partly due to increasing capillary permeability which is caused by cytokine release leading to extracellular edema. The edema is the most common pathology of RIBI is just sustained by endothelial dysfunction, tissue hypoxia as well as subsequent necrosis. Consequently, it is a logical option to block the vascular endothelial growth factor (VEGF) at an early stage to reduce the development of radiation necrosis and thus decrease the vascular permeability. After the patient with radiation-induced necrosis was treated with an anti-VEGF antibody (bevacizumab), the improvement neurologic signs and symptoms in accordance with the decrease in T1-weighted fluid-attenuated inversion recovery signals put bevacizumab as a treatment direction for patients with RIBI [68].

5.12. Hyperbaric Oxygen Treatment (HBOT)

HBOT is proven to be able to stimulate angiogenesis and restore the regional blood supply by reaching the goal of increasing parenchymal oxygen concentration. HBOT treatment has been demonstrated to be beneficial in pediatric patients with radiation necrosis [69]and in smaller series and case reports [70, 71]. However, Jun L et al. reported that HBOT treatment did not reduce visual loss or blindness in patients with RION [44]. As single institution studies vary widely due to patient selection bias, it would be necessary to conduct more randomized trials to delineate the true benefit of HBOT. [72]

6. Problems and prospects

Although a great many treatment strategies have eliminated acute and early delayed brain injury as well as most delayed demyelination and white matter necrosis, radiotherapy is still carries a risk of RIBI which may seriously affect the life quality of survivors. This risk is further exacerbated while the patient need to use chemotherapeutic agents at the same time [2].

To get more knowledge about the mechanism of RIBI is the key to the solution. Although many theories have been proposed, it is likely that the pathogenesis in long term survivors of various tumors like small cell lung cancer, NPC, low-grade glioma, non-parenchymal tumors, primary brain tumors and metastatic brain tumors are different just because they were treated differently. There is not a solely theory that can be used to fully answer this question.

As a result, it is imperative to detect the pathological change non-invasively as early as possible. However, there still a lot of difficulties which need to be solved in clinical practice. It is explicit that the most important issue is to differentiate radiation necrosis and tumor progression. Fortunately, there are multiple radiological and nuclear medicine techniques available to help us even these anatomic and metabolic imaging techniques all have inherent limitations in sensitivity and specificity.

Researchers all over the world have tried hard but have had only modest success in modulating RIBI to date. However, the future looks promising since we have attached importance to RIBI and find some innovative treatments such as the NECs or anti-VEGF therapy which can be the alternative offer [72].

Over the next decade, we will continue paying more attention to the investigation that how radiation-induced brain injury develops and how it can be treated [2].

Acknowledgements

We are grateful for support from the National Natural Science Foundation of China (no. 81372919) and the Natural Science Foundation of Guangdong Province, China(no. S2013010013964).

Author details

Zhihua Yang[1], Shoumin Bai[2], Beibei Gu[3], Shuling Peng[3], Wang Liao[4] and Jun Liu[4*]

*Address all correspondence to: docliujun@hotmail.com

1 Department of Neurology, the First Affiliated Hospital, Guangzhou Medical University, Guangdong, China

2 Department of Oncology, Sun Yat-Sen Memorial Hospital, Sun Yat-Sen University, Guangdong, China

3 Department of Anesthesiology, Sun Yat-Sen Memorial Hospital, Sun Yat-Sen University, Guangdong, China

4 Department of Neurology, Sun Yat-Sen Memorial Hospital, Sun Yat-Sen University, Guangdong, China

References

[1] Tsao, M.N., et al., Radiotherapeutic management of brain metastases: a systematic review and meta-analysis. Cancer Treat Rev, 2005. 31(4): p. 256-73.

[2] Greene-Schloesser, D., et al., Radiation-induced brain injury: A review. Front Oncol, 2012. 2: p. 73.

[3] Roman, D.D. and P.W. Sperduto, Neuropsychological effects of cranial radiation: current knowledge and future directions. Int J Radiat Oncol Biol Phys, 1995. 31(4): p. 983-98.

[4] Sheline, G.E., Radiation therapy of brain tumors. Cancer, 1977. 39(2 Suppl): p. 873-81.

[5] Schultheiss, T.E. and L.C. Stephens, Invited review: permanent radiation myelopathy. Br J Radiol, 1992. 65(777): p. 737-53.

[6] Yan, L., Z. Xi and B. Drettner, Epidemiological studies of nasopharyngeal cancer in the Guangzhou area, China. Preliminary report. Acta Otolaryngol, 1989. 107(5-6): p. 424-7.

[7] Brown, W.R., et al., Capillary loss precedes the cognitive impairment induced by fractionated whole-brain irradiation: a potential rat model of vascular dementia. J Neurol Sci, 2007. 257(1-2): p. 67-71.

[8] Lee, A.W., et al., Factors affecting risk of symptomatic temporal lobe necrosis: significance of fractional dose and treatment time. Int J Radiat Oncol Biol Phys, 2002. 53(1): p. 75-85.

[9] Ruben, J.D., et al., Cerebral radiation necrosis: incidence, outcomes, and risk factors with emphasis on radiation parameters and chemotherapy. Int J Radiat Oncol Biol Phys, 2006. 65(2): p. 499-508.

[10] Liu, Y., et al., An experimental study of acute radiation-induced cognitive dysfunction in a young rat model. AJNR Am J Neuroradiol, 2010. 31(2): p. 383-7.

[11] Zhou, H., et al., Fractionated radiation-induced acute encephalopathy in a young rat model: cognitive dysfunction and histologic findings. AJNR Am J Neuroradiol, 2011. 32(10): p. 1795-800.

[12] Ansari, R., et al., Anti-TNFA (TNF-alpha) treatment abrogates radiation-induced changes in vacular density and tissue oxygenation. Radiat Res, 2007. 167(1): p. 80-6.

[13] Zhao, Z.Y., et al., Edaravone protects HT22 neurons from H2O2-induced apoptosis by inhibiting the MAPK signaling pathway. CNS Neurosci Ther, 2013. 19(3): p. 163-9.

[14] Monje, M.L., et al., Irradiation induces neural precursor-cell dysfunction. Nat Med, 2002. 8(9): p. 955-62.

[15] Gorman, A.M., et al., Oxidative stress and apoptosis in neurodegeneration. J Neurol Sci, 1996. 139 Suppl: p. 45-52.

[16] Pettmann, B. and C.E. Henderson, Neuronal cell death. Neuron, 1998. 20(4): p. 633-47.

[17] Ramanan, S., et al., Role of PPARs in Radiation-Induced Brain Injury. PPAR Res, 2010. 2010: p. 234975.

[18] Li, Y.Q., et al., Endothelial apoptosis initiates acute blood-brain barrier disruption after ionizing radiation. Cancer Res, 2003. 63(18): p. 5950-6.

[19] Monje, M.L., H. Toda and T.D. Palmer, Inflammatory blockade restores adult hippocampal neurogenesis. Science, 2003. 302(5651): p. 1760-5.

[20] Zhou, H., et al., Fractionated radiation-induced acute encephalopathy in a young rat model: cognitive dysfunction and histologic findings. AJNR Am J Neuroradiol, 2011. 32(10): p. 1795-800.

[21] Wilson, C.M., et al., Radiation-induced astrogliosis and blood-brain barrier damage can be abrogated using anti-TNF treatment. Int J Radiat Oncol Biol Phys, 2009. 74(3): p. 934-41.

[22] Conner, K.R., et al., Effects of the AT1 receptor antagonist L-158,809 on microglia and neurogenesis after fractionated whole-brain irradiation. Radiat Res, 2010. 173(1): p. 49-61.

[23] Moore, A.H., et al., Radiation-induced edema is dependent on cyclooxygenase 2 activity in mouse brain. Radiat Res, 2004. 161(2): p. 153-60.

[24] Lee, W.H., et al., Irradiation induces regionally specific alterations in pro-inflammatory environments in rat brain. Int J Radiat Biol, 2010. 86(2): p. 132-44.

[25] Zhao, W. and M.E. Robbins, Inflammation and chronic oxidative stress in radiation-induced late normal tissue injury: therapeutic implications. Curr Med Chem, 2009. 16(2): p. 130-43.

[26] Persson, H.L., et al., Radiation-induced cell death: importance of lysosomal destabilization. Biochem J, 2005. 389(Pt 3): p. 877-84.

[27] Schultheiss, T.E. and L.C. Stephens, Invited review: permanent radiation myelopathy. Br J Radiol, 1992. 65(777): p. 737-53.

[28] Zhao, W., et al., Administration of the peroxisomal proliferator-activated receptor gamma agonist pioglitazone during fractionated brain irradiation prevents radiation-induced cognitive impairment. Int J Radiat Oncol Biol Phys, 2007. 67(1): p. 6-9.

[29] Zhao, W., D.I. Diz and M.E. Robbins, Oxidative damage pathways in relation to normal tissue injury. Br J Radiol, 2007. 80 Spec No 1: p. S23-31.

[30] Tofilon, P.J. and J.R. Fike, The radioresponse of the central nervous system: a dynamic process. Radiat Res, 2000. 153(4): p. 357-70.

[31] Nakata, H., et al., Early blood-brain barrier disruption after high-dose single-fraction irradiation in rats. Acta Neurochir (Wien), 1995. 136(1-2): p. 82-6; discussion 86-7.

[32] Palmer, T.D., J. Takahashi and F.H. Gage, The adult rat hippocampus contains primordial neural stem cells. Mol Cell Neurosci, 1997. 8(6): p. 389-404.

[33] Gage, F.H., et al., Multipotent progenitor cells in the adult dentate gyrus. J Neurobiol, 1998. 36(2): p. 249-66.

[34] Machida, M., G. Lonart and R.A. Britten, Low (60 cGy) doses of (56)Fe HZE-particle radiation lead to a persistent reduction in the glutamatergic readily releasable pool in rat hippocampal synaptosomes. Radiat Res, 2010. 174(5): p. 618-23.

[35] Sundgren, P.C. and Y. Cao, Brain irradiation: effects on normal brain parenchyma and radiation injury. Neuroimaging Clin N Am, 2009. 19(4): p. 657-68.

[36] Ji-yong, Q., Diagnosis, prevention and treatment of radiation brain damage of nasopharyngeal carcinoma patients treated by radiotherapy, L.K.J. Yun-he, L.K.J. Yun-he^Editors. 2006. p. 942-943.

[37] Gu, B., et al., Radiation-induced Brachial Plexus Injury After Radiotherapy for Nasopharyngeal Carcinoma. Jpn J Clin Oncol, 2014. 44(8): p. 736-42.

[38] Flickinger, J.C., et al., Development of a model to predict permanent symptomatic postradiosurgery injury for arteriovenous malformation patients. Arteriovenous Malformation Radiosurgery Study Group. Int J Radiat Oncol Biol Phys, 2000. 46(5): p. 1143-8.

[39] Kondziolka, D., et al., Radiosurgery with or without whole-brain radiotherapy for brain metastases: the patients' perspective regarding complications. Am J Clin Oncol, 2005. 28(2): p. 173-9.

[40] Sundgren, P.C. and Y. Cao, Brain irradiation: effects on normal brain parenchyma and radiation injury. Neuroimaging Clin N Am, 2009. 19(4): p. 657-68.

[41] Herman, M.A., et al., Neurocognitive and functional assessment of patients with brain metastases: a pilot study. Am J Clin Oncol, 2003. 26(3): p. 273-9.

[42] Chang, E.L., et al., Neurocognition in patients with brain metastases treated with radiosurgery or radiosurgery plus whole-brain irradiation: a randomised controlled trial. Lancet Oncol, 2009. 10(11): p. 1037-44.

[43] Rong, X., et al., Radiation-induced cranial neuropathy in patients with nasopharyngeal carcinoma. A follow-up study. Strahlenther Onkol, 2012. 188(3): p. 282-6.

[44] Zhao, Z., et al., Late-onset radiation-induced optic neuropathy after radiotherapy for nasopharyngeal carcinoma. J Clin Neurosci, 2013. 20(5): p. 702-6.

[45] Qiu, S.J., et al., Proton magnetic resonance spectroscopy for radiation encephalopathy induced by radiotherapy for nasopharyngeal carcinoma. Nan Fang Yi Ke Da Xue Xue Bao, 2007. 27(3): p. 241-6.

[46] Rabin, B.M., et al., Radiation-induced changes in the central nervous system and head and neck. Radiographics, 1996. 16(5): p. 1055-72.

[47] Khong, P.L., et al., White matter anisotropy in post-treatment childhood cancer survivors: preliminary evidence of association with neurocognitive function. J Clin Oncol, 2006. 24(6): p. 884-90.

[48] Dellani, P.R., et al., Late structural alterations of cerebral white matter in long-term survivors of childhood leukemia. J Magn Reson Imaging, 2008. 27(6): p. 1250-5.

[49] Shaw, P.J. and D. Bates, Conservative treatment of delayed cerebral radiation necrosis. J Neurol Neurosurg Psychiatry, 1984. 47(12): p. 1338-41.

[50] Glantz, M.J., et al., Treatment of radiation-induced nervous system injury with heparin and warfarin. Neurology, 1994. 44(11): p. 2020-7.

[51] He, F., et al., Effect of edaravone on Abeta1-40 induced enhancement of voltage-gated calcium channel current. CNS Neurosci Ther, 2012. 18(1): p. 89-90.

[52] Tang, Y., et al., Psychological disorders, cognitive dysfunction and quality of life in nasopharyngeal carcinoma patients with radiation-induced brain injury. PLoS One, 2012. 7(6): p. e36529.

[53] Sezen, O., et al., Vitamin E and L-carnitine, separately or in combination, in the prevention of radiation-induced brain and retinal damages. Neurosurg Rev, 2008. 31(2): p. 205-13; discussion 213.

[54] Brown, W.R., et al., Vascular damage after fractionated whole-brain irradiation in rats. Radiat Res, 2005. 164(5): p. 662-8.

[55] Liu, Y., et al., An experimental study of acute radiation-induced cognitive dysfunction in a young rat model. AJNR Am J Neuroradiol, 2010. 31(2): p. 383-7.

[56] Moulder, J.E., B.L. Fish and E.P. Cohen, ACE inhibitors and AII receptor antagonists in the treatment and prevention of bone marrow transplant nephropathy. Curr Pharm Des, 2003. 9(9): p. 737-49.

[57] Molteni, A., et al., Control of radiation-induced pneumopathy and lung fibrosis by angiotensin-converting enzyme inhibitors and an angiotensin II type 1 receptor blocker. Int J Radiat Biol, 2000. 76(4): p. 523-32.

[58] Jenrow, K.A., et al., Ramipril mitigates radiation-induced impairment of neurogenesis in the rat dentate gyrus. Radiat Oncol, 2010. 5: p. 6.

[59] Lee, T.C., et al., Chronic administration of the angiotensin-converting enzyme inhibitor, ramipril, prevents fractionated whole-brain irradiation-induced perirhinal cortex-dependent cognitive impairment. Radiat Res, 2012. 178(1): p. 46-56.

[60] Shaw, E.G., et al., Phase II study of donepezil in irradiated brain tumor patients: effect on cognitive function, mood, and quality of life. J Clin Oncol, 2006. 24(9): p. 1415-20.

[61] Robbins, M.E., et al., The AT1 receptor antagonist, L-158,809, prevents or ameliorates fractionated whole-brain irradiation-induced cognitive impairment. Int J Radiat Oncol Biol Phys, 2009. 73(2): p. 499-505.

[62] Acharya, M.M., et al., Rescue of radiation-induced cognitive impairment through cranial transplantation of human embryonic stem cells. Proc Natl Acad Sci U S A, 2009. 106(45): p. 19150-5.

[63] Joo, K.M., et al., Trans-differentiation of neural stem cells: a therapeutic mechanism against the radiation induced brain damage. PLoS One, 2012. 7(2): p. e25936.

[64] Gutierrez, A.N., et al., Whole brain radiotherapy with hippocampal avoidance and simultaneously integrated brain metastases boost: a planning study. Int J Radiat Oncol Biol Phys, 2007. 69(2): p. 589-97.

[65] Barani, I.J., et al., Neural stem cell-preserving external-beam radiotherapy of central nervous system malignancies. Int J Radiat Oncol Biol Phys, 2007. 68(4): p. 978-85.

[66] Munck, A.R.P., et al., Photon and proton therapy planning comparison for malignant glioma based on CT, FDG-PET, DTI-MRI and fiber tracking. Acta Oncol, 2011. 50(6): p. 777-83.

[67] Wang, X., C. Hu and A. Eisbruch, Organ-sparing radiation therapy for head and neck cancer. Nat Rev Clin Oncol, 2011. 8(11): p. 639-48.

[68] Matuschek, C., et al., Bevacizumab as a treatment option for radiation-induced cerebral necrosis. Strahlenther Onkol, 2011. 187(2): p. 135-9.

[69] Chuba, P.J., et al., Hyperbaric oxygen therapy for radiation-induced brain injury in children. Cancer, 1997. 80(10): p. 2005-12.

[70] Bui, Q.C., et al., The efficacy of hyperbaric oxygen therapy in the treatment of radiation-induced late side effects. Int J Radiat Oncol Biol Phys, 2004. 60(3): p. 871-8.

[71] Kishi, K., et al., Preferential enhancement of tumor radioresponse by a cyclooxygenase-2 inhibitor. Cancer Res, 2000. 60(5): p. 1326-31.

[72] Siu, A., et al., Radiation necrosis following treatment of high grade glioma--a review of the literature and current understanding. Acta Neurochir (Wien), 2012. 154(2): p. 191-201; discussion 201.

3

BMI Transcription Factor as a Novel Target for the Treatment of Brain Tumors

Mohammad M. Hossain, Bárbara Meléndez,
Juan A. Rey, Javier S. Castresana and Mehdi H. Shahi

1. Introduction

Recent studies have hypothesized that brain tumor stem cells (BTSCs) are responsible for the poor survival outcome of brain tumor patients. Sonic hedgehog (Shh) is one of the crucial signaling pathways to regulate stem cell self-renewable capacity. Disruption of this pathway activate Gli transcription factors, which further activate other downstream target genes including BMI1 to promote brain tumor development (medulloblastoma and glioblastoma among other tumors) (Leung *et al.*, 2004; Bruggeman *et al.*, 2007; Godlewski *et al.*, 2008). BMI1 is a polycomb complex protein also known as polycomb group RING finger protein 4 (PCGF4) or RING finger protein 51 (RNF51). BMI1 gene (B cell-specific Moloney Murin leukemia virus integration site 1) is located on human chromosome 10 (10p13). Interestingly, BMI1 showed high expression in medulloblastoma and glioblastoma (Leung *et al.*, 2004; Natsume *et al.*, 2011). Shh treatment induced both BMI1 and Gli1 expression. Gli1 overexpression also promoted high expression of BMI1. High expression of BMI1 in tumor cells indicates high capacity of self-renewing characteristics (Hemmati *et al.*, 2003). Most of the BTSCs showed high expression of BMI1. Inhibition of Gli with specific inhibitor GANT61 and Gli siRNAs mediated knock-down inhibited brain tumor cell proliferation and also decreased the expression of BMI1 in medulloblastoma and glioblastoma (Shahi *et al.*, unpublished). Therefore, all these studies suggest that BMI1 would be a novel therapeutic transcription factor to target BTSCs and enhance the survival of brain tumor patients.

2. BMI1: An oncogene and stem cell marker

BMI1 is one of the crucial genes for the development of various tissues including the nervous system. This gene is located at chromosome 10p13 in humans. BMI1 was initially identified as a murin leukemia viral oncogene [1]. BMI1 was the first gene reported to belong to the Polycomb-group of genes [2]. These genes express the proteins which form a large multimeric structure to silence other genes via modification in chromatin organization [3]. Polycomb repressive complexes are divided into two groups.

Polycomb repressive complex 1 (PRC1)

Polycomb repressive complex 2 (PRC2)

PRC1 includes BMI1, and PRC2 includes enhancer of zeste homolog 2 (EZHZ) to facilitate stable silencing of gene expression [4]

3. Role of BMI1 in normal development

BMI1 polycomb protein is essential for the self-renewal of stem cells of different tissues of the body besides the central nervous system (CNS) [5]. One study showed that Nestin-BMI1-GFP transgenic mice cells increased the development of neural stem cell colonies and the self-renewal capability of fetal and adult CNS cells (He et al., 2009). Ink4a and Arf genes encode tumor suppressor proteins p16Ink4a and p19Arf respectively, which are involved in the inhibition of cell cycle progression [6]. Interestingly, BMI1 promotes the maintenance of CNS stem cells from the embryonic stage to adulthood by suppressing Ink4a and Arf genes [5]. BMI1 is also involved in Shh signaling mediated postnatal cerebellar neurogenesis by binding to the promoter of p21waf1/cip1 [7]. Moreover, BMI1 is a crucial gene for the development of embryonic and adult stem cells and brain tumors. Interestingly, selective conditional knockout of BMI1 based on Cre/LoXP in transgenic mouse showed that BMI1 has potential to induce neural stem cells proliferation and self-renewal both in vitro and in vivo [8]. In this process BMI1 down-regulates both Ink4a/ARF and p21/FoxG1. Moreover, increased ectopic expression of BMI1 in progenitors committed to a neuronal lineage during embryonic cortical development, triggered apoptosis via a survivin-mediated mechanism, and caused a reduction in brain size [8]. However, the self-renewable capability of adult neural stem progenitor cells is independent of FoxG1, while apoptosis resistance of neural progenitor cells depends on high expression of BMI1 [8].

4. Role of BMI1 in glioblastoma development

Gliomas are the most common brain tumors of the central nervous system comprising astrocytic gliomas, oligodendrogliomas, or a mixture of both. The most malignant glioma is glioblastoma multiforme (GBM) (WHO grade IV) comprising about 50% of glioma. Post-therapy survival rate of GBM patients is 24% for 1 year and 12% for 2 years only [9]. There are ample amount of evidence suggesting that gliomas have stem-like cells called glioma initiating cells (GICs). These cells have self-renewal capability and cause gliomagenesis. The GICs are under the regulation of several signaling pathways including Shh, Notch, Wnt and BMI1. Effective targeting of GICs could become a novel strategy to target glioma [10]. The 10p13 region is highly significant in brain tumorigenesis especially glioblastoma. BMI1 is part of the polycomb repressive complex 1, which epigenetically regulates gene expression by acetylation, methylation, and mono-ubiquitination of histones [11]. These modifications cause transcriptional repression of differentiation and pluripotency of embryonic stem cells [12]. BMI1 is essential for the proliferation and transformation of primary glial cells. BMI1 deficient glial cells have less proliferating and tumorigenic capacities. BMI1 is also involved in pathways including proliferation, adhesion, and differentiation. All these pathways play a significant contribution to stem cell renewal and glioblastoma development [13]. One report demonstrates a high copy number of BMI1 in glioma samples [11]. Even, a murine tumor model showed a role for BMI1 in the genesis of glioma and high fold expression of BMI1 in high-grade gliomas [13]. BMI1 shows functional diversity in different cell types including embryonic stem cells and mature neurons [12]. Moreover, BMI1 sometimes behaves as a tumor suppressor gene or oncogene in different tumors. According to one study most of the glioma samples showed BMI1 gene allelic imbalance. BMI1 negatively regulates p16 in astrocytoma. However, they also suggest that BMI1 is not very significant for prognosis of astrocytic tumors [2]. Interestingly, BMI1 is considered as a transgene, which helps MYC to promote hematopoietic malignancies [14-16]. High expression of BMI1 has been noted in brain tumors irrespective of tumor grades [5]. BMI1 has a role in glioma and glioma stem cell growth which is both dependent and independent of InK4a-Arf [13]. GBM showed an association of BMI1 overexpression and enrichment in CD133+ cells [Xia et al., 2012]. Stable knockdown of BMI1 in GBM reveals that BMI1 prevented the clonogenic nature of GBM cells and also these cells were not able to develop brain tumors in vivo. Accordingly, BMI1 is a potent inhibitor of apoptosis in CD133+ cells and of differentiation into neurons and astrocytes [17]. BMI1 is also capable to inhibit alternate tumor suppressor pathways that attempt to compensate for INK4A-ARF/p53 deletion and hyperactivity of the PI3K/AKT pathway [17]. Interestingly, one study suggests that BMI1 causes apoptotic resistance to glioma cells through the activation of IKK-Nuclear factor-kB pathway and could therefore be a good prognostic factor for glioma [20]. IKK-Nuclear factor-kB pathway is very active in high grade GBM and glioma cell lines [18, 19]. High expression of BMI1 protects brain tumor cells from cytotoxic reagents-induced apoptosis, while attenuated BMI1 expression promotes apoptosis inducer factors. BMI1 also controls apoptosis in glioma cell lines by activation of the IKK-NF-kB pathway and promoting antiapoptotic genes [20]. Co-expression of BMI1 and p65 protein, a subunit of NF-kB in glioma is in favour of BMI1 and NF-kB pathways involvement in glioma chemoresistance. GBM is resistant to all types of therapies. It has been postulated that most CD133+ cells are resistant to gamma radiation via activation of DNA double-strand break (DSB) response mechanism, including the participation of the ataxia-telangiectasia-mutated kinase gene (ATM). After purification of BMI1 with DNA DSB responsive factors and nonhomologous end joining (NHEJ) repair proteins in GBM cells [21], a BMI1 enrichment was observed after irradiation, being colocalized and co-purified with ATM and histone gammaH2AX. Deficient BMI1 glioma cells showed inactive DNA DSB response, which promoted sensitivity of radiation in glioma cells. Overexpressed BMI1 modulated the neural stem cells radiation resistance by enhancing the ATM activity. Therefore, a combined effect of BMI1 inhibition together with radiation therapy might efficiently target GBM stem cells [21]. Interestingly, a recent report suggested that expression of BMI1 and c-Myc correlated in glioma. This finding further reveals that c-Myc, either directly or indirectly, activates several epigenetic modulators including acetylase GCN5 and polycomb-group (PcG) gene BMI1 [22, 23]. It is interesting to know that BMI1 promoter contains functional E-box and c-Myc binding regions [24, 25]. Moreover, c-Myc was able to activate BMI1; and BMI1 further facilitated the oncogenic expression of c-Myc in glioblastoma development [17]. It has been speculated that c-Myc and BMI1 might be good biomarkers of glioblastoma due to their high expression and involvement in gliomagenesis. Inhibition of both genes could give glioblastoma a greater sensitivity to combined anticancer therapy. A recent study revealed that Tamoxifen (TAM) has the ability to reduce the expression of neural stem cell markers, like Nestin, Bmi1 and Vimentin, in glioma cell lines. Moreover, the action of TAM in glioma cells apotosis is assisted by prostate apoptosis response-4(par-4) [26]. It has been published that AR-A 014418 inhibits GSK3 beta kinase activation which further regulates the cancer escape pathway via downregulation of anti-apoptotic gene BMI1 [27].

5. BMI1 and miRNAs

Low expression of miRNA-128 was reported in GBM samples. High expression of miRNA-128 in GBM down-regulates ARP5 (ANGPTL 6), BMI1 and E2F-3a, factors which are key regulator for brain cell proliferation [28]. miRNA-128 also targets BMI1 and down-regulates its expression. Most of the glioma samples show less expression of miRNA-128. Overexpression of miRNA-128 shows inhibition of GICs proliferation and self-renewable capacity [10]. Normal brain has abundant expression of miRNA-124, however, miRNA-124 expression is diminished during the development of glioma. Interestingly, overexpression of miRNA-124 reduced the formation of neurospheres, the CD133+ cell subpopulation, and the expression of stem cells markers like BMI1, Nanog and Nestin [29]. Smoothened inhibitor NPV-LDE-225 (Erismodegib) inhibits BMI1 in GICs via upregulation of miRNA-128, miRNA-21 and miRNA-200 [30]. Interestingly, NPV-LDE-225 was used in topical cream for basal cell carcinoma treatment and it inhibited the Shh pathway [31]. A recent study suggested that NPV-LDE-225 mediated inhibition of Shh signaling downregulates Bmi1 via upregulation of miRNA-128 [30]. Another study also suggested that polycomb repressor complex BMI1 is targeted by miRNA-128 in glioma stem cells [32]. Another miRNA-218 also inhibited the expression of BMI1 which further retarded glioma invasion, migration, and glioma stem cell renewal capability. Most gliomas showed less expression of miRNA-218 and overexpression of miRNA-128, which further inhibited glioma tumor characteristics. It was assumed that BMI1 is the downstream target gene of miRNA-218. miRNA-218 regulates many genes which are involved in glioma tumorigenesis [33]. Interestingly, we illustrate a model diagram for the role of BMI1 in gliomagenesis (Figure 1).

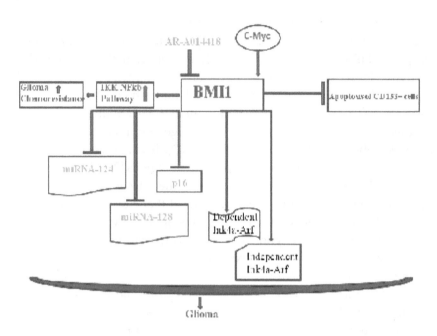

Figure 1. BMI1 networking in gliomagenesis

6. Role of BMI1 in medulloblastoma

Medulloblastoma is a primitive neuroectodermal tumor of the cerebellum. Medulloblastoma is the most common pediatric malignant brain tumor, representing 20% of newly identified CNS tumors in children [34]. Medulloblastoma is driven by several signaling pathways, among which, Shh plays a critical role for the majority of these tumors [35, 36]. Mutations of the Shh pathway regulators are present in about 20-25% of medulloblastomas [37]. Shh-driven medulloblastoma showed high expression of BMI1. A recent study reveals the role of BMI1 in Shh-driven medulloblastoma. Transgenic mice showed the expression of Shh signaling activator SmoA1 with the help of glial fibrillary acidic protein (GFAP) promoter. They found that SmoA1/BMI1+/+; SmoA1/BMI1+/-postnatal mice (p=26) between days P14 to P26 showed prominent potential to develop medulloblastoma compared to SmoA1/BMI1-/-post natal mice (n=6) [38]. Interestingly, cells with BMI1 deficiency BMI1-/- even in the presence of SmoA1 were non-proliferative compared to BMI1+/+ cells [38]. Two down-stream genes which are inversely regulated by BMI1 in Shh-driven medulloblastoma development were reported. Cyclin D1 expression was downregulated and cyclin-dependent kinase inhibitor p19Arf was upregulated. Moreover, it was concluded that BMI1 is crucial for the Shh-driven medullo-blastoma development and that BMI1 facilitates medulloblastoma development de novo [38]. During embryonic development Shh signaling pathway regulates proliferation of granular neuron precursors (GNPs). GNPs are progenitors for medulloblastoma development, com-prising the transient external granular layer of cerebellum [39]. BMI1 seems to promote the expression of downstream target genes during cerebellum development [40]. BMI1-null mice developed reduced cerebellum and impaired production of granular neurons. Altered expression of BMI1 in medulloblastoma as well as correlation of BMI1 expression and Shh activation was reported in medulloblastoma [38, 41]. It was suggested that polycomb gene expression could be used as a predictor of poor clinical outcome in medulloblastoma [42]. BMI1 overexpression caused cell proliferation and assisted Shh signaling driven tumorigenesis [43]. BMI1 expression and Shh ligand concentration were positively correlated during development. Chromatin immunoprecipitation experiments revealed that Shh signaling pathway main transcriptional activator Gli1 preferentially binds to the promoter regions of BMI1. Moreover, overexpression and downregulation of Gli1 controls high and low expression of BMI1 respectively. Interestingly, BMI1 is not only a Shh-Gli1 downstream target gene but also promotes a feedback mechanism which further activates Shh-Gli1 signaling. This finding suggested that both BMI1 and Shh signaling pathways are mutually indispensable pathways in brain tumor initiating cells (BTICs) of medulloblastoma [43]. One study reported that overexpressed BMI1 was unable to induce tumors in mice from granule cell progenitors (GCPs). Therefore, it was concluded that overexpression of BMI1 in GCP-derived human medulloblastoma, could promote later stages of tumorigenesis and further sustain tumor cell survival [44]. Apart from cell proliferation other characteristic of tumors include anti-apoptotic nature and sustaining of high metabolic rate, both supported by high BMI1 and low TP53 levels of expression which are characteristic of group 4 human medulloblastoma [44]. BMI1 overexpression alone was not sufficient to induce medulloblastoma; however BMI1 overexpression and loss of p53 induced medulloblastoma in mice, producing similar tumors to group 4 human medulloblastomas [44]. Recently, medulloblastomas have been categorized in 4 subgroups on the basis of prognosis and predicted therapeutics (Kool et al., 2012, Ramaswamy et al., 2013 and Gottardo et al., 2014). Group 1 and group 2 are under the good clinical outcome and regulated by Shh and Wnt signaling, respectively [45]. Groups 3 and 4 medulloblastoma are not Shh/Wnt signaling mediated tumors, have metastatic potential, and poor patient outcome and lack of known molecular pathways. Current gene expression analysis is unable to detect self-renewal gene and brain tumor-initiating cells (BTIC) in group 3 and group 4 medulloblastoma. BTICs constitute a minority of the tumor mass, and their detection can be difficult in medulloblastoma. High BTIC promoted tumors to increase tumor aggressiveness and poor patient outcome. They investigated the potential stem cells candidate genes among the different subgroups of 251 human medulloblastoma samples from the 4 overlapping MB transcriptional data bases (Amsterdam, Memphis, Toronto and Boston) and 74 nano-string sub-grouped medulloblastoma (Vancouver) [45]. This analysis showed two crucial genes BMI1 and FoxG1, which presented abundant expression in non-Shh/wnt medulloblastoma groups. These genes are responsible to promote MB stem cells and tumor initiation in mice [45]. We also depicted a model for the different group of medulloblastoma development on the basis of cell signaling pathways and gene expression profile (Figure 3). This study also identified a reciprocal promoter in CD15+ medulloblastoma stem cells. The finding could be used as a novel target therapy against BTIC self-renewal. They also found BMI1 is a downstream target of FoxG1 and further promotes tumorigenicity. BMI1 also exerts feedback to FoxG1 expression and facilitates *in vivo* tumor malignancy and enhances in vitro stem cell self-renewal capability. Moreover, high expression of BMI1 can be considered as a strong molecular prognostic marker in pediatric brain tumors. We attempted to show a model for the role of BMI1 in medulloblastoma development (Figure 2).

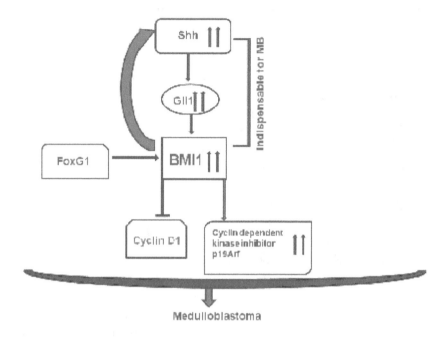

Figure 2. BMI1 networking in medulloblastoma development

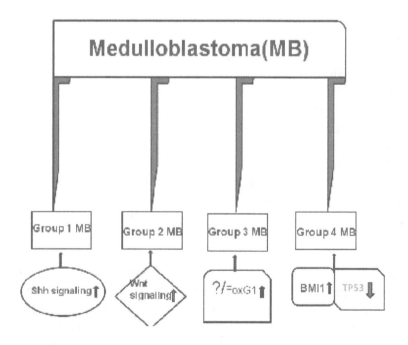

Figure 3. Division of medulloblastoma on the basis of gene and cell signaling expression

7. Conclusion

BMI1 is a very significant stem cell marker gene which contributes to the development of glioblastoma and medulloblastoma. Therefore, the treatment of glioblastoma and medulloblastoma would improve with the addition of BMI1 inhibitors. Moreover, high expression of BMI1 could be used as one of the earliest markers to diagnose brain tumors.

Acknowledgements

Authors are thankful to all members of Interdisciplinary Brain Research Centre, Aligarh Muslim University, Aligarh, India for their constant supports.

Author details

Mohammad M. Hossain[1], Bárbara Meléndez[2], Juan A. Rey[3], Javier S. Castresana[4] and Mehdi H. Shahi[1*]

*Address all correspondence to: mehdihayat@gmail.com

1 Interdisciplinary Brain Research Centre, Faculty of Medicine, Aligarh Muslim University,Aligarh, , India

2 Molecular Pathology Research Unit, Virgen de la Salud Hospital, Toledo, Spain

3 IdiPaz Research Unit, La Paz University Hospital, Madrid, Spain

4 Department of Biochemistry and Genetics, University of Navarra School of Sciences, Pamplona, Spain

References

[1] Jacobs, J.J., et al., *The oncogene and Polycomb-group gene bmi-1 regulates cell proliferation and senescence through the ink4a locus.* Nature, 1999. 397(6715): p. 164-8.

[2] Tirabosco, R., et al., *Expression of the Polycomb-Group protein BMI1 and correlation with p16 in astrocytomas an immunohistochemical study on 80 cases.* Pathol Res Pract, 2008. 204(9): p. 625-31.

[3] Sparmann, A. and M. van Lohuizen, *Polycomb silencers control cell fate, development and cancer.* Nat Rev Cancer, 2006. 6(11): p. 846-56.

[4] Dellino, G.I., et al., *Polycomb silencing blocks transcription initiation.* Mol Cell, 2004. 13(6): p. 887-93.

[5] He, S., et al., *Bmi-1 over-expression in neural stem/progenitor cells increases proliferation and neurogenesis in culture but has little effect on these functions in vivo.* Dev Biol, 2009. 328(2): p. 257-72.

[6] Lowe, S.W. and C.J. Sherr, *Tumor suppression by Ink4a-Arf: progress and puzzles.* Curr Opin Genet Dev, 2003. 13(1): p. 77-83.

[7] Subkhankulova, T., et al., *Bmi1 directly represses p21Waf1/Cip1 in Shh-induced proliferation of cerebellar granule cell progenitors.* Mol Cell Neurosci, 2010. 45(2): p. 151-62.

[8] Yadirgi, G., et al., *Conditional activation of Bmi1 expression regulates self-renewal, apoptosis, and differentiation of neural stem/progenitor cells in vitro and in vivo.* Stem Cells, 2011. 29(4): p. 700-12.

[9] Zhou, Y.H., et al., *Establishment of prognostic models for astrocytic and oligodendroglial brain tumors with standardized quantification of marker gene expression and clinical variables.* Biomark Insights, 2010. 5: p. 153-68.

[10] Natsume, A., et al., *Glioma-initiating cells and molecular pathology: implications for therapy.* Brain Tumor Pathol, 2011. 28(1): p. 1-12.

[11] Hayry, V., et al., *Copy number alterations of the polycomb gene BMI1 in gliomas.* Acta Neuropathol, 2008. 116(1): p. 97-102.

[12] Spivakov, M. and A.G. Fisher, *Epigenetic signatures of stem-cell identity.* Nat Rev Genet, 2007. 8(4): p. 263-71.

[13] Bruggeman, S.W., et al., *Bmi1 controls tumor development in an Ink4a/Arf-independent manner in a mouse model for glioma.* Cancer Cell, 2007. 12(4): p. 328-41.

[14] Haupt, Y., et al., *bmi-1 transgene induces lymphomas and collaborates with myc in tumorigenesis.* Oncogene, 1993. 8(11): p. 3161-4.

[15] Jacobs, J.J., et al., *Bmi-1 collaborates with c-Myc in tumorigenesis by inhibiting c-Myc-induced apoptosis via INK4a/ARF.* Genes Dev, 1999. 13(20): p. 2678-90.

[16] van Lohuizen, M., et al., *Sequence similarity between the mammalian bmi-1 proto-oncogene and the Drosophila regulatory genes Psc and Su(z)2.* Nature, 1991. 353(6342): p. 353-5.

[17] Abdouh, M., et al., *BMI1 sustains human glioblastoma multiforme stem cell renewal.* J Neurosci, 2009. 29(28): p. 8884-96.

[18] Lefranc, F., J. Brotchi, and R. Kiss, *Possible future issues in the treatment of glioblastomas: special emphasis on cell migration and the resistance of migrating glioblastoma cells to apoptosis.* J Clin Oncol, 2005. 23(10): p. 2411-22.

[19] Nagai, S., et al., *Aberrant nuclear factor-kappaB activity and its participation in the growth of human malignant astrocytoma.* J Neurosurg, 2002. 96(5): p. 909-17.

[20] Li, J., et al., *Oncoprotein Bmi-1 renders apoptotic resistance to glioma cells through activation of the IKK-nuclear factor-kappaB Pathway.* Am J Pathol, 2010. 176(2): p. 699-709.

[21] Facchino, S., et al., *BMI1 confers radioresistance to normal and cancerous neural stem cells through recruitment of the DNA damage response machinery.* J Neurosci, 2010. 30(30): p. 10096-111.

[22] Cole, M.D. and V.H. Cowling, *Transcription-independent functions of MYC: regulation of translation and DNA replication.* Nat Rev Mol Cell Biol, 2008. 9(10): p. 810-5.

[23] Martinato, F., et al., *Analysis of Myc-induced histone modifications on target chromatin.* PLoS One, 2008. 3(11): p. e3650.

[24] Guney, I., S. Wu, and J.M. Sedivy, *Reduced c-Myc signaling triggers telomere-independent senescence by regulating Bmi-1 and p16(INK4a).* Proc Natl Acad Sci U S A, 2006. 103(10): p. 3645-50.

[25] Guo, W.J., et al., *Mel-18, a polycomb group protein, regulates cell proliferation and senescence via transcriptional repression of Bmi-1 and c-Myc oncoproteins.* Mol Biol Cell, 2007. 18(2): p. 536-46.

[26] Jagtap, J.C., et al., *Expression and regulation of prostate apoptosis response-4 (Par-4) in human glioma stem cells in drug-induced apoptosis.* PLoS One, 2014. 9(2): p. e88505.

[27] Yadav, A.K., et al., *AR-A 014418 Used against GSK3beta Downregulates Expression of hnRNPA1 and SF2/ASF Splicing Factors.* J Oncol, 2014. 2014: p. 695325.

[28] Cui, J.G., et al., *Micro-RNA-128 (miRNA-128) down-regulation in glioblastoma targets ARP5 (ANGPTL6), Bmi-1 and E2F-3a, key regulators of brain cell proliferation.* J Neurooncol, 2010. 98(3): p. 297-304.

[29] Xia, H., et al., *Loss of brain-enriched miR-124 microRNA enhances stem-like traits and invasiveness of glioma cells.* J Biol Chem, 2012. 287(13): p. 9962-71.

[30] Fu, J. and W. Hsu, *Epidermal Wnt controls hair follicle induction by orchestrating dynamic signaling crosstalk between the epidermis and dermis.* J Invest Dermatol, 2013. 133(4): p. 890-8.

[31] Skvara, H., et al., *Topical treatment of Basal cell carcinomas in nevoid Basal cell carcinoma syndrome with a smoothened inhibitor.* J Invest Dermatol, 2011. 131(8): p. 1735-44.

[32] Peruzzi, P., et al., *MicroRNA-128 coordinately targets Polycomb Repressor Complexes in glioma stem cells.* Neuro Oncol, 2013. 15(9): p. 1212-24.

[33] Tu, Y., et al., *MicroRNA-218 inhibits glioma invasion, migration, proliferation, and cancer stem-like cell self-renewal by targeting the polycomb group gene Bmi1.* Cancer Res, 2013. 73(19): p. 6046-55.

[34] Packer, R.J., et al., *Medulloblastoma: clinical and biologic aspects*. Neuro Oncol, 1999. 1(3): p. 232-50.

[35] Goodrich, L.V., et al., *Altered neural cell fates and medulloblastoma in mouse patched mutants*. Science, 1997. 277(5329): p. 1109-13.

[36] Wetmore, C., D.E. Eberhart, and T. Curran, *The normal patched allele is expressed in medulloblastomas from mice with heterozygous germ-line mutation of patched*. Cancer Res, 2000. 60(8): p. 2239-46.

[37] Ellison, D.W., et al., *What's new in neuro-oncology? Recent advances in medulloblastoma*. Eur J Paediatr Neurol, 2003. 7(2): p. 53-66.

[38] Michael, L.E., et al., *Bmi1 is required for Hedgehog pathway-driven medulloblastoma expansion*. Neoplasia, 2008. 10(12): p. 1343-9, 5p following 1349.

[39] Marino, S., *Medulloblastoma: developmental mechanisms out of control*. Trends Mol Med, 2005. 11(1): p. 17-22.

[40] Leung, C., et al., *Bmi1 is essential for cerebellar development and is overexpressed in human medulloblastomas*. Nature, 2004. 428(6980): p. 337-41.

[41] Glinsky, G.V., O. Berezovska, and A.B. Glinskii, *Microarray analysis identifies a death-from-cancer signature predicting therapy failure in patients with multiple types of cancer*. J Clin Invest, 2005. 115(6): p. 1503-21.

[42] Zakrzewska, M., et al., *Polycomb genes expression as a predictor of poor clinical outcome in children with medulloblastoma*. Childs Nerv Syst, 2011. 27(1): p. 79-86.

[43] Wang, X., et al., *Sonic hedgehog regulates Bmi1 in human medulloblastoma brain tumor-initiating cells*. Oncogene, 2012. 31(2): p. 187-99.

[44] Behesti, H., et al., *Bmi1 overexpression in the cerebellar granule cell lineage of mice affects cell proliferation and survival without initiating medulloblastoma formation*. Dis Model Mech, 2013. 6(1): p. 49-63.

[45] Manoranjan, B., et al., *FoxG1 interacts with Bmi1 to regulate self-renewal and tumorigenicity of medulloblastoma stem cells*. Stem Cells, 2013. 31(7): p. 1266-77.

4

Techniques to Improve the Extent of Brain Tumor Resection — Awake Speech and Motor Mapping, and Intraoperative MRI

Todd W. Vitaz

1. Introduction

It has long been believed by many neurosurgeons that maximizing tumor resection improved patient outcome for patients with high-grade gliomas. Over the past decade the impact of maximizing tumor resection has been clearly shown to be a favorable prognostic factor in the treatment of many types of brain tumors in clinical studies [1-11]. This holds true not only for GBM and other high-grade gliomas but also for lower grade lesions as well [11-13]. In addition, complete tumor resection has also been long known to be potentially curative for many "benign" intracranial lesions such as meningiomas and pituitary tumors with much higher rates of progression free survival for these types of lesions when complete resection has been performed [14].

Even for the most experienced surgeon visual inspection and surgical judgment are not enough to determine when complete resection has been obtained [3,15,16]. Too little resection increases the chances for earlier recurrence and disease progression and overly aggressive resection leads to an increased risk of potential neurological and cognitive deficits. As a result of this many technological advances have been developed to try to assist the surgeon with determining when complete resection has been obtained. These developments included intraoperative ultrasound, frame based and frameless navigation systems, intraoperative MRI, and intraoperative fluorescence with 5-aminolevulinic acid (5-ALA).

In addition, the utilization of awake mapping procedures also allows surgeons to maximize tumor resection by enabling them to monitor the patient's neurological status (motor or speech) throughout a resection. This real-time feedback enables surgeons to maximize tumor resection in lesions near eloquent cortex while minimizing the development of neurological deficits [17].

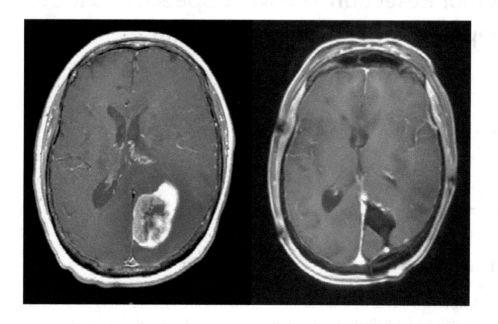

Figure 1. T1 Weighted post contrast preoperative and intraoperative MRI scans illustrating complete resection of a left parietal GBM

2. Literature review of positive prognostic effect for extent of resection (EOR)

One of the original studies to clearly show a survival advantage for extent of resection was a large retrospective endeavor by LaCroix and the MD Anderson Group [1]. They showed a survival advantage for extent of resection greater than 90% and an even greater advantage when resection was over 97%. A 2012 review by Sanai found five studies which used volumetric imaging to compare pre and postoperative MRIs for the EOR of contrast enhancement for patients undergoing surgical treatment of primary GBM. Three of these studies showed a survival advantage of between 2-8 months for patients undergoing complete resections compared to subtotal resections [18]. He also found that seventeen out of twenty eight nonvolumetric studies also found a survival advantage for extent of resection on univariate analysis [18]. Fourteen of these twenty eight studies also performed multivariate analysis to attempt to control for patient age, KPS and other factors. All fourteen of these papers found extent of resection to be a positive prognostic factor using this type of analysis [18].

In 2011 Sanai et al. [2] published a retrospective review evaluating extent of resection from a retrospective series of 500 consecutive newly diagnosed GBM patients treated at the University of California San Francisco Brain Tumor Center. Not only did they find a survival advantage based on extent of resection; but they also showed that a resection threshold greater than 78% was associated with a significant survival advantage. Although this study was retrospective in nature, the large patient volume adds significantly to its importance and illustrates that even in cases where complete resection may not be deemed safe that a significant debulking of greater than 78% likely conveys a survival advantage versus less aggressive resections [2].

Finally Marko et al. [19] recently published another retrospective review of 721 primary GBM patients treated at MD Anderson. They used an Accelerated Failure Time computer modeling system to evaluate the effects of various parameters on patient outcome. They once again showed a significant survival advantage for patients based on extent of resection. Unlike previous studies they felt that there was an advantage across all levels compared to biopsy alone and therefore felt that surgery should not be withheld based on preoperative assumptions of only obtaining a subtotal resection. In addition, they also showed the strength of such systems in reliably modelling outcome based on numerous patient and treatment parameters and suggest possible uses for this system in determining personalized outcome models as well as more appropriately stratifying patients for future clinical studies [19].

3. Elderly patients with GBM

At many institutions older patients with GBMs are not treated as aggressively as their younger counterparts. Part of this problem is associated with higher rates of medical comorbidities which may make more aggressive surgical interventions riskier. However, another bias is the belief that elderly patients will not tolerate more aggressive procedures and subsequent adjuvant treatments. Osvald et al. [20] performed a retrospective review of a large prospectively collected database to evaluate the impact of patient age on treatment. They found that 72% of patients younger than 65 were treated with resection vs. 55% of the older patients ($p<0.001$). Elderly patients had lower KPS and significantly more medical comorbidities. However, of the patients undergoing resection there was no statistical difference in the percent that had gross total resection when the two groups were compared. Elderly patients had a significantly decreased overall survival (9.1 months vs. 14.9 months), but subgroup analysis of patients undergoing resection showed no difference in overall survival based on age (13.0 months for elderly vs. 13.3 months in younger patients) [20].

Grossman et al. [21] evaluated the effect of age on a group of patients undergoing awake craniotomy for high-grade gliomas. They found perioperative morbidity (3.3% vs 0.59%) as well as length of stay (6.6 vs 4.9 days) higher in the elderly group (age >65 years). The EOR was not significantly different between the two groups (77.25 vs 81.9%).

4. Recurrent GBM

The value of extent of resection for patients with recurrent GBM is even more difficult to determine. Part of the issue in evaluating these patients is secondary to the bias created in evaluating patients who are candidates for surgery, as less than 30% of patients are typically deemed candidates for additional surgery. Factors in determining surgical eligibility include patient performance, tolerance to previous treatments, patient wishes, and tumor factors such as timing, size and location of recurrence [2,22-26].

Subgroup analysis of the Lacroix [1] paper showed a survival advantage for patients with recurrent GBM who had maximal tumor resection at time of recurrence. In addition Bloch et al. [7] evaluated the importance of extent of resection at the time of repeat surgery on a group of 107 patients who underwent multiple resections at USCF. They found that if patients had gross total resection at time of initial surgery than the extent of resection at recurrence did not affect outcome; however, in patients who had subtotal resections at time of initial surgery than the extent of resection at time of recurrence did impact overall survival. In addition, they found that in patients who had an initial subtotal resection had a complete resection at recurrence than there was no difference between them and patients who had complete resection initially and were candidates for additional surgery regardless of extent of resection [7].

Oppenlander et al. [22] published results of 170 patients who were treated with recurrent GBM at Barrow Neurological Institute. They found a distinct survival advantage based on an extent of resection of 80% or greater in these patients. The median interval between initial and subsequent surgery was 8.6 months (range 1.1-93.1 months) [22]. While these data do once again show level 3 data of a survival advantage for these patients it is important to approach this subgroup of patients with great care. First of all, early recurrence (less than 4-6 months) should be approached with great hesitancy. Many of these patients harbor "treatment effect" or pseudo-progression which can be managed medically in most of these patients. Secondly patients who have true progression in this very short time frame often have very aggressive tumor subtypes and are likely to progress despite further surgical interventions. My personal practice is to typically withhold additional cytoreductive surgery in patients who have disease progression prior to 6 months unless surgery is planned as a salvage intervention for symptom management in an otherwise healthy individual, for tissue diagnosis, or to obtain tissue for enrollment in a clinical trial. Finally, the incidence of wound healing and neurological complications is much higher in this patient population. The Barrow group [22] reported preoperative motor and language deficits in 33 and 31% respectively. Additionally they found new or worsened deficits in 19% and 13% postoperatively at one week which only decreased to 15% and 9% at one month [22]. These lesions are not curable and thus patient quality of life is of paramount importance. Every effort should be made to minimize neurological worsening in this patient population and thus judicious evaluation should be performed when determining who is a candidate for additional cytoreductive surgery.

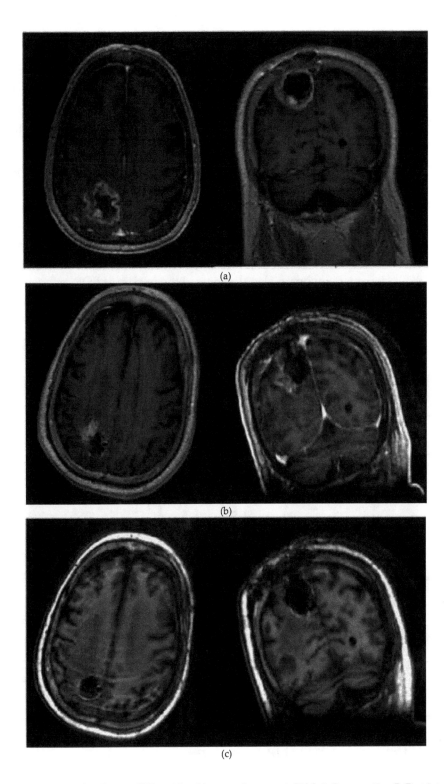

(a)

(b)

(c)

Figure 2. Post contrast axial and coronal T1-weighted images of recurrent GBM, A. Preoperative; B. First intraoperative (showing residual tumor along the lateral wall); C. Second intraoperative MRI scans

5. Low grade gliomas

Once again in Sanai's 2012 review [18] he found three papers which evaluated EOR for low grade gliomas using volumetric analysis and all three of these showed a significant increase in 5 year survival. He also reviewed eight nonvolumetric studies and once again found an advantage in five year survival in 7 of these 8 studies. Five year survival was shown to increase from 50-70% in cases with subtotal resection to 80-95% in total resections.

Several recent studies have also shown that increasing the extent of resection in low grade gliomas may also decrease the rate of malignant transformation in these tumors. Typically only pilocytic gliomas and other infrequent subtypes such as Ganglioglioma can be cured with complete surgical resection. For the remainder of these lesions recurrence and often progression to a higher grade lesion is the norm. Smith et al. [11] in their review of 216 low grade lesions found that increased EOR was associated with increased malignant progression free survival (MPFS). However, Snyder et al [12] reviewed the impact of EOR on overall survival and MPFS in 93 pure grade II oligodendrogliomas treated at their institution. They found that an increased EOR was associated with an improved OS but did not influence the rate or timing of progression in these patients as MPFS was not influenced by EOR [12].

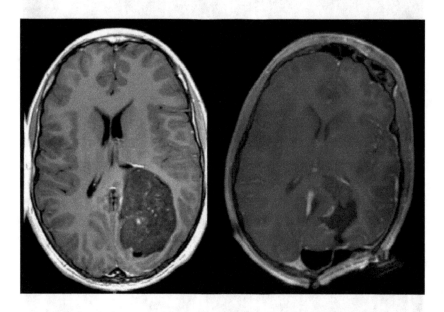

Figure 3. Axial T1-weighted preoperative and intraoperative scans showing low-grade non-enhancing tumor with residual tumor positioned next to atrium on intraoperative scan, that was subsequently resected.

6. Methods to increase extent of resection

Despite the growing body of evidence leaning towards significant survival advantage in both low and high grade gliomas, complete resection is often only obtained between 17-47% of cases

[1,27-33]. Numerous intraoperative adjuncts have been trialed to help increase the EOR in these procedures. Intraoperative frameless navigation is a mainstay in most North American Brain Tumor Centers. This technology which is based on a preoperatively obtained imaging set has been shown to be ineffective in increasing the EOR in a prospective randomized trial [34]. Upon opening the dura and proceeding with CSF drainage and tumor resection considerable brain shift can occur which makes the information obtained from preoperative datasets inaccurate (figure 4)[35].

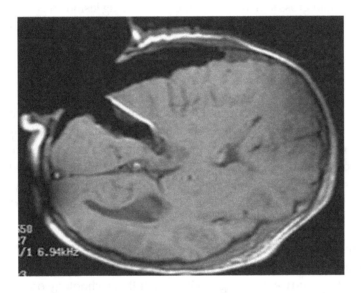

Figure 4. Axial T1 weighted intraoperative MRI scan illustrating the extreme degree of brain shift that can occur with opening the dura, drainage of CSF and tumor resection.

Orringer et al. [27] evaluated patient and tumor characteristics that might effect EOR in GBM patients. Interestingly they found that based on postoperative MRI scans complete resection was obtained in only 17% of cases despite the surgeon's belief that GTR had been obtained based on intraoperative assessments. They also found that larger tumors, lesions touching the ventricles and lesions in or near eloquent cortex were associated with lower extent of resection [27]. Of the 17 cases where complete resection was felt to be possible based on blinded review of two experienced surgeons this was only obtained in four patients (23%)[27]. This study clearly shows that the surgeon's impression alone is not enough to maximize tumor resections for these patients.

6.1. Ultrasound

Ultrasound was introduced as a surgical tool in the 1960s. This technology which typically utilized low frequencies was extremely limited secondary to poor image resolution and cumbersome intraoperative probes. The sensitivity and specificity of findings was limited especially for highlighting small tumor remnants or differentiating tumor from edematous brain. In addition, it was even more difficult to differentiate tumor from surrounding normal brain in low grade gliomas [36,37]. However, newer developments in ultrasound technology; with the use of higher frequency devices, has created a recent resurgence in this technology. New smaller light-weight probes can be placed within a resection cavity and give a much better spatial resolution of surrounding areas. The use of higher frequencies improves image resolution however this has a tradeoff of lower tissue penetration [38]. Serra et al. [38] performed a retrospective review of 22 patients with high grade lesions (mixed pathology) who they felt to be good candidates for gross total resection based on preoperative imaging findings. High frequency intraoperative ultrasound was used for all patients. They found that 21 of the 22 patients had gross total resection of the enhancing lesion on postoperative imaging; however, as the study was retrospective they were unable to determine how many patients underwent additional imaging based on ultrasound findings.

6.2. Fluorescence guided resections

5-aminolevulinic acid (5-ALA) is an orally administered pro-drug which is metabolized intracellularly to protoporphyrin IX which gives off a red-violet fluorescent signal to blue light. This agent preferentially accumulates in certain tumor types and thus can be used to help differentiate tumor from normal surrounding brain tissue [39]. The oral agent is administered 3 hours prior to surgery and then the operative field can be intermittently interrogated for evidence of fluorescence throughout the procedure by switching back and forth between white and blue light on the operative microscope.

Several prospective studies have been performed evaluating the benefits of 5-ALA in patients undergoing surgical resection of high-grade gliomas [39]. Stummer et al [40] performed a phase IIIa prospective study evaluating the impact of this technology on patients with high-grade gliomas. The study was terminated early because interim analysis showed a significant benefit in the study arm. Gross total resection was seen in 65% of patients in the 5-ALA arm vs. 36% in the control group [40]. The utility of this technology only seems beneficial in patients with high-grade lesions as significant accumulation has not been shown to occur in low grade gliomas [41,42].

6.3. Intraoperative MRI

Intraoperative MRI (iMRI) was first used in Boston in the mid 1990's. Since then numerous revisions and variations of the technology have been performed. While significant expansion in the number of centers with this technology has occurred in the past decade, cost is still the limiting factor. The current technology can be divided into two categories based on magnet strength. Low field systems such as the original 0.5 Tesla GE Signa SP (GE Medical Systems, Milwaukee, WI) the 0.12 Tesla Odin Polestar table mounted system (Odin Technologies, Yokneam, Israel); versus high-field systems which consist of 1.5 or 3.0 Tesla magnets. The high-field systems all require cessation of the surgical procedure for imaging. Two subgroups exist in this category. One in which the magnet is moved from a storage facility into the operating theater via an overhead crane system (IMRIS Inc., Winnipeg Canada) and the other in which the patient is moved from the operating theater into an adjacent ferrous free imaging zone (figure 5). This use of this technology allows for intraoperative imaging for evaluation and confirmation of the anticipated surgical results. In addition, it also allows for intraoperative updating of the navigation system to offset the changes that result from tumor resection and brain shift. Each system has its own advantages and tradeoffs in terms of cost, ease of use and image resolution [43].

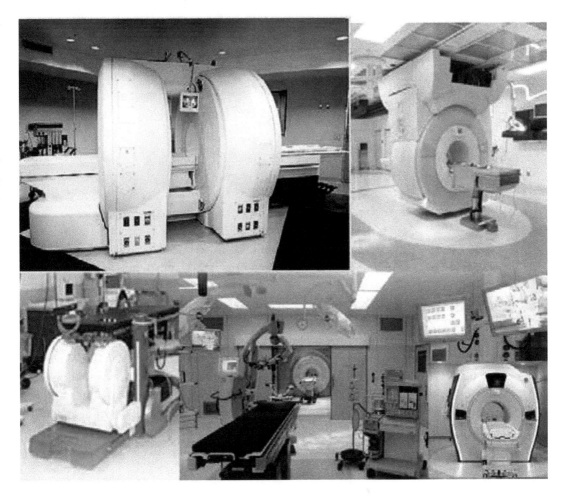

Figure 5. Various Intraoperative MRI concepts (clockwise from top left: GE Signa SP double doughnut, IMRIS mobile ceiling mounted system (scanner moves to patient), GE hybrid OR concept (inset shows close up of scanner; patient moves to scanner), Odin table mounted system.

I [44] previously reviewed the results for treatment of GBM using the older GE Signa SP system at Norton Healthcare (Louisville, KY) and found that additional surgical resection was performed in 71.4% of cases based on intraoperative imaging results. The average EOR in this patient group was 93.7% and was limited secondary to tumor location and vascular anatomy in cases where EOR was less than 95%. Numerous other authors have shown the value of such systems in increasing EOR [15,16,45-50].

Senft [6] performed a randomized controlled study looking at the utility of iMRI for treatment of gliomas. All patients were felt to be candidates for complete resection based on preoperative imaging findings. Patients were randomized to undergo surgery with conventional microsurgical techniques vs iMRI using the Odin Polestar system. In the study group the use of iMRI led to additional tumor resection in 33% of patients with 96% of patients in the iMRI group obtaining complete resection vs 68% in the control arm. Six month progression free survival was 67% in the iMRI group compared to 36% in the control arm (p<0.05).

Roder et al. [51] compared a group of 117 patients treated with iMRI (IMRIS Visius System) vs. a control arm treated with microsurgical techniques plus 5-ALA in some patients. 5-ALA was used in 70% of iMRI patients and 60% of patients in the control arm. Complete tumor resection was seen in 74% of the iMRI group vs 34% for the conventional group. Subgroup analysis of the control group showed that complete resection in the conventional group increased to 45% and mean residual volume decreased for patients who had 5-ALA fluorescence as part of their procedure.

These studies all show a significant advantage for the use of this technology not only for high-grade gliomas as outlined above but also for low-grade gliomas and pituitary tumors [16,43,52-54]. However, despite the use of this technology complete resection is sometimes still not possible. This can be secondary to tumor location in or near eloquent cortex, tumor adjacent to the ventricle or tumor extending into deep or midline structures or associated around major vascular structures[27,35,55,56]. Image interpretation during intraoperative procedures can also lead to its own challenges. Tissue can become distorted and damaged secondary to surgical trauma. This can lead to a disruption of the blood-brain barrier and thus increased contrast enhancement. In addition, blood products and air in the surgical cavity can also distort the imaging findings [35,43,44]. Finally the administration of contrast agents for preoperative navigational studies the morning of surgery can also affect intraoperative imaging results. As a result of these issues we routinely review all intraoperative imaging scans alongside an experienced neuroradiologist in the iMRI control room during all procedures. Intraoperative scans are directly compared to preoperative studies and when necessary any areas of questionable residual tumor are directly investigated after the new dataset is downloaded to the navigation system. Careful review of the imaging findings are necessary as overly aggressive resections can lead to increased risk of new neurological deficits.

7. Awake mapping techniques

Regardless of the surgical techniques used for tumor resection the goal for extensive tumor removal must always be tempered with the potential risk of inducing new or worsened neurological injuries, as the patients postoperative neurological status is strongly correlated with overall outcome. For lesions located in or near motor or speech centers intraoperative mapping via electro-cortical stimulation can effectively identify these eloquent areas.

Newer developments in preoperative imaging such as functional MRI (fMRI) and diffusion tensor imaging based fiber tracking (DTI-FT) can help to grossly localize the location of eloquent cortex and their corresponding deep white matter tracts; however the accuracy of exact localization is more reliably determined with intraoperative cortical and subcortical mapping techniques [57-64]. A meta-analysis of over 8000 patients who underwent craniotomy for resection of intracranial glioma showed that patients who underwent intraoperative mapping had a greater than two fold reduction in permanent neurological deficits [65].

Motor mapping can be performed either with the patient awake or under general anesthesia (without muscle paralysis) while speech mapping requires the use of an awake anesthesia technique at least during the mapping portion. Remifentanil and propofol or dexmetomidate infusions are often used for these procedures as they have very short half-lives [17,55]. The use of longer acting narcotics should be minimized as patients can become agitated and unco-operative with the over use of sedatives or narcotics. In addition an extensive local field block of all regional nerves with a combination of a short and long-acting local anesthetic also helps significantly with patient comfort and cooperation [17]. Patient selection is of paramount importance as patients with severe edema, or significant pulmonary or airway issues may not tolerate such a procedure. Time should be taken with the patient preoperatively to address and concerns and thus minimize anxiety as well as to prepare the patient for their involvement for the procedure. Complete details regarding the anesthesia for this technique are available elsewhere [17,55]. I prefer to conduct all of my mapping procedures with an awake technique regardless of whether speech function is being interrogated as having the ability to converse with the patient and readily assess their neurological function is as important as localizing the area of eloquent cortex. I have my anesthesiologist or operating room nurse regularly assess the patients motor function throughout tumor resection, if speech cortex is involved we routinely employ the assistance of a trained speech and language therapist who also assists the patient in carrying on a conversation during tumor resection after mapping and stimulation have been completed.

Mapping is routinely performed using a bipolar stimulation probe with 5 mm spacing between the electrodes. Stimulation is performed at increasing amplitudes until a positive result in encountered or after discharges are seen on electrocorticography or a upper threshold limit is reached. The use of surface EEG is of great importance as it can minimize the risk of generalized seizure activity induced by the stimulation and can verify that the stimulation system in functioning adequately. A constant current generator is used to provide square biphasic wave pulses for 1-4 seconds at 60Hz frequency (figure 6) [17,55,66]. Unlike epilepsy surgery where positive stimulation results are almost always obtained the growing trend among tumor surgeons is to perform smaller more tailored craniotomies for these cases. In these instances negative stimulation results (with appropriate artifact on surface recordings) can be interpret-ed as absence of eloquent tissue [18]. Most authors recommend keeping a border of at least 0.8-1.0 cm of tissue between resection site and any site showing positive stimulation results [17,18,55,66].

Subcortical stimulation can be performed using the same equipment and settings. The surgeon must frequently alternate between deep white matter tract stimulation and tumor resection. Resection is continued until either positive stimulation results are obtained or complete tumor resection has been achieved. Higher rates of postoperative neurological deficits have been shown in cases where positive motor stimulation is obtained during subcortical mapping, likely secondary to manipulation in close proximity of these pathways [55,67].

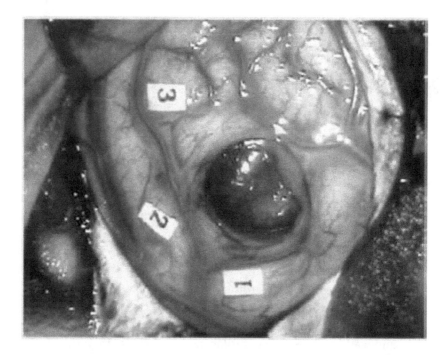

Figure 6. Picture of intraoperative mapping case; #1 corresponds to area of lower extremity stimulation, #2 hand stimulation, #3 face stimulation, lesion is seen just anterior to #2 on surface of the brain.

In appropriately selected patients awake mapping procedures can be performed safely with minimal patient anxiety or discomfort. The information obtained from mapping and intraoperative neurological assessment allows the surgeon to make a well informed decision regarding the safety of continued resection vs. the risk of inducing new neurological deficits (figure 7).

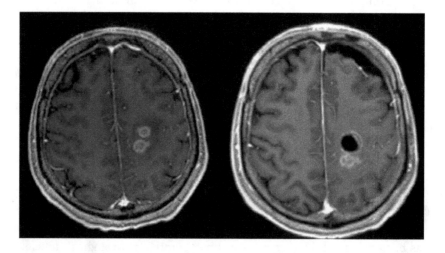

Figure 7. Preoperative and intraoperative axial T1-weighted post contrast scans; subcortical stimulation was positive along the lateral and posterior border of the resection cavity thus a portion of the tumor was not resected.

8. Conclusion: Combining technologies to obtain maximal safest results

I and several other authors have had experience combining several of these advanced technologies together for the treatment of high risk patients undergoing treatment of intracranial gliomas [44,45,56,68]. Select patients with lesions near or in eloquent cortex can undergo awake mapping procedures with frequent neurological assessment to ensure the absence of generating new neurological deficits. Intraoperative imaging can be performed once maximal tumor resection has been performed to verify that the anticipated results have been obtained (figure 8). If significant residual tumors remains than the surgeon can immediately determine whether further resection is deemed safe and continue with additional tumor removal while constantly assessing the patients function or evaluating subcortical stimulation results. In cases where the patient may be sedated but not intubated than transport of the patient into the scanner does carry additional risks as the anesthesiologist has even more limited access to the patient and their airway during imaging; however, I am unaware of any serious complications as a result of performing iMRI on a mildly sedated non-intubated patient.

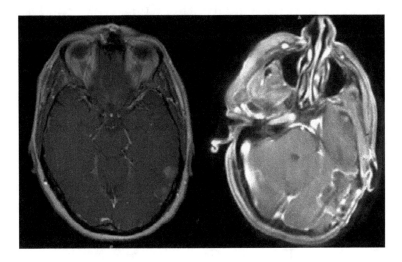

Figure 8. Preoperative and intraoperative axial T1-weighted post contrast images showing complete resection of a posterior left temporal lesion that was removed using an awake mapping technique in the intraoperative MRI.

One of the main drawbacks of the current high-field iMRI systems is the time required for patient transport and scanning. For a majority of our cases we conduct only a single intraoperative scan, typically if any residual tumor exists than further resection is performed based off of updated neuronavigation results. In a minority of cases, typically those with large volumes of residual tumor on the first scan, than a second confirmatory scan is performed. The use of 5-ALA plus iMRI in patients with high-grade gliomas can further decrease the need for additional scans. By maximizing the EOR based on the intraoperative fluorescence findings, there is a higher likelihood of satisfactory results on the first scan, thus eliminating the need for subsequent imaging. Any small or deep areas of residual tumor not appreciated with 5-ALA can be seen on the iMRI images and resected with updated neuronavigation [51].

Author details

Todd W. Vitaz*

Address all correspondence to: todd.vitaz@spectrumhealth.org

Department of Clinical Neurosciences Spectrum Health Medical Group, and College of Human Medicine, Michigan State University, Grand Rapids, Michigan, USA

References

[1] Lacroix M, Abi-Said D, Fourney DR, Gokaslan ZL, Shi W, DeMonte F, et al. A multivariate analysis of 416 patients with glioblastoma multiforme: prognosis, extent of resection, and survival. Journal of Neurosurgery 2001;95: 190-198.

[2] Sanai, N, Mei-Yin P, McDermott MW, Parsa AT, Berger MS. An extent of resection threshold for newly diagnosed glioblastomas. Journal of Neurosurgery 2011;115: 3-8.

[3] Senft C, Franz K, Blasel S, Osvald A, Rather J, Seifert V, Gasser T. Influence of iMRI-guidance on the extent of resection and survival of patients with glioblastoma multiforme. Technology in Cancer Research and Treatment 2010;9: 339-346.

[4] Hassaneen W, Levine NB, Suki D, Salaskar AL, de Moura Lima, McCutcheon IE, et al. Multiple craniotomies in the management of multifocal and multicentric glioblastoma. Journal of Neurosurgery 2011;114: 576-584.

[5] De Bonis P, Anile C, Pompucci A, Fiorentino A, Balducci M, Chiesa S, et al. The influence of surgery on recurrence pattern of glioblastoma. Clinical Neurology and Neurosurgery 2013;115: 37-43.

[6] Senft C, Bink A, Franz K, Vatter H, Gasser T, Seifert V. Intraoperative MRI guidance and extent of resection in glioma surgery: a randomized, controlled trial. The Lancet Oncology 2011;12: 997-1003.

[7] Bloch O, Han SJ, Cha S, Sun M, Aghi MK, McDermott MW et al. Impact of extent of resection for recurrent glioblastoma on overall survival. Journal of Neurosurgery 2012;117: 1032-1038.

[8] McGirt MJ, Chaichana KL, Gathinji M, Attenello FJ, Than K, Olivi A et al. Independent association of extent of resection with survival in patients with malignant brain astrocytoma. Journal of Neurosurgery 2009;110: 156-162.

[9] Laws ER, Parney IF, Huang W, Anderson F, Morris AM, Asher A, et al. Survival following surgery and prognostic factors for recently diagnosed malignant glioma: data from the glioma outcomes project. Journal Neurosurgery 2003;99: 467-473.

[10] Murkami R, Hirai T, Nakamura H, Furusawa M, Nakaguchi Y, Uetani H, et al. Recurrence patterns of glioblastoma treated with postoperative radiation therapy: relationship between extent of resection and progression-free survival. Japanese Journal of Radiology 2012;30: 193-197.

[11] Smith JS, Chang EF, Lamborn KR, Chang SM, Prados MD, Cha S, et al. Role of extent of resection in the long-term outcome of low-grade hemispheric gliomas. Journal of Clinical Oncology 2008;26:1338-1345.

[12] Snyder LA, Wolf AB, Oppenlander ME, Bina R, Wilson JR, Ashby L, et al. The impact of extent of resection on malignant transformation of pure oligodendrogliomas. Journal of Neurosurgery 2014;120: 309-314.

[13] Yordanova YN, Moritz-Gasser S, Duffau H. Awake surgery for WHO grade II gliomas within "noneloquent" areas in the left dominant hemisphere: toward a "supratotal" resection. Journal of Neurosurgery 2011;115:232-239.

[14] Bumrungrachpukdee P, Pruphetkaew N, Phukaoloun M, Pheunpathom N. Recurrence of intracranial meningioma after surgery: analysis of influencing factors and outcome. Journal of the Medical Association of Thailand 2014;97(4): 399-406.

[15] Schneider JP, Trantakis C, Rubach M, Schulz T, Dietrich J, Winkler D, et al. Intraoperative MRI to guide the resection of primary supratentorial glioblastoma multiforme-a quantitative radiological analysis. Neuroradiology 2005;47: 489-500.

[16] Bohinski RJ, Kokkino AK, Warnick RE, Gaskill-Shipley MF, Kormos DW, Lukin RR, et al. Glioma resection in a shared resource magnetic resonance operating room after optimal image guided frameless stereotactic resection. Neurosurgery 2001;48: 731-742.

[17] Vitaz TW, Marx W, Victor JD, Gutin PH. Comparison of conscious sedation and general anesthesia for motor mapping and resection of tumors located near motor cortex. Neurosurgical Focus 2003;15: article 8.

[18] Sanai N. Emerging operative strategies in neurosurgical oncology. Current Opinion in Neurology 2012;25: 756-766.

[19] Marko NF, Weil RJ, Schroeder JL, Lang FF, Suki D, Sawaya RE. Extent of resection of glioblastoma revisited: personalized survival modeling facilitates more accurate survival prediction and supports a maximum-safe-resection approach to surgery. Journal of Clinical Oncology 2014;32: 774-782.

[20] Osvald A, Guresir E, Setzer M, Vatter H, Senft C, Seifert V, Franz K. Glioblastoma therapy in the elderly and the importance of the extent of resection regardless of age. Journal Neurosurgery 2012;116:357-364.

[21] Grossman R, Nossek E, Sitt R, Hayat D, Shahar T, Barzilai O, et al. Outcome of elderly patients undergoing awake-craniotomy for tumor resection. Annals of Surgical Oncology 2013;20: 1722-1728.

[22] Oppenlander ME, Wolf AB, Snyder LA, Bina R, Wilson JR, Coons SW, et al. An extent of resection threshold for recurrent glioblastoma and its risk for neurological morbidity. Journal of Neurosurgery 2014; 120:846-853.

[23] Barker FG, Chang SM, Gutin PH, Malec MK, McDermott MW, Prados MD, et al. Survival and functional status after resection of recurrent glioblastoma multiforme. Neurosurgery 1998;42:709-723.

[24] Chaichana KL, Zadnik P, Weingart JD, Olivi A, Gallia GL, Blakeley J, et al. Multiple resections for patients with glioblastoma: prolonging survival. Journal of Neurosurgery 2013;118: 812-820.

[25] Helseth R, Helseth E, JohannesenTB, Langberg CW,Lote K, Ronning P, et al. Overall survival, prognostic factors, and repeated surgery in a consecutive series of 516 patients with glioblastoma multiforme. Acta Neurologica Scandinavia 2010;122: 159-167.

[26] Zinn PO, Colen RR, Kasper EM, Burkhardt JK. Extent of resection and radiotherapy in GBM: a 1973 to 2007 surveillance, epidemiology and end results analysis of 21,783 patients. International Journal of Oncology 2013;42: 929-934.

[27] Orringer D, Lau D, Khatri S, Zamora-Berridi GJ, Zhang K, Wu C et al. Extent of resection in patients with glioblastoma: limiting factors, perception of resectability, and effect on survival. Journal Neurosurgery 2012;117: 851-859.

[28] Chen X, Xu BN, Meng X, Zhang J, Yu X, Zhou D. Dual-room 1.5T intraoperative magnetic resonance imaging suite with a movable magnet: implementation and preliminary experience. Neurosurgical Review 2012;35: 95-109.

[29] Senft C, Seifert V, Hermann E, Franz K, Gasser T. Usefulness of intraoperative ultra-low-field magnetic resonance imaging in glioma surgery. Neurosurgery 2008;63: 257.

[30] Kuhnt D, Becker A, Ganslandt O, Bauer M, Buchfelder M, Nimsky C. Correlation of the extent of tumor volume resection and patient survival in surgery of glioblastoma multiforme with high-field intraoperative MRI guidance. Neuro Oncology 2011;13: 1339-1348.

[31] Chicoine MR, Lim CC, Evans JA, Singla A, Zipfel GJ, Rich KM, et al. Implementation and preliminary clinical experience with the use of ceiling mounted mobile high-field intraoperative magnetic resonance imaging between two operating rooms. Intraoperative Imaging. Acta Neurochirgica Supplemental 2011;109: 97-102.

[32] Nimsky C, Fujita A, Ganslandt O, Von Keller B, Fahlbusch R. Volumetric assessment of glioma removal by intraoperative high-field magnetic resonance imaging. Neurosurgery 2004;55: 358-370.

[33] Hatiboglu MA, Weinberg JS, Suki D, Rao G, Prabhu SS, Shah K, et al. Impact of intraoperative high-field magnetic resonance imaging guidance on glioma surgery: a prospective volumetric analysis. Neurosurgery 2009;64: 1073-1081.

[34] Willems PWA, Taphoorn MJB, Burger H, van der Sprenkel JWB, Tulleken CAF. Effectiveness of neuronavigation in resecting solitary intracerebral contrast-enhancing tumors: a randomized controlled trial. Journal of Neurosurgery 2006;104: 360-368.

[35] Kubben PL, terMeulen KJ, Schijns OEMG, ter Laak-Poor MP, van Ovenbeeke JJ, van Santbrink H. Intraoperative MRI-guided resection of glioblastoma multiforme: a systemic review. Lancet Oncology 2011;12:1062-1070.

[36] Erdogan N, Tucer B, Mavili E, Menkü A, Kurtsoy A. Ultrasound guidance in intracranial tumor resection: correlation with postoperative magnetic resonance findings. Acta Radiology 2005;46: 743-749.

[37] Gerganov VM, Samii A, Akbarian A, Stieglitz L, Samii M, Fahlbusch R. Reliability of intraoperative high-resolution 2D ultrasound as an alternative to high-field strength MR imaging for tumor resection control: a prospective comparative study. Journal of Neurosurgery 2009;111: 512-519

[38] Serra C, Stauffer A, Actor B, Burkhardt JK, Ulrich NH, Bernays RL, Bozinov O. Intraoperative high frequency ultrasound in intracerebral high-grade tumors. Ultrasound in Medicine 2012;33: 306-312.

[39] Tykocki T, Michalik R, Bonicki W, Nauman P. Fluorescence-guided resection of primary and recurrent malignant gliomas with 5-aminolevulinic acid. Preliminary results. Neurology and Neurosurgery Poland 2012;46: 47-51.

[40] Stummer W, Pichlmeier U, Meinel T, Wiestler OD, Zanella F, Reulen HJ, et al. Fluorescence-guided surgery with 5-aminolevulinic acid for resection of malignant glioma: a randomized controlled multicenter phase III trial. Lancet Oncology 2006;7: 392-401.

[41] Ishihara R, Katayama Y, Watanabe T, Yoshino A, Fukushima T, Sakatani K. Quantitative spectroscopic analysis of 5-aminolevulinic acid-induced protoporphyrin IX fluorescence intensity in diffusely infiltrating astrocytomas. Neurologia medico-chirurgica 2007;47: 53-57.

[42] Floeth FW, Sabel M, Ewelt C, Stummer W, Felsberg J, Reifenberger G, et al. Comparison of (18)F-FET PET and 5-ALA fluorescence in cerebral gliomas European Journal of Medical Molecular Imaging 2011;38: 731-417.

[43] Ram Z, Hadani M. Intraoperative imaging-MRI. Acta Neurchirgica Supplemental 2003;88: 1-4.

[44] Lenaburg HJ, Inkabi KE, Vitaz TW. The use of intraoperative MRI for the treatment of glioblastoma multiforme. Technology in Cancer Research and Treatment 2009;8: 159-162.

[45] Senft C, Forster MT, Bink A, Mittelbronn M, Franz K, Seifert V, Szelenyi A. Optimizing the extent of resection in eloquently located gliomas by combining intraoperative

MRI guidance with intraoperative neurophysiological monitoring. Journal Neurooncology 2012;109: 81-90.

[46] Black PMcL, Moriarty T, Alexander ER, Stieg P, Woodard EJ, Gleason PL, et al. Development and implementation of intraoperative magnetic resonance imaging and
its neurosurgical applications. Neurosurgery 1997;41: 831-842.

[47] Sutherland GR, Kaibara T, Louw D, Hoult DI, Tomanek B, Saunders J. A mobile
high-field magnetic resonance imaging system for neurosurgery. Neurosurgical Focus 1999;6: article 6.

[48] Hirschberg H, Samset E, Hol PK, Tillung T, Lote K. Impact of intraoperative MRI on
the surgical results for high-grade gliomas. Minimally invasive Neurosurgery
2005;48: 77-84.

[49] Schulder M, Carmel PW. Intraoperative magnetic resonance imaging: impact on
brain tumor surgery. Cancer Control 2003;10: 115-124.

[50] Nimsky C, Fujita A, Ganslandt O, Von Keller B, Fahlbusch R. Volumetric assessment
of glioma removal by intraoperative high-field magnetic resonance imaging. Neurosurgery 2004;55: 358-370.

[51] RoderC, Bisdas S, Ebner FH, Honegger J, Naegel T,Ernemann U, Tatagiba M. Maximizing the extent of resection and survival benefit of patients in glioblastoma surgery: High-field iMRI versus conventional and 5-ALA-assisted surgery. European
Journal of Surgical Oncology 2014;40: 297-304.

[52] Vitaz TW, Inkabi KE, Carruba CJ. Intraoperative MRI for transphenoidal procedures:
short-term outcome for 100 consecutive cases. Clinical Neurology and Neurosurgery
2011;113: 731-735.

[53] Anand VK, Schwartz TH, Hiltzik DH, Kacker A. Endoscopic transphenoidal pituitary surgery with real-time intraoperative magnetic resonance imaging. American
Journal of Rhinology 2006;20: 401-405.

[54] Lu J, Wu J, Yao C, Zhang D, Qiu T, Hu X et al. Awake language mapping and 3-Tesla
intraoperative MRI-guided volumetric resection for gliomas in language areas. Journal of Clinical Neuroscience 2013;20: 1280-1287.

[55] Carrabba G, Fava E, Giussani C, Acerbi F, Portaluri F, Songa V, et al. Cortical and
subcortical motor mapping in rolandic and perirolandic glioma surgery: impact on
postoperative morbidity and extent of resection.

[56] Sanai N, Berber MS. Extent of Resection influences outcome for patients with gliomas. Neurology Review 2011;167: 648-654.

[57] Vassal F, Schneider F, Nuti C. Intraoperative use of diffusion tensor imaging-based
tractography for resection of gliomas located near the pyramidal tract: comparison

with subcortical stimulation mapping and contribution to surgical outcomes. British Journal of Neurosurgery 2013;27: 668-75.

[58] Roux FE, Ibarrola D, Tremoulet M, Lazorthes Y, Henry P, Sol JC, Berry I. Methodological and technical issues for integrating functional magnetic resonance imaging data in a neuronavigational system. Neurosurgery 2001;49: 1145-1156.

[59] Sunaert S. Presurgical planning for tumor resection. Journal Magnetic Resonance Imaging 2006;23: 887-905.

[60] Vlieger EJ, Majoie CB, Leenstra S, den Heeten GJ. Functional magnetic resonance imaging for neurosurgical planning in neurooncology. European Journal of Radiology 2004;14: 1143-1153.

[61] Berman JI, Berger MS, Mukherjee P, Henry RG. Diffusion tensor imaging-guided tracking of fibers of the pyramidal tract combined with intraoperative cortical stimulation mapping in patients with gliomas. Journal Neurosurgery 2004;101: 66-72.

[62] Clark CA, Barrick TR, Murphy MM, Bell BA. White matter fiver tracking in patients with space-occupying lesions of the brain: a new technique for neurosurgical planning? Neurological Imaging 2003;20: 1601-1608.

[63] Hendler T, Pianka P, Sigal M, Kafri M, Ben-Bashat D, Constantini S, et al. Delineating gray and white matter involvement in brain lesions: three-dimensional alignment of functional magnetic resonance and diffusion-tensor imaging. Journal Neurosurgery 2003;99: 1018-1027.

[64] Nimsky C, Ganslandt O, Hastreiter P, Wang R, Benner T, Sorensen AG, Fahlbusch R. Preoperative and intraoperative diffusion tensor imaging-based fiber tracking in glioma surgery. Neurosurgery 2005;56: 130-137.

[65] De Witt Hamer PC, Gil Robles S, Zwinderman AH, Duffau H, Berger MS. Impact of intraoperative stimulation brain mapping on glioma surgery outcome: a meta-analysis. Journal Clinical Oncology 2012;10: 2559-2565.

[66] Sanai N, Berger MS. Operative Techniques for gliomas and the value of extent of resection. Neurotherapeutics 2009;6:478-486.

[67] Keles GE, Lundin DA, Lamborn KR, Chang EF, Ojemann G, Berger MS. Intraoperative subcortical stimulation mapping for hemispherical perirolandic gliomas located within or adjacent to the descending motor pathways: evaluation of morbidity and assessment of functional outcome in 294 patients. Journal Neurosurgery 2004;100: 369-375.

[68] Hatiboglu MA, Weinberg JS, Suki D, Tummala S, Rao G, Sawaya R, Prabhu S. Utilization of intraoperative motor mapping in glioma surgery with high-field intraoperative magnetic resonance imaging. Stereotactic and Functional Neurosurgery 2009;88: 345-352.

5

Metalloproteinases in Brain Tumors

Krzysztof Siemianowicz, Wirginia Likus and
Jarosław Markowski

1. Introduction

Metalloproteinases (MMPs) were first described by Gross more than fifty years ago. They are a family of zinc-dependent endopeptidases. They comprise a group of 25 enzymes. MMPs were first described as proteases degrading extracellular matrix (ECM) proteins such as collagens, elastin, proteoglycans and laminins, hence they were named matrix metalloproteinases. MMPs were divided according to their substrate specificity into collagenases, gelatinases, stromolysins and matrilysins. This classification was later replaced by numbering the enzymes according to the chronology of their identification.

Four metalloproteinases (MMP-14, MMP-15, MMP-16 and MMP-24) have a transmembrane and cytosolic domains. They constitute a subgroup of membrane-type metalloproteinases (MT-MMPs). Recently an intracellular, nuclear localization and functions of metalloproteinases have been discovered [1-4].

2. Physiological role of metalloproteinases

MMP-1 (collagenase 1) hydrolyzes collagen types I, II, III, VII, VIII, X and XI, as well as gelatin, fibronectin, vitronectin, laminin, tenascin, aggrecan, links protein, myelin basic protein and versican. MMP-2 (gellatinase) degrades collagen types I, II, III, IV, V, VII, X and XI, gelatin, elastin, fibronectin, vitronectin, laminin, entactin, tenascin, SPARC and aggrecan, links protein, galectin-3, versican, decanin and myelin basic protein. One of the most important differences between these two metalloproteinases is the possibility of the hydrolysis of elastin and collagen type IV by MMP-2, but not by MMP-1. Researchers have also focused their interest on MMP-9 which can degrade collagen types IV, V, VII, X and XIV, fibronectin, laminin, nidogen, proteoglycan link protein and versican.

For a long time metalloproteinases have been viewed solely as enzymes of matrix proteins breakdown. Results of researches performed in recent years indicate that there is a group of non-matrix proteins which can be substrates for various MMPs. Metalloproteinases are involved in the activation of latent forms of effective proteins. For example, MMP-2, MMP-3 and MMP-9 can activate interleukin 1β (IL-1β). They can also act on active cytokines, IL-1β undergoes subsequent degradation catalyzed by MMP-3. Metalloproteinases can alter cell surface proteins such as receptors and act on microbial peptides.

Metalloproteinases are not indiscriminately released by cells. They are secreted to or anchored to cell membrane. MT-MMPs have a specific transmembrane domain placing them in a certain position. Other metalloproteinases can be bound by specific cell-MMP interactions. This phenomenon allows an exact localization of their proteolytic activity [1-3].

3. Activation of metalloproteinases

Metalloproteinases are encoded as inactive proenzymes, zymogens. They undergo proteolytic activation. This process can take place either intracellulary or extracellulary. One third of MMPs are activated by intracellular serine protease, furin. This process takes place in trans-Golgi network. A number of MMPs has a cleavage site for other metalloproteinases. MMP-3 activates proMMP-1 and pro-MMP-7. Some metalloproteinases have been described to be activated by kallikrein or plasmin.

In vivo studies indicate that reactive oxygen species (ROS) generated by neutrophils can both activate and subsequently inactivate MMPs. Hypochlorus acid (HClO) generated by neutrophil myeloperoxidase and hydroxyl radicals can activate proMMP-1, proMMP-7 and proMMP-9, whereas peroxynitrate can activate proenzymes of MMP-1, MMP-2 and MMP-9. This process enables a control of burst of proteolytic activity within an inflammatory setting.

Like some other proteases, activity of MMPs is controlled also by two other mechanisms, regulation of gene expression and specific inhibitors. MMP-2 is constitutively expressed and regulation of its activity occurs by either activation or inhibition. Expression of a number of metalloproteinases is up-regulated during various pathological conditions. Among them inflammation is the most studied setting. MMPs are inhibited by α-2 macroglobulin and tissue inhibitors of metalloproteinases (TIMPs). There are four TIMPs. Their secretion is also regulated and represents another point in a network of control of the activity of metallopro-teinases. TIMP-3 is primarily bond to ECM and allows a regulation of MMPs' activity in the very site of their action. The network of the control of the activity of metalloproteinases is complex and very precise. Sometimes TIMP interacts with proMMP and inactivate other MMP, e.g. a complex of TIMP-1 and proMMP-9 inactivates MMP-3.

Protection from MMP degradation represents the next step in this sophisticated network of diverse interactions. Neutrophil gelatinase-associated lipocalin (NGAL) bounds to MMP-9 protecting this metalloproteinase from its degradation [1-3].

4. Metalloproteinases in central nervous system

Metalloproteinases in central nervous system can be produced by cells constituting it, by cells of blood vessels' wall or by blood cells. The production of MMPs in central nervous system under normal conditions is low, however it can be augmented in several neoplastic and non-neoplastic conditions. The expression of MMP-14 (MT1-MMP) in microglia is very low under physiological conditions. It can be increased in neurodegenerative and neuroinflammatory pathologies, e.g. Alzheimer's disease, multiple sclerosis, amyotrophic lateral sclerosis (ALS) or even in a stroke. Astrocytes were reported to secrete MMP-2 and MMP-9 [5,6].

For a long time MMPs were thought to be enzymes acting exclusively in extracellular compartment. Studies carried in last few years have revealed nontraditional roles for MMPs in extracellular space as well as in the cytosol and nucleus. MMP-2 and MMP-9 which were largely studied in central nervous system have been shown to present an increased activity in cortex neuronal nuclei after focal cerebral ischemia. These two MMPs, MMP-2 and MMP-9, are also termed gelatinase A and gelatinase B. The increased gelanolytic activity in nucleus occurs to be linked with MMP-dependent cell death triggering neuroinflammatory reactions. MMP-13, named also collagenase-3, was found to be activated mostly in neurons and oligodendrocytes. Its function in cell nucleus may be linked to the apoptosis cascade following ischemic stimulus. MMPs localized in cell nucleus can have a different set of target proteins than MMPs acting in extracellular space. Poly-ADP-ribose polymerase-1 (PARP-1) and X-ray cross-complementary factor-1 (XRCC-1) can be the substrates for MMP-dependent cleavage [4].

5. Metalloproteinases in brain tumors

Gliomas are the most common malignant tumors in the brain, and the overall prognosis for patients suffering from this neoplasm is poor. Glioblastoma multiforme (GBM) is the most aggressive type of glioma. Molecular mechanisms of invasiveness of this neoplasm have been most widely studied. Many factors are involved in the migration and invasiveness of GBM. MMPs have gained a large interest of researchers. The role of MMPs is significant in the degradation of ECM, thereby facilitating tumor cell invasion into surrounding stroma. Neoplastic cell invades in three steps. The first one is the attachment of tumor cell to the basement membrane through binding of neoplastic cell receptors to the basement membrane receptors. The next one is the secretion of hydrolytic enzymes, MMPs, which locally degrade ECM by extracellular proteolysis. The third step comprises the movement of the tumor cell to the free space obtained by degradation of ECM. MMP-13 is involved in the initiation of progression of invasion due to its proteolytic activity. Expression of MMP-13 is higher in glioma than in the surrounding normal brain tissue. High expression of this MMP is more often detected in advanced grades of glioma. Some researchers suggest that MMP-13 can be used as a biomarker of GBM progression. A study of Hsieh *et al.* revealed that GBM cells express higher amount of endothelin-1 receptors ET$_A$ and ET$_B$. The stimulation of one of the most invasive glioma cell lines *in vivo*, U251, with endothelin resulted in an increased expression of MMP-13, MMP-9 and increased cell migration. The addition of MMP-13 and MMP-9 inhibitors attenuated this increased cell migration [7-9].

Other scientists have shown that GBM cells can present an increased expression of other metalloproteinases: MMP-1, MMP-2, MMP-3, MMP-7, MMP-9 and MMP-14. Some researchers tried to reveal the molecular markers of invasiveness in gliomas. In the results of their studies various MMPs can be found. Bakalova *et al.* found that patients in terminal stages of brain tumors had elevated plasma levels of MMP-2 and MMP-9. Mariani *et al.* measured levels of MMP-2 and MMP-9 in cerebrospinal fluid (CSF) of dogs with intracranial tumors. Latent, but not active form of MMP-2 was found in all samples. MMP-9 was found in CSF of a minority of studied animals. Xu *et al.* analyzed brain samples obtained from patients undergoing surgery for GBM and non-malignant condition, epilepsy. Overexpression of both MMP-1 and vascular endothelial growth factor-1 (VEGF-1) was an independent poor prognostic factor in gliomas. Wang and co-workers analyzed frozen glioma samples and found out an increased expression of stromal periostin (POSTN) gene. This protein took part in both cell invasion and migration. In glioma cells POSTN signaling led to increased MMP-9 expression. The expression of POSTN correlated with both grade and progression of glioma being a poor prognostic factor [10-13].

MT1-MMP (MMP-14) activates directly proMMP-2 and indirectly MMP-2 and MMP-9. Expression of MMP-14 was shown to correlate with invasiveness of glioma and to increase with glioma grade. MMP-14 expression was also shown to correlate with brain tumor progression. This metalloproteinase, MMP-14, has been proposed as a biomarker to determine the type and grade of specific tumor. MMP-14 has a very interesting set of digested proteins. Apart from ECM proteins it can hydrolyze the most potent central nervous myelin inhibitory proteins, including BN-220. MMP-14 can also digest some proteins having adhesion functions. MMP-14 can also be involved in some intracellular processes. It can be trafficked along the tubulin cytoskeleton and be involved in intracellular recycling pathway. MMP-14 expression abnormalities were linked to mitotic spindle aberrations and chromosome instability leading to malignant transformation of neoplastic cells. MMP-14 may also be involved in regulation of VEGF-A expression. VEGF-A induces angiogenesis and inhibits apoptosis. MMP-14 seems to promote malignant glioma transformation, invasion and metastasis through intracellular signaling pathways [14].

6. Metalloproteinases and intracellular signaling pathways

Increased expression of various MMPs observed in brain tumors is a result of multiple intracellular events which may be termed as dysregulated pathways. These intracellular molecular mechanisms leading to increased invasion of neoplasmatic cells have focused scientists' interest. Understanding these complex mechanisms may be a key to design a molecular targeted therapy for patients with brain tumors. Signaling pathways leading to increased expression of MMPs are of special interest.

Tsai *et al.* observed that inhibition of focal adhesion kinase (FAK) phosporylation by osthole reduced MMP-13 expression in human glioma cells. This inhibition led to a reduction of cells migration even in a subgroup of glioma cells selected for high migratory ability. Lee *et al.* observed GMB U251 cell line presented increased FAK activation which led to an augmented expression of MMP-2. This study also revealed that examined GBM cells had an increased Bcl-w (B-cell lymphoma-w) expression. This protein is a prosurvival member of Bcl-2 family. The augmented expression of this protein is associated with infiltration properties and aggressiveness of various cancers. Bcl-w promotes the mesenchymal traits of glioblastoma cells by inducing vimentin expression of transcription factors, β-catenin, Twist1 and Snail. The increased expression of MMP-2 is accompanied by and results from the FAK activation, i.e. phosphorylation, via the PI3K-p-Akt-p-GSK3β-β-catenin pathway. The role of Bcl-w in promoting invasiveness of GBM by increasing MMP-2 activation was also confirmed in another study of this researchers team which proposed Bcl-w induced activation of β-catenin, also termed specificity protein-1 (Sp1), as a putative marker for aggressiveness of GBM. Nuclear factor of activated T cell (NFAT) family has been identified as a group of regulators of oncogenic transformation in several human malignancies. NFAT1 (NFATc2) is the prevalent family member expressed in peripheral T lymphocytes and many other cells outside the immune system. It is associated with tumor cell survival, apoptosis, migration and invasion. Clustering analysis of microarray data revealed that in glioma cells the expression of invasion related genes, cyclooxygenase-2 (COX-2), MMP-7 and MMP-9, was correlated with the expression of NFAT1. In vitro analysis confirmed the role of NFAT1, as in a specific NFAT1 knock down in U87 glioma cell line led to a marked reduction of COX-2, MMP-7 and MMP-9 expression [7,15-17].

MMP-2 has been discovered to posses intracellular activity and play some role in cell nucleus. A study by Kesanakurti *et al.* put new light on a role of MMP-2 in molecular mechanisms engaged in aggressiveness of glioma cells. p21 activated kinase 4 (PAK4) is one of down stream effectors of small GTPases Rac1 and Cdc42 which have diverse cellular functions by regulating cytoskeletal reorganization, cell survival and angiogenesis. Abberant PAK4 expression was found to be associated with enhanced tumor progression in various carcinomas. MMP-2 directly interacts with PAK-4 and augments the activation of αvβ3-mediated phospho-epidermal growth factor receptor (phospho-EGFR) in GBM. MMP-2 is supposed to bind to PAK4 and the complex PAK4/MMP-2 is supposed to regulate integrin mediated pathways in gliomas. Earlier study of Kesanakurti study group revealed that MMP-2 knock down glioma cells entered on apoptosis pathway [18-20].

Understanding the molecular pathways enhancing aggressiveness of glioma cells may lead to introducing a complex therapy focused on several targets which may give a better effectiveness.

7. Metalloproteinases in other cells supporting tumor and metastasis development

In last few years scientists have paid more attention to interactions between glioma cells and microglia as well as on inreactions between metastatic cancer cells and astrocytes. Ellert-

Miklaszewska *et al.* observed that glioma attracted microglia and polarized them into tumor-supporting cells that participated in matrix-remodeling, invasion, angiogenesis and suppression of adaptative immunity. In her experiment rat microglial cultures exposed to glioma conditioned medium polarized into pro-inflammatory or alternatively activated cells. Glioma derived factors increased cell motility, phagocytosis and sustained proliferation. Glioma induced activation of microglia was associated with induction of expression of several genes. One of them was MT1-MMP. Vinnakota *et al.* also observed that microglia promoted glioma through upregulation of MT1-MMP. This conversion of microglia into glioma supportive phenotype was dependent on activation of Toll-like receptor 2 (TLR 2) along with TLR 1 and or TLR 6 signaling [21, 22].

Brain metastasis is a defining component of tumor pathophysiology and underlying mechanisms urgently need deeper elucidation. The relationship between metastatic cells and astrocytes is crucial for tumor cell sustenance in brain. Some researchers postulate that tumor cell metastasis to the brain are influenced by astrocyte secretome and astrocytes play a direct role in tumor metastasis. Wang *et al.* revealed that astrocyte conditioned tumor cells displayed highly invasive and metastatic behavior both *in vitro* and *in vivo* as well. MMP-2 and MMP-9 were two factors in the astrocyte secretome that were responsible for that response. Blocking these MMPs proteins partially prevented the invasion and metastasis of tumor cells both *in vitro* and *in vivo* as well. A very important question arises. What are the mechanisms by which MMPs secreted by astrocytes trigger invasion of tumor cells? MMP-2 and MMP-9 may increase the permeability of blood-brain barrier and allow the transfer of metastatic cells reaching brain via blood stream. The alternative hypothesis is that latent MMPs substrates on tumor cells or cells of tumor microenvironment may be activated upon cleavage by astrocyte secreted MMP-2 and MMP-9 leading to an invasive phenotype. The precise elucidation of these interactions is urgent as astrocytes may be a novel target for therapy aimed at prevention of brain metastases in patients with various cancers [21-23].

8. Blocking MMPs expression and/or activity

Scientists have widely studied the possibilities of attenuating MMPs expression and activity in order to reduce the invasiveness of gliomas. They efforts have combined various directions.

Atorvastatin is a well known statin, an inhibitor of β-hydroxy-β-methylglutaryl-CoA reductase. By inhibiting the key enzyme in a mevalonate synthesis pathway atorvastatin has pleiotropic effects. The main mode of action of this drug is the inhibition of *de novo* cholesterol synthesis. However, this drug has some other advantages resulting in its pleiotropic antiatherogenic properties due to the inhibition of synthesis of other biologically important mevalonate pathway derivates: dolichol, ubichinon, farnesyl and geranyl residues. This inhibition leads to disturbances in some signaling pathways. The possible anticancer properties of statins have been postulated since a long time.

Yongjun and co-workers have observed that atorvastatin reduced pro-tumorigenic effects of microglia on glioma migration and invasion by reducing microglial expression of MT1-MMP

(MMP-14). Mohebbi *et al.* observed that atorvastatin 40 mg administered twice daily seven from days before till three weeks after the neurosurgical procedure led to better outcome after the neurosurgical treatment of brain tumors and raised significantly Karnofsky score. The biochemical analysis showed that two weeks after the surgical treatment patients on atorvastatin therapy had significantly reduced plasma level of MMP-9 compared to patients receiving placebo [24,25].

Locatelli *et al.* evaluated a composition of polymeric nanoparticles containing a composition of two cytotoxic agents, drug alisertib and nanosilver conjugated with chlorotoxin, a peptide binding specifically to MMP-2. Their experimental *in vitro* and *in vivo* studies showed the tumor reduction [26].

Researchers are trying to investigate drugs aimed at inhibiting MT1-MMP (MMP-14). DX-2400, a fully human antibody was shown to reduce MMP-14 activity, retard tumor progression, metastasis, migration and invasion. Two natural isoflavonoid phytoestrogens, genistein and biochain A, were shown to reduce MMP-14 activity in a dose dependent manner in U87MG cell line. The green tea polyphenol, (Q)-epigallocatechin gallate (EGCg), has been found to inhibit MMP-14 mediated cell migration. This compound also disrupted proMMP-2 activation via downregulation of MMP-14 gene expression. Marimastat, an orally administered MMP inhibitor, was tested in two clinical trials in GBM patients after neurosurgery or irradiation. Marimastat alone did not improve survival, but in conjunction with cytotoxic chemotherapy gave promising results [27-30].

The next point of scientists interest are microRNAs (miRNAs). These small, non-coding RNA molecules containing 18-25 nucleotides in length can inhibit gene expression by binding to the 3' untranslated region of their target genes and suppress translation. Several studies have shown that various miRNAs can inhibit expression of MMP-14, MMP-2 and inhibit tumor cell adhesion, migration, invasion and angiogenesis [31-35].

Lei *et al.* proposed a new strategy combining a cytotoxic drug paclitaxel and RNA interference suppressing MMP-2 expression. This conception was aimed at blocking tumor growth and proliferation by Paclitaxel and blocking tumor angiogenesis and invasion by inhibiting MMP-2 expression [36].

9. Conclusions

In last few years MMPs have been shown to exert new biochemical properties. Their extracellular mode of action as well as intracellular, intranuclear activities were shown to be involved in invasiveness of brain tumors, especially gliomas. Inhibiting their expression may be a new therapeutical approach. So far some drugs being MMPs inhibitors have some serious adverse effects. Inhibiting MMPs expression and activity seems to be rather a supplement to chemotherapy, radiotherapy or neurosurgical procedures than a new single method of treatment of brain tumors.

Author details

Krzysztof Siemianowicz[1*], Wirginia Likus[2] and Jarosław Markowski[3]

*Address all correspondence to: ksiem@mp.pl

1 Department of Biochemistry, School of Medicine in Katowice, Medical University of Silesia, Poland

2 Department of Human Anatomy, School of Medicine in Katowice, Medical University of Silesia, Poland

3 Department of Laryngology, School of Medicine in Katowice, Medical University of Silesia, Poland

Sections 1-3 contain text originally published in [3].

References

[1] Pearce WH, Shively VP. Abdominal aortic aneurysm as a complex multifactorial disease. Annals of New York Academy of Sciences 2006;1085 117-132.

[2] Ra H-J, Parks WC. Control of matrix metalloproteinase catalytic activity. Matrix Biology 2007;26: 587-596.

[3] Siemianowicz K. The role of metalloproteinases in the development of aneurysm. in: „Aneurysm" (ed.) Yasuo Murai, Rijeka, InTech, 2012, p65-74.

[4] Mannello F, Medda V. Nuclear localization of matrix metalloproteinases. Progress in Histochemistry and Cytochemistry 2012;47 27-58.

[5] Langenfurth A, Rinnenthal JL, Vinnakota K, Prinz V, Carlo AS, Stadelmann C, Siffrin V, Peaschke S, Endres M, Heppner F, Glass R, Wolf SA, Kettenmann H. Membrane-type 1 metalloproteinase is upregulated in microglia/brain macrophages in neurodegenerative and neuroinflammatory diseases. Journal of Neuroscience Research 2014;92(3) 275-286.

[6] Wang L, Cossette SM, Rarick KR, Gershan J, Dwinell MB, Harder DR, Ramchandran R. Astrocytes directly influence tumor cell invasion and metastasis *in vivo*. PLoS ONE 8(12): e80933, doi: 10.1371/journal.pone.0080933.

[7] Tsai CF, Yeh WL, Chen JH, Lin C, Huang SS, Lu DY. Osthole suppresses the migratory ability of human glioblastoma multiforme cells via inhibition of focal adhesion kinase-mediated matrix metalloproteinase-13 expression. International Journal of Molecular Sciences 2014;15 3889-3903.

[8] Wang J, Li Y, Li C, Yu K, Wang Q. Increased expression of metalloproteinase-13 in glioma is associated with poor overall survival of patients. Medical Oncology 2012; 29, 2432-2437.

[9] Hsieh WT, Yeh Wl, Cheng RY, Lin C, Tsai CF, Huang BR, Wu CY, Lin HY, Huang SS, Lu DY. Exogenous endothelin-1 induces cell migration and matrix metalloproteinase expression in U251 glioblastoma multiforme. Journal of Neuro-Oncology 2014;118(2) 257-69.

[10] Bakalova R, Zhelev Z, Aoki I, Saga T. Tissue redox activity as a hallmark of carcinogenesis: from early to terminal stages of cancer. Clinical Cancer Research 2013;19(9) 2503-2517.

[11] Mariani CL, Boozer LB, Braxton AM, Platt SR, Vernau KM, McDonnell JJ, Guevar J. Evaluation of matrix metalloproteinase-2 and -9 in the cerebrospinal fluid of dogs with intracranial tumors. American Journal of Veterinary Research 2013;74(1) 122-129.

[12] Xu Y, Zhong Z, Yuan J, Zhang Z, Wei Q, Song W, Chen H. Collaborative overexpression of matrix metallloproteianse-1 and vascular endothelial growth factor-C predicts adverse prognosis in patients with gliomas. Cancer Epidemiology 2013;37(5) 697-702.

[13] Wang H, Wang Y, Jiang C. Stromal protein periostain identified as a progression associated and prognostic biomarker in glioma via inducing an invasive and proliferative phenotype. International Journal of Oncology 2013;42(5) 1716-1724.

[14] Ulasof I, Yi R, Guo D, Sarvaiya, Cobbs C. The emerging role of MMP-14 in brain tumorigenesis and future therapeutics. Biochimica et Biophysica Acta 2014;1846 113-120.

[15] Lee WS, Woo EZ, Kwon J, Park MJ, Lee JS, Han YH, Bae IH. Bcl-w enhances mesenchymal changes and invasiveness of glioblastoma cells by inducing nuclear accumulation of β-catenin. PLoS ONE 8(6): e68030. doi: 10.1371/journal.pone.0068030.

[16] Lee SL, Kwon J, Yun DH, Lee YN, Woo EY, Park MJ, Lee JS, Han YH, Bae IH. Specifity protein 1 expression contributes to Bcl-w-induced aggressiveness in glioblastoma multiforme. Molecules and Cells 2014;37(1) 17-23.

[17] Tie X, Han S, Meng L, Wang Y, Wu A. NFAT1 is highly expressed in, and regulates the invasion of, glioblastoma multiforme cells. PLoS ONE 2013;8(6): e66008. doi: 10.1371/journal.pone.0068008.

[18] Kesanakurti D, Chetty C, Maddirela DR, Gujrati M, Rao JS. Functional cooperativity by direct interaction between PAK4 and MMP-2 in the regulation of anoikis resistance, migration and invasion in glioma. Cell Death and Disease 2012;3, e445; doi: 10.1038/cddis.2012.182.

[19] Kesanakurti D, Chetty C, Bhoopathi P, Lakka SS, Gorantla B, Tsung AJ, Rao JS. Suppression of MMP-2 attenuates TNF-alpha induced NF-kappaB activation and leads to JNK mediated cell death in glioma. PLoS One 2011; 6: e19341.

[20] Kesanakurti D, Chetty C, Dinh DH, Gujrati M, Rao JS. Role of MMP-2 in the regulation of IL-6/Stat3 survival signaling via interaction with a5b1 integrin in glioma. Oncogene 2013;32(3) 327-40.

[21] Ellert-Miklaszewska A, Dabrowski M, Lipko M, Sliwa M, Maleszewska M, Kaminska B, Molecular definition of the pro-tumorigenic phenotype of glioma-activated microglia. Glia 2013;61(7) 1178-1190.

[22] Vinnakota K, Hu F, Ku MC, Georgieva PB, Szulzewsky F, Polhmann A, Waiczies S, Waiczies H, Niedorf T, Lehnardt S, Hanisch S, Synowitz M, Markovic D, Wolf SA, Glass R, Kettenmann H. Toll-like receptor-2 mediates microglia/brain macrophage MT1-MMP expression and glioma expansion. Neuro-Oncology 2013;15(11) 1457-1468.

[23] Wang L, Cossette SM, Rarick KR, Gershan J, Dwinell MB, Harder DR, Ramchandran R. Astrocytes directly influence tumor cell invasion and metastasis in vivo. PLos ONE 2013;8(12): e80933. doi:10.1371/journal.pone.0080933.

[24] Yongjun Y, Shuyun H, Lei C, Xiangrong C, Zhilin Y, Yiquan K. Atorvastatin suppresses glioma invasion and migration by reducing microglial MT1-MMP expression. Journal of Neuroimmunology 2013;260(1-2) 1-8.

[25] Mohebbi N, Khoshnevisan A, Naderi S, Abdollahzade S, Salamzadeh J, Javadi M, Mojtahezadeh M, Gholami K. Effects of atorvastatin on plasma matrix metalloproteinase-9 concentration after glial tumor resection; a randomized, double blind, placebo controlled trial. Daru. Journal of Pharmaceutical Sciences 2014;7;22(1): 10. doi: 10.1186/2008-2231-22-10.

[26] Locatelli E, Naddaka M, Uboldi C, Loudos G, Fragogeorgi E, Molinari V, Pucci A, Tsotakos T, Psimadas D, Ponti J, Franchini MC. Targeted delivery of silver nanoparticles and alisertib: in vitro and in vivo synergistic effect against glioblastoma. Nanomedicine (Lond) 2014;9(6) 839-49.

[27] Devy L, Huang L, Naa L, Yanamandra N, Pieters H, Frans N, Chang E, Tao Q, Vanhove M, Lejeune A, van Gool R, Sexton DJ, Kuang G, Rank D, Hogan S, Pazmany C, Ma YL, Schoonbroodt S, Nixon AE, Ladner RC, Hoet R, Henderikx P, Tenhoor C, Rabbani SA, Valentino ML, Wood CR, Dransfield DT. Selective inhibition of matrix metalloproteinase-14 blocks tumor growth, invasion, and angiogenesis. Cancer Research 2009;69 1517-1526.

[28] Puli S, Lai JC, Bhushan A. Inhibition of matrix degrading enzymes and invasion in human glioblastoma (U87MG) cells by isoflavones. Journal of Neuro-Oncology 2006;79 135-142.

[29] Annabi B, Lachambre MP, Bousquet-Gagnon N, Page M, Gingras D, Beliveau R. Green tea polyphenol (–)-epigallocatechin 3-gallate inhibits MMP-2 secretionand MT1-MMP-driven migration in glioblastoma cells, Biochim. Biophys. Acta 2002;1542 209-220.

[30] Groves MD, Puduvalli VK, Hess KR, Jaeckle KA, Peterson P, Yung WK, Levin VA. Phase II trial of temozolomide plus the matrix metalloproteinase inhibitor, marimastat, in recurrent and progressive glioblastoma multiforme. Journal of Clinical Oncology 2002;20(5) 1383-1388.

[31] Zhang H, Qi M, Li S, Qi T, Mei H, Huang K, Zheng I, Tong Q. microRNA-9 targets matrix metalloproteinase 14 to inhibit invasion, metastasis, and angiogenesis of neuroblastoma cells. Molecular Cancer Therapeutics 2012;11 1454-1466.

[32] Hu X, Chen D, Cui Y, Li Z, Huang J. Targeting microRNA-23a to inhibit glioma cell invasion via HOXD10. Scientific Reports 2013; 3 : 3423 DOI: 10.1038/srep03423.

[33] Pratt J, Annabi B. Induction of autophagy biomarker BNIP3 requires a JAK2/STAT3 and MT1-MMP signaling interplay in Concavalin-A-activated U87 glioblastoma cells. Cellular Signalling 2014; 26(5) 917-924.

[34] Dontula R, Dinasarapu A, Chetty C, Pannuru P, Herbert E, Ozer H, Lakka S. MicroRNA 203 modulates glioma cell migration via Robo I/ERK/MMP-9 signaling. Genes & Cancer 2013;4(7-8) 285-296.

[35] Yang TQ, Lu XJ, Wu TF, Ding DD, Zhao ZH, Chen GL, Xie XS, LI B, Wei YX, Guo LC, Zhang Y, Huang YL, Zhou YX, Du ZW. MicroRNA-16 inhibits glioma cell growth and invasion through suppression of BCL2 and the nuclear factor-κB1/MMP-9 signaling pathway. Cancer Science 2014;105(3) 265-71.

[36] Lei C, Cui Y, Zheng L, Chow PK, Wang CH. Development of a gene/drug dual delivery system for brain tumor therapy: potent inhibition via RNA interference and synergistic effects. Biomaterials 2013;34(30) 7483-7494.

6

Understanding Mitochondrial DNA in Brain Tumorigenesis

Abdul Aziz Mohamed Yusoff, Farizan Ahmad,
Zamzuri Idris, Hasnan Jaafar and
Jafri Malin Abdullah

1. Introduction

In developed countries, most studies reveal that the number of people who develop brain tumors and die from them has increased. Brain tumor, one of the most devastating central nervous system pathologies, is the leading cause of solid tumor death in children under the age of 15, and the second leading cause of cancer death in male adults ages 20-39. So far, researches on genesis and development of tumor are intensively focused and studied on alteration of the gene in nucleus and brain tumors is the one where most were reported arise as the result of progressive nuclear genetic alterations. Multiple genetic events have been identified in brain tumor cells involving some well-known susceptibility genes such as tumor suppressor and oncogenes that are encoded by the nuclear DNA (nDNA). For instance, the p53 tumor suppressor gene is frequently mutated and often detected altered or lost early in brain tumor mainly in astrocytic tumors formation [1-3]. Similarly, mutations or loss of PTEN (phosphatase and tensin homolog), p16, RB (retinoblastoma) and amplification of EGFR (epidermal growth factor receptor), MDM2, CDK4, CDK6 (cyclin-dependent kinase) are also involved in the pathogenesis of brain tumor [4,5].

Although, it is well established that multiple alterations in the nuclear-encoded genes are associated with tumor development, it is reasonable to consider and postulate that there is another factor or genome yet to be investigated. The involvement of the mitochondrial genome in tumorigenesis and cancer progression remains controversial to date. Mitochondria are cytoplasmic organelles in eukaryotic cell and recognized as "the power houses of the cell", thus one of their principal functions is providing cellular energy, adenosine triphosphate

(ATP) through the oxidative phosphorylation (OXPHOS) [6]. OXPHOS can be defined as the oxidation of electron transfer chain by oxygen and the concomitant transduction of this energy into ATP. The OXPHOS system is composed of five protein complexes: NADH-ubiquinone oxidoreductase as complex I, succinate-ubiquinone oxidoreductase as complex II, ubiquinone-cytochrome c oxidoreductase as complex III, cytochrome c oxidase as complex IV and ATP synthase as complex V.

In addition to energy production, mitochondria are also key components in calcium signalling, regulation of cellular metabolism, haem synthesis, steroid synthesis and, perhaps most importantly, the initiation and execution of apoptosis [7,8]. Over the last 25 years, mitochondrial abnormalities that associated with mitochondrial DNA (mtDNA) alterations, has been identified in human disease, including seizure, ataxia, ophthalmoplegia, optic atrophy, short stature, sensorineural hearing loss, cardiomyopathy, diabetes mellitus and kidney failure [9,10]. Accumulation of altered mtDNA has also been widely believed to play the pivotal role in aging and the development of various age-related degenerative diseases [11]. In recent years, more attention has been directed towards the role of mitochondrial dysfunction in various cancer due to genetic defects of OXPHOS system [12-17]. Proteins that take part in the proper functioning of the OXPHOS system are encoded by both nDNA and mtDNA. Similar to nDNA, mtDNA mutations and deletions have been identified in a wide variety of cancers including brain tumor [18-26], although it is unclear whether these are causal or a consequence of the neoplastic process.

This chapter begins with a general overview of basic mitochondrial structure and OXPHOS system functions and then outlines more specifically the link between mitochondrial reactive oxygen spices (ROS) and apoptosis with tumorigenesis and genetic alterations in mitochondria associated with human cancers mainly brain tumor.

2. Mitochondrial structure

Mitochondria are seen by electron microscopy to be intracellular oblong or ovoid shaped organelles with a transverse diameter of 0.1-0.5 μm and a variable length [27]. The structure of mitochondria is shown in Figure 1. Most eukaryotic cells contain many mitochondria, which cover up to 25% of the volume of the cytoplasm. The number of mitochondria within a cell increases with the amount of substrate and oxygen. Mitochondria are large enough to be observed under a light microscope, but the detail of their structure can be viewed only with the electron microscope.

Initial studies based on electron microscopy investigations by two researchers Palade and Sjöstrand, revealed that mitochondria contain more than one membrane system with the existence of an outer membrane and of a highly folded inner membrane [28,29]. The baffle model which was coined by Palade has been accepted and currently depicted as a model of mitochondria structure in all the textbooks [28]. The baffle model describes mitochondria as having four compartments (Figure 1). The first compartment is termed the outer membrane. This smooth membrane surrounds with a very convoluted or folded inner membrane. The

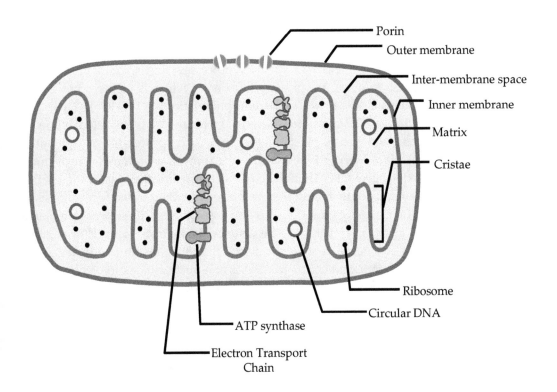

Figure 1. The structure of a mitochondrion

inner membrane is folded to create cristae. The outer and inner membranes have very different properties. Together they create two compartments, namely the intermembrane space (the space between the outer and inner membranes), and the matrix (closed by the inner membrane- the very interior of the mitochondria).

Nowadays, the baffle model has been shown to be inaccurate. Based on the investigations of 3-D structure of mitochondrial morphology by electron microscope tomography, the inner membrane is believed to be further divided into two distinct domains: an inner boundary membrane and cristae membranes [27, 30-32]. The inner boundary membrane is located close to the outer membrane and makes close contact with it at numerous positions. Cristae membranes protrude into the matrix compartment and are connected to the inner boundary membrane by narrow tubular structures called cristae junctions.

The outer bilayer lipid membrane contains channels made of voltage dependent anion channels called porins and are permeable to molecules < 10,000 Da. It is composed of approximately 50% lipids and 50% proteins. The inner bilayer lipid membrane is folded and impermeable to most molecules and protons. It is built up of 70% protein. The inner membrane is also the site of the electron transport chain and contains transport proteins for OXPHOS system. Within the matrix a large number of enzymes and other proteins and peptides, including DNA-polymerase, chaperones (heat shock proteins), ribosomes, mRNAs, tRNAs, and the mtDNA are located.

3. Mitochondrial function: OXPHOS system

Mitochondria play a central role in energy conversion processes (respiration) within the cell through the electron transport chain, the primary function of which is ATP synthesis via a complex mechanism referred to as "oxidative phosphorylation" (OXPHOS) (Figure 2). OXPHOS is the production of ATP using energy derived from the transfer of electrons in an electron transport system and occurs by chemiosmosis. As the process of mitochondrial electron transport takes place, energy is released in the form of a proton electrochemical gradient that can be used to make ATP. Though, the details regarding the conservation of this released energy are still being debated, most scientists accept the chemiosmotic hypothesis as the general mechanism for the energy transfer. The chemiosmotic hypothesis was formulated in the 1960s by Peter Mitchell [33,34]. This hypothesis states that hydrogen ions (H+or protons) are transferred from mitochondrial matrix out across the inner membrane to the inter-membrane space as electron transport occurs by a series of reduction-oxidation reactions that establish an electrochemical gradient. The membrane is impermeable to protons, which flow back down the proton gradient through a large enzyme called ATP synthase or complex V, the energy from which is subsequently used to produce ATP.

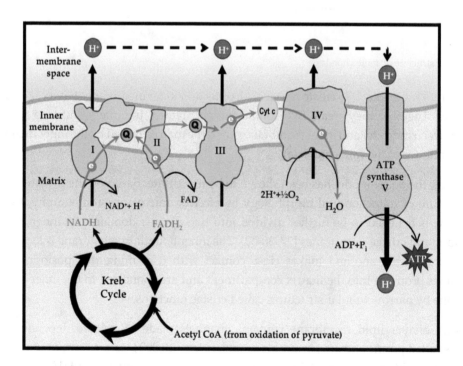

Figure 2. A schematic representation of the mitochondrial OXPHOS system

For achieving the whole process, in first stage pyruvate, which is generated in the cytosol during glycolysis, is transported across the double mitochondrial membranes and enters the matrix. The pyruvate molecules are produced by the breakdown of glucose molecules from carbohydrates via glycolysis. Once inside the matrix, pyruvate molecules are converted to the two carbon compound acetyl coenzyme A (acetyl CoA). This oxidative decarboxylation reaction is catalyzed by the pyruvate dehydrogenase complex. The acetyl CoA is then taken into a sequence of enzymatically catalyzed reactions known as the citric acid cycle which completes the oxidation of carbon and regenerates an electron acceptor to keep the cycle going. The oxidation of acetyl CoA in the citric acid cycle (which is also called the Krebs cycle or tricarboxylic acid cycle) is catalyzed by a set of enzymes localized in the mitochondrial matrix. During this process, the released electrons are transferred to co-enzymes, NAD^+ and FAD to form the reduced molecules NADH and $FADH_2$. Later, NADH and $FADH_2$ transfer electrons to acceptor molecules in the electron transport chain, in the inner mitochondrial membrane. Coenzyme Q (ubiquinone) and cytochrome c are also involved in mitochondrial respiration, serving as 'electron shuttles' or mobile electron carriers between the complexes.

Electrons donated from NADH to Complex I or from $FADH_2$ to Complex II are passed to coenzyme Q. Electrons then flow from coenzyme Q to Complex III which transfers the electrons to cytochrome c. From cytochrome c the electrons move to Complex IV and finally to $\frac{1}{2}$ O_2 to produce H_2O [35]. As electrons pass through these complexes in a series of oxidation-reduction reactions, the energy that is released by this electron transport chain is used to pump protons out from the mitochondrial matrix to the inter membrane space via Complexes I, III and IV creating the electrochemical gradient. The electrochemical gradient allows protons to drive back into the matrix through a pore in Complex V (ATP synthase), using the released energy to catalyze the synthesis of ATP from ADP and phosphate.

4. Mitochondrial genome

Mitochondria have a genetic system of their own, separate from the nuclear one, with all the machinery necessary for its expression; that is, to replicate, transcribe and translate the genetic information they contain. The mitochondrial deoxyribonucleic acid (mtDNA) was discovered in 1963 [36] and the near complete sequence for human mtDNA was available in 1981 [37] and was minimally revised in 1999 [38]. Human mtDNA is mostly a double-stranded, closed circular molecule composed of 16,569 base pairs.

Figure 3 shows the human mitochondrial genome. It is very compact, containing little non-coding sequence, essentially just the 1.1 kb D-loop (displacement loop or non-coding) region, and having even some overlapping genes. The non-coding region that includes the D-loop is located between genes encoding tRNA phenylalanine (F) and proline (P). The two strands of mtDNA have been named light strand (L-strand, rich in cytosines) and heavy strand (H-strand, rich in guanines) according to their buoyancy through a denaturing caesium chloride gradient [39].

The D-loop region of mtDNA contains the origin of replication for H-strand synthesis as well as both mitochondrial transcription promoters (the light strand promoter, LPS and two heavy strand promoters, HSP1 and HSP2), and serves as the main site for mitochondrial genomic replication and transcription [40,41]. Between different mammalian species, the mtDNA is about the same size and has the similar organization and content of genes [42-44]. The mitochondrial genome has been sequenced and mapped for many species yet the regulation of its expression is poorly understood.

The human mtDNA contains 37 genes coding mRNAs for 13 polypeptides that are part of four of the five multi-enzymatic complexes in the OXPHOS system, 22 tRNAs (that are able to decode all open reading frames) and 2 rRNAs (components of the specific mitochondrial ribosomes) necessary for synthesis of the polypeptides. Unlike nuclear DNA, mtDNA coding sequences have no introns. Seven of those polypeptides, ND1 to ND6 and ND4L are subunits of Complex I; one, cytochrome b, is part of Complex III; three, COX I, COX II and COX III, are the catalytic subunits of Complex IV, and ATPase 6 and 8 are subunits of Complex V (F_0F_1 ATP synthase). The heavy strand is the main coding strand, and codes for 2 rRNAs, 14 tRNAs and 12 polypeptides. The light strand codes for remaining 8 tRNAs and only one polypeptide, the ND6 subunit (NADH-dehydrogenase) [6].

Mammalian mitochondria are not self-supporting entities in the cell. Replication and transcription depend upon *trans*-acting nuclear-encoded factors. All proteins of mitochondrial ribosomes and their associated translation factors and, indeed, all other mitochondrial proteins including the components of the mitochondrial import machinery are encoded by the nuclear DNA. For instance, mitochondrial tRNAs are charged by imported aminoacyl-tRNA synthetases from nuclear genes.

There are approximately hundreds or thousands copies of mitochondrial genome in each somatic cell. Normally, all of the mitochondrial DNAs within the cells of an individual are identical, which is termed homoplasmy. However, in the presence of a mitochondrial DNA mutation, the affected individual cells will usually harbour a mixture of mutated and wild-type mitochondrial DNA. The condition of these two populations of mitochondrial DNA molecules is called heteroplasmy [45]. As cells divide, the mutant and wild-type mitochondrial DNA are randomly distributed to the daughter cells, so the proportion of mutant to wild-type mitochondrial DNA may increase or decrease with each subsequent generation of the cell line. If that proportion increases past a certain level, the cellular energy capacity will decline, and clinical signs appear. This is referred to as the threshold effect. The threshold may vary from tissue to tissue because the percent of mutant mitochondrial DNA needed to cause cell dysfunction varies according to the oxidative requirements of the tissue and the severity of the mutation. It has often been claimed that tissues with high requirements for oxidative energy metabolism, such as muscle and brain, have relatively low thresholds and are particularly vulnerable to mitochondrial DNA mutation.

Human mitochondrial DNA is a 16,569 base pair circle of double-stranded DNA that encodes 13 essential respiratory chain subunits. ND1–ND6 and ND4L encode seven complex I (NADH–ubiquinone oxidoreductase) subunits, CYT b encodes one subunit of complex III (ubiquinol:cytochrome c oxidoreductase), COX I–COX III encode the three major catalytic subunits of complex IV, and ATPase6 and ATPase8 encode two subunits of complex V (ATP synthase). Also shown are the two ribosomal RNA (12S rRNA and 16S rRNA) genes and the 22 transfer RNA genes (red spheres, depicted by single letter amino acid code abbreviation) required for mitochondrial protein synthesis. tRNAs are F, Phenylalanine; V, Valine; L, Leucine; I, Isoleucine; Q, Glutamine; M, Methionine; W, Tryptophan; A, Alanine; N, Asparagine; C, Cysteine;

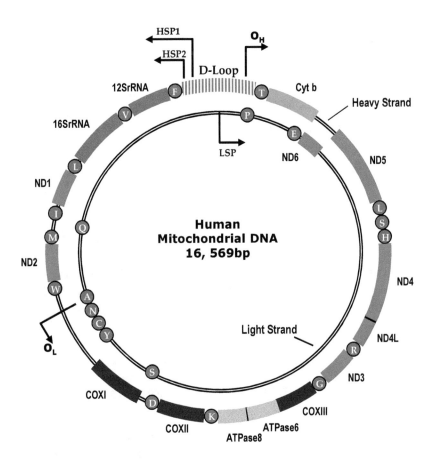

Figure 3. The human mitochondrial genome

Y, Tyrosine; S, Serine; D, Aspartic acid; K, Lysine; G, Glycine; R, Arginine; H, Histidine; E, Glutamic acid; T, Threonine; P, Proline. The genome is highly organised and shows little redundancy of its coding sequence. The displacement loop (D-loop), or non-coding control region contains the promoters for transcription of the L (LSP) and H strands (HSP1 and HS2) and the origin of replication of the H strand (O_H). The origin of light-strand replication is shown as O_L.

5. Warburg theory and mitochondrial dysfunction in cancer cells

In the 1930s, the German scientist, Dr. Otto H. Warburg pioneered the research specifically targeted to the alterations of mitochondrial respiration in the aspect of cancer. He reported that cancer cells exhibited a high glycolysis rate even in the presence of abundant oxygen. This phenomenon was known as the "Warburg effect". Cancer cells had to depend on anaerobic glycolysis rather than respiration to generate ATP [46]. He further proposed that defects in energy metabolism, especially due to mitochondrial malfunction, are involved in the initiation or progression of cancer. Dr. Warburg's discovery encouraged many scientists to realize the potential role of mitochondria in cancer cells.

Since then, alterations of mitochondria in the number, shape and function have been reported in various cancers [47]. The conversion of ATP production from mitochondrial OXPHOS to glycolysis has been suggested to be the bioenergetic hallmark of cancer cells [48]. Furthermore, it has been shown that mitochondrial dysfunction is able to initiate critical signaling pathways that modulate cell proliferation or growth [49,50]. A study done by Pelicano's group found that mitochondrial respiration defects promoted to increased level of NADH, which could inactivate PTEN via a redox modification mechanism [51]. PTEN deactivation could lead to activation of the protein kinase B (Akt) survival pathway [51]. Akt was show to stimulate glycolysis and also trigger an increase in cell survival of cancer cells [52,53]. In addition, Lopez-Rios and colleagues showed that inhibition of OXPHOS activity by incubation of lung cancer cells with oligomycin could trigger a rapid increase in aerobic glycolysis [54]. This finding demonstrates that suppression of mitochondrial energy production can lead tumor cells become glycolytic [54]. However, when glycolysis was inhibited, tumor cells were unable to sufficiently upregulate mitochondrial OXPHOS and this indicating was due to partial mito-chondrial impairment [55].

6. Reactive Oxygen Spices (ROS) and tumorigenesis

ROS such as superoxide anion radical (O_2^-), hydrogen peroxide (H_2O_2) and hydroxyl radical (OH) are constantly generated during metabolic process in all living species [56]. Mitochon-drial respiratory chain is a major intracellular source or producer of ROS generation, as some of the electrons passing to molecular oxygen are instead leaked out of the chain. Under normal physiological conditions, cellular ROS generation is counterbalanced by the action of the endogenous systems include mainly antioxidant enzymes for instance superoxide dismutases (SODs), cytosolic copper/zinc SOD (CuZnSOD) and mitochondrial manganese SOD (MnSOD). Low levels of ROS regulate cellular signaling and are essential in proliferation of normal cell. However, overproduction of ROS will lead to various cellular components injury, such as damage to DNA, proteins and lipids. Recent studies have demonstrated a role of ROS in promoting tumor development. The exposure of normal cells to ROS led to an increase in proliferation [57] and expression of growth-related genes [58-60]. Furthermore, cancer cells are commonly known to generate more ROS than normal cells [61,62]. These observations suggest that the stimulation of ROS may be an important contributing factor in the initiation, maintenance and development of cancer *in vivo*.

ROS are highly active and can also cause damage to mitochondrial genome [63,64]. It has been proposed that damage to mtDNA, if not repaired properly, could initiate tumorigenesis and promote cancer development [65,66]. Mutations in mtDNA may lead to a decreased efficiency of the OXPHOS system and increased leakage electrons as well as enhanced more mitochon-drial and cellular ROS production. This situation may result in creating oxidative stress which will further accumulate more total damage to mtDNA because the location of mtDNA is in close proximity to the ROS-generating electron transport system. Thus, it is possible that persistent oxidative stress on cells may favour the neoplastic process through induction of mtDNA damage which leads to mutations [67].

Moreover, in contrast to nDNA, mtDNA does not contain intronic sequences and not cover up with protective proteins such as histones. Due to these reasons, it has been suggested that most mtDNA mutations occur in coding sequences. However, more recent data shows that mtDNA can be almost completely covered by the DNA binding protein Tfam (mitochondrial transcription factor A) [68]. In addition, mtDNA also harbors limited effective DNA repair mechanisms. All these conditions are believed may contribute to the increased sensitivity of mitochondrial genome to damage, and ultimately leads to mutations. Whether mutations in mtDNA are a cause or a consequence of cancer is still debatable and need to be worked out. However, it is proven that mutations of mtDNA induced by oxidative damage could contribute significantly to OXPHOS defects and genetic instability in tumours and thereby promoting a higher propensity for tumour cell growth and progression [69]. This can be suggested that mutation of mtDNA may worsen oxidative stress or vice versa.

7. Apoptosis and tumorigenesis

Apoptosis, also called programmed cell death, is a crucial physiological process in the development and homeostasis of multicellular organisms which requires the involvement of mitochondria. Mitochondria have long been recognized for their essential role in regulating apoptotic signaling pathways [70,71]. Defects in apoptotic cell-death pathways are believed to contribute to genomic instability and tumorigenesis [72]. Study recently conducted shows that the mitochondrial respiratory chain has the ability to modulate apoptosis [73]. Respiratory chain dysfunction has been shown to either promote or suppress apoptotic cell death, relying on the specific alteration of electron flux [73]. Stimulation of ROS production can initiate apoptosis in the mitochondria. Mitochondrial defects normally can lead to reduced phosphorylation with low ATP generation and high cytosolic calcium and theses situations become a signal which triggers the apoptotic cell death [74]. Mitochondrial respiration defects in cancer cells can lead to activation of the Akt survival pathway which promotes cell death resistance. As mentioned earlier, this activation of Akt was suggested to result from increased level of NADH and inactivation of PTEN through a redox modification mechanism [51]. More interestingly, another study has elucidated the role of mitochondrial chaperones in modulating mitochondrial function for the survival of cancer cells [75,76]. Molecular chaperone heat shock protein 60 (Hsp60) was shown to orchestrate a broad cell survival program centered on stabilization of mitochondria and also to restrain p53 function [75]. Another chaperone, Hsp90 and its mitochondrial-related molecule, TRAP-1, were suggested to interact with cyclophilin D to suppress cell death [76].

8. Mitochondrial DNA mutations in cancer

Over 300 mtDNA mutations and even more mtDNA deletions have been reported that are associated with human diseases, since the first diseases caused by mtDNA damage were described 25 years ago [77-79]. Diseases that have been shown to be linked with mitochondrial dysfunction are diabetes mellitus, Parkinson's disease, Alzheimer's disease, epilepsy, sensorineural deafness and a variety of syndromes involving muscles and the central nervous system as well as a variety of forms of cancer [80-83]. The same mutation or different mutations in the same mtDNA gene may present with very different clinical manifestations, while the same clinical phenotype may be caused by different mutations (DiMauro and Schon, 2003). A large number of mtDNA mutations have been associated to a wide variety of clinical manifestations/phenotypes of mitochondrial diseases include mitochondria encephalomyopathy, lactic acidosis and stroke-like syndrome (MELAS), myoclonic epilepsy and ragged red fiber disease (MERRF), Lebers hereditary optic neuropathy (LHON), Leigh's syndrome, Kearns-Sayre syndrome, chronic progressive external ophthalmoplegia (CPEO), neuropathy, ataxia, retinitis pigmentosa (NARP).

Although the role of nDNA mutations in carcinogenesis is well established, the importance of mtDNA alterations in the development and maintenance of cancers is only now beginning to be focused by researchers. Alterations in mtDNA which may lead to OXPHOS system destabilization seem to be particularly crucial because 13 proteins encoded by mtDNA are essential for complex I, and III–V respiratory chain assembly and these enzymatic complexes defects have been reported in human solid tumours [85]. There is considerable evidence suggesting that mitochondria may serve as potential contributors to carcinogenesis even though the exact mechanism of how mitochondria involved is still debatable and is not well-documented. Thus, mtDNA is now being targeted organelle by an increasing number of laboratories in order to investigate its potential role as biomarker for tumorigenesis in various types of tissues [86,87].

DNA alterations in mitochondria are believed to become fast hotspots of cancer research. Indeed, numerous mutations in mtDNA has now been observed in multiple cancer types (88-90] since the first somatic mtDNA mutation was detected 15 years ago by Bert Vogelstein's group in human colorectal cancer cells [91]. After these initial findings, mtDNA mutations or alterations have also been identified in bladder cancer [92], breast cancer [93-96], esophageal cancer [97-99], head and neck cancer [100], hepatocellular carcinoma [101-103], lung cancer [104-106], ovarian cancer [107,108], prostate cancer [109-111], renal cancer [112], thyroid cancer [113] and a number of blood cancers [114,115]. More recently, various types of molecular abberations in mtDNA such as point mutations, polymorphisms, depletion, insertions, microsatellite instability and changes in mtDNA copy number have been characterized throughout the mitochondrial genome in human cancers [89,90,116].

9. Somatic mitochondrial DNA alterations and brain tumors

Although there have been studies reporting about the association of mtDNA mutations with brain tumors, it is still no clear evidence whether mitochondrial abnormalities are contributing factors in brain tumorigenesis. Several types of somatic mtDNA alterations have been identified in brain tumors. These mtDNA alterations include point mutations, deletions, insertions, mtMSI (mitochondrial microsatellite instability) and copy number changes.

9.1. Point mutations

A number of studies have detected mtDNA point mutations in cancer of the brain and other central nervous system, including gliomas, astrocytomas, gliomatosis cerebri, medulloblastoma, meningiomas, schwannomas, and neurofibromas [19,20,117-120]. Mitochondrial genome somatic point mutations were most frequently found in the D-loop region, especially in a poly-cytosine (poly-C) mononucleotide repeat tract located between 303 and 315 nucleotides known as D310. This location has been identified as a hot spot region for somatic mtDNA mutations in various human cancers, including in brain cancer. In 2005, Montanini's groups analyzed the D-loop region of mtDNA in 42 patients affected by malignant gliomas and found sequence alterations in 36% of the patients including 16 somatic mutations, mostly in the D310 area. The authors suggested that mtDNA mutations were easily amplified from post-surgical tumor cavities and could be used for the clinical follow-up of malignant gliomas [121].

Instead of focusing on D-loop region, the complete of mitochondrial genome was also examined by various researchers in brain cancer patients. In a study that involved the entire mtDNA mutation scanning by temporal temperature gel electrophoresis (TTGE) in medulloblastomas, 40% of the cases (6/15) were found to have at least one somatic mutation [20]. Seven matched cerebrospinal fluid (CSF) samples were also analyzed to detect mtDNA mutations, where some of them were harbored mtDNA mutations in the tumors. This study suggests that somatic mtDNA mutations in CSF shows some promise as potentially useful biomarkers for disease prognosis. On the other hand, Lueth's group (2010) also reported the existence of somatic mtDNA mutations in 6 of 15 medulloblastoma patients. These results are in support of their previous findings on frequency of somatic mitochondrial mutations in medulloblastoma [23]. Before investigation on medulloblastoma patients, Lueth and colleagues have sequenced entire mitochondrial genome of tumor tissue and matched blood samples from 19 pilocytic astrocytomas patients and identified somatic mutations in as many as 16 (84%) cases [22].

In the cases of neurofibromas, Kurtz and team (2004) analyzed the whole mitochondrial genome in 37 neurofibromatosis type 1 patients and found somatic mutations in 7 individuals with cutaneous neurofibromas (37%) and 9 patients with plexiform neurofibromas (50%) [119]. All of the mtDNA somatic mutations detected in this study occurred in the D-loop region. The reason of most genetic mutations to occur in non-coding regions of the mitochondrial genome is currently unknown. However, mutations in the D-loop are believed to influence the origin of replication and promoter region and thus may lead to impair mitochondrial biogenesis and defective transcription and protein expression [122,123].

9.2. Deletion

Amongst the large-scale deletions identified in the mitochondrial genome, the 4977-bp deletion is the most common mtDNA deletion detected in various types of cancers including thyroid tumors, esophageal carcinoma, hepatocellular carcinoma, gastric cancer, and breast cancer [124-128]. This deletion recognized as "common deletion" removes all 5 tRNA genes and 7 genes encoding 4 complex I subunits, 1 complex IV subunit, 2 complex V subunits, which are essential for maintaining normal mitochondrial OXPHOS function. The consequence of this deletion could cause a complete failure of ATP production and abnormal ROS generation [129]. Although the 4977-bp deletion has been implicated in the process of carcinogenesis, the involvement or role of this deletion in brain tumors has not yet been investigated. Besides no study to date on the brain tumors, Wallace's group examined the existence of 4977-bp deletion in the aging process using brain normal individuals [130]. They found a significant increase in the 4977-bp deletion from young to old individuals, in different regions of the brain between cortex, putamen and cerebellum. Therefore, it was suggested that this mtDNA deletion might contribute to the neurological impairment associated with ageing. The 4977-bp deletion was also detected in the autopsied brains of patients with bipolar disorder [131].

9.3. Mitochondrial microsatellite instability

In 1999, Kirches and colleagues revealed high mtDNA sequence variants in 12 astrocytic tumors [117]. Two years later, the same group extended the study by examining 55 gliomas specimens for mtDNA instability in the poly-C tract of mitochondrial D-loop using a combination of laser microdissection and PCR technique [19]. They found a lower frequency of 9% of specimens with the poly-C tract alterations. In addition, they also sequenced the entire D-loop in 17 frozen glioblastoma samples and corresponding blood samples for detecting somatic mutation. In 2003, a follow up study of mitochondrial genome instability was carried out and the author later determined that poly-C tract of the hypervariable region (HVR2) as a clonal marker in gliomatosis cerebri patients [118].

Most recently, Yeung's team investigated the contribution of mitochondrial genome variants in glioblastoma multiforme (GBM) [132]. In this study, mtDNA variants were analysed in a series of GBM cell lines using a combination of next generation sequencing and high resolution melt (HRM) analysis. They reported a greatest frequency of mtDNA variants in the D-loop and origin of light strand replication in non-coding regions. Moreover, in coding region, ND4 and ND6 were the most affected genes to mutation which both of them encode subunits of complex I of the electron transport chain. The author concluded that these novel variants at the mitochondrial genome offer an advantage to cells for promoting GBM tumorigenesis [132].

9.4. Copy number changes

In addition to mtDNA mutations and deletion, changes in the mtDNA copy number have been studied in gliomas [133,134]. As first previously reported by Liang (1996), 15 of low-grade were assessed with cDNA homologous to mtDNA at position 1,679-1,946 and 2,017-2,057 and the results revealed that these tumors had increased mtDNA copy number when compared to normal brain tissue controls [133]. In a separate study done by Liang and Hays (1999), 39 out of 45 (87%) examined gliomas, both low-grade and high-grade specimens, had increased up to 25-fold in mtDNA copy numbers [134]. They claimed that this frequency was much higher than erb-b gene amplification which was present in only 18% of these tumors.

9.5. Mitochondrial gene expression changes

In 2005, Dmitrenko's group screened cDNA libraries of human fetal glioblastoma and normal human brain samples and revealed 80 differentially expressed genes [135]. They identified 30 were corresponded to mitochondrial genes for ATP6, COXII, COXIII, ND1, ND4 and 12S rRNA. According to their data, all these mitochondrial transcripts were expressed at lower level in glioblastomas as compared to tumor-adjacent histologically normal brain [135].

10. Conclusion

The role of mtDNA mutations in cancer remains largely unclear and therefore more studies and attentions should been given before a clear conclusion could be achieved. There is a lot of evidence suggesting that some mtDNA mutations do play a role in certain stages of cancer development, but further research is needed to clarify this possible link. There are still multiple potential experimental pitfalls and weaknesses, thus relevant caution and basic guidelines in research should be followed in order to obtain the best results [136,137]. Based on our ongoing research and previous studies from other researchers, it could be suggested that mtDNA mutations could be a genetic aberration target in cancer development, instead of nuclear oncogenes and tumor suppressor genes. Cancer cells are very mutagenic in the early stage either due to exposure to high levels of carcinogenic substances or conditions or because of lack of repair mechanism. Thus, mtDNA simply seem to be more prone to mutation at this stage and has a limited ability to repair itself.

Mitochondria produce energy and their genome is responsible for regulating OXPHOS function. Aberrations in mtDNA may interrupt this process and ultimately lead to abnormal function of the cell. The unique properties of mtDNA, including its high copy number, high susceptibility to mutations, and quantitative and qualitative changes in cancer, stimulate researchers to closely be involved in the clinical relevance investigation of mtDNA alterations in cancers. In addition, the screening of mtDNA mutations is more easy and cost-effective than nDNA analysis, due to several advantages that mtDNA have such as a simple circular structure with a short sequence length. It has been shown that the existence of mtDNA mutations in cancer cells is particularly consistent with the intrinsic sensitivity of mtDNA to accumulate oxidative damage. Impairment of mitochondrial OXPHOS activity and mtDNA damage seem to be a common feature of malignant cells. Instability and abnormality in DNA and protein of mitochondria have been identified in various solid tumors and hematologic malignancies. However, up to now many studies have been directed toward identifying and characterizing the altered mtDNA. There have been only limited studies, mainly in relation to its functional consequences and clinical relevance. The functional aspects of mtDNA mutations in cancer development will provide a mechanistic link between mitochondria and carcinogenesis and also will translate into some useful prevention and therapeutic strategies of cancer in the future research.

Although to date mutations, polymorphisms, and variants of mtDNA have been described in brain tumors, there are more studies that need to be done to fully understand the role of mtDNA in these tumor cells. Further studies which include the assessment of the different types and stages of brain tumor need to be carried out. It is very crucial because perhaps that only certain stages and types will be sensitive to the effects of mtDNA mutations. Based on available evidence suggests that mtDNA may play a key role in the development and modulation of different steps of carcinogenesis. They could be used in the future as new potential target markers for rapid and effective early detection of brain tumorigenesis.

Acknowledgements

This work was supported in part by the Research University Grant for Individual (RUI) from Universiti Sains Malaysia 1001/PPSP/812110.

Author details

Abdul Aziz Mohamed Yusoff[1*], Farizan Ahmad[1], Zamzuri Idris[1], Hasnan Jaafar[2] and Jafri Malin Abdullah[1,3]

*Address all correspondence to: azizmdy@yahoo.com

1 Department of Neurosciences, School of Medical Sciences, Universiti Sains Malaysia, Health Campus, Kubang Kerian, Kelantan, Malaysia

2 Department of Pathology, School of Medical Sciences, Universiti Sains Malaysia, Health Campus, Kubang Kerian, Kelantan, Malaysia

3 Center for Neuroscience Services and Research, Universiti Sains Malaysia, Health Campus, Kubang Kerian, Kelantan, Malaysia

References

[1] Louis DN. The p53 gene and protein in human brain tumors. Journal of Neuropathology & Experimental Neurology 1994;53(1) 11-21.

[2] Nozaki M, Tada M, Kobayashi H, Zhang CL, Sawamura Y, Abe H, Ishii N, Van Meir EG. Roles of the functional loss of p53 and other genes in astrocytoma tumorigenesis and progression. Neuro-Oncology 1999;1(2) 124-137.

[3] Yusoff AA, Abdullah J, Abdullah MR, Mohd Ariff AR, Isa MN. Association of p53 tumor suppressor gene with paraclinical and clinical modalities of gliomas patients in Malaysia. Acta Neurochirurgica (Wien). 2004;146(6) 595-601.

[4] Louis DN. Molecular pathology of malignant gliomas. Annual Review of Pathology. 2006;1 97-117.

[5] Ohgaki H, Kleihues P. Genetic pathways to primary and secondary glioblastoma. American Journal of Pathology 2007;170(5) 1445-1453.

[6] Attardi G, Schatz G. Biogenesis of mitochondria. Annual Review of Cell Biology 1988;4 289-333.

[7] Galluzzi L, Kepp O, Kroemer G. Mitochondria: master regulators of danger signalling. Nature Reviews Molecular Cell Biology 2012;13(12) 780-788.

[8] Wallace DC. Mitochondria and cancer. Nature Reviews Cancer 2012;12(10) 685-698.

[9] Wallace DC. Mitochondrial DNA in aging and disease. Scientific American 1997;277(2) 40-47.

[10] DiMauro S, Schon EA. Mitochondrial DNA mutations in human disease. American Journal of Medical Genetics 2001;106(1) 18-26.

[11] Wallace DC. A mitochondrial paradigm for degenerative diseases and ageing. Novartis Foundation Symposia 2001;235 247-263; discussion 263-246

[12] Kaipparettu BA, Ma Y, Wong LJ. Functional effects of cancer mitochondria on energy metabolism and tumorigenesis: utility of transmitochondrial cybrids. Annals of the New York Academy of Sciences 2010;1201:137-146. doi: 10.1111/j. 1749-6632.2010.05621.x.

[13] Kim HS, Patel K, Muldoon-Jacobs K, Bisht KS, Aykin-Burns N, Pennington JD, van der Meer R, Nguyen P, Savage J, Owens KM, Vassilopoulos A, Ozden O, Park SH, Singh KK, Abdulkadir SA, Spitz DR, Deng CX, Gius D. SIRT3 is a mitochondria-localized tumor suppressor required for maintenance of mitochondrial integrity and metabolism during stress. Cancer Cell 2010;17(1) 41-52.

[14] Mullen AR, Wheaton WW, Jin ES, Chen PH, Sullivan LB, Cheng T, Yang Y, Linehan WM, Chandel NS, DeBerardinis RJ. Reductive carboxylation supports growth in tumour cells with defective mitochondria. Nature 2011;481(7381) 385-388.

[15] Owens KM, Kulawiec M, Desouki MM, Vanniarajan A, Singh KK. Impaired OXPHOS complex III in breast cancer. PLoS One 2011;6(8) e23846.

[16] Cook CC, Kim A, Terao S, Gotoh A, Higuchi M. Consumption of oxygen: a mito-chondrial-generated progression signal of advanced cancer. Cell Death and Disease 2012; 3:e258. doi: 10.1038/cddis.2011.141.

[17] Chen PL, Chen CF, Chen Y, Guo XE, Huang CK, Shew JY, Reddick RL, Wallace DC, Lee WH. Mitochondrial genome instability resulting from SUV3 haploinsufficiency leads to tumorigenesis and shortened lifespan. Oncogene 2013;32(9) 1193-1201.

[18] Baysal BE, Ferrell RE, Willett-Brozick JE, Lawrence EC, Myssiorek D, Bosch A, van der Mey A, Taschner PE, Rubinstein WS, Myers EN, Richard CW 3rd, Cornelisse CJ, Devilee P, Devlin B. Mutations in SDHD, a mitochondrial complex II gene, in heredi-tary paraganglioma. Science 2000;287(5454) 848-851.

[19] Kirches E, Krause G, Warich-Kirches M, Weis S, Schneider T, Meyer-Puttlitz B, Ma-wrin C, Dietzmann K. High frequency of mitochondrial DNA mutations in glioblas-toma multiforme identified by direct sequence comparison to blood samples. International Journal of Cancer 2001;93(4) 534-538.

[20] Wong LJ, Lueth M, Li XN, Lau CC, Vogel H. Detection of mitochondrial DNA muta-tions in the tumor and cerebrospinal fluid of medulloblastoma patients. Cancer Re-search 2003;63(14) 3866-3871.

[21] Dai JG, Xiao YB, Min JX, Zhang GQ, Yao K, Zhou RJ. Mitochondrial DNA 4977 BP deletion mutations in lung carcinoma. Indian Journal of Cancer 2006;43(1) 20-25.

[22] Lueth M, Wronski L, Giese A, Kirschner-Schwabe R, Pietsch T, von Deimling A, Henze G, Kurtz A, Driever PH. Somatic mitochondrial mutations in pilocytic astrocy-toma. Cancer Genetics and Cytogenetics 2009;192(1) 30-35.

[23] Lueth M, von Deimling A, Pietsch T, Wong LJ, Kurtz A, Henze G, Driever PH. Me-dulloblastoma harbor somatic mitochondrial DNA mutations in the D-loop region. Journal of Pediatric Hematology/Oncology 2010; 32(2) 156-159.

[24] Li LH, Kang T, Chen L, Zhang W, Liao Y, Chen J, Shi Y. Detection of mitochondrial DNA mutations by high-throughput sequencing in the blood of breast cancer pa-tients. International Journal of Molecular Medicine 2014;33(1) 77-82.

[25] Larman TC, DePalma SR, Hadjipanayis AG; Cancer Genome Atlas Research Net-work, Protopopov A, Zhang J, Gabriel SB, Chin L, Seidman CE, Kucherlapati R, Seid-man JG. Spectrum of somatic mitochondrial mutations in five cancers. Proceedings of the National Academy of Sciences USA 2012;109(35) 14087-14091.

[26] Yin PH, Wu CC, Lin JC, Chi CW, Wei YH, Lee HC. Somatic mutations of mitochon-drial genome in hepatocellular carcinoma. Mitochondrion 2010;10(2) 174-182.

[27] Frey TG, Mannella CA. The internal structure of mitochondria. Trends in Biochemi-cal Sciences 2000;25(7) 319-324.

[28] Palade G. The fine structure of mitochondria. Anatomical Record. 1952;114(3) 427-451.

[29] Sjöstrand FS. The ultrastructure of cells as revealed by the electron microscope. International Review of Cytology 1956; 5: 455-533.

[30] Perkins G, Renken C, Martone ME, Young SJ, Ellisman M, Frey T. Electron tomography of neuronal mitochondria: three dimensional structure and organization of cristae and membrane contacts. Journal of Structural Biology 1997;119(3) 260-272.

[31] Perkins GA, Frey TG. Recent structural insight into mitochondria gained by microscopy. Micron 2000;31(1) 97-111.

[32] Frey TG, Renken CW, Perkins GA. Insight into mitochondrial structure and function from electron tomography. Biochimica et Biophysica Acta 2002;1555(1-3) 196-203.

[33] Mitchell P. Coupling of phosphorylation to electron and hydrogen transfer by chemiosmotic type mechanism. Nature 1961;191: 144-148.

[34] Mitchell P, Moyle J. Chemiosmotic hypothesis of oxidative phosphorylation. Nature 1967;213(5072) 137-139.

[35] Voet D, Voet JG, Pratt CW. 2002. Fundamentals of Biochemistry. John Wiley & Sons,Inc., New York

[36] Nass S, Nass MMK. Intramitochondrial fibres with DNA characteristics. Journal of Cell Biology 1963;19: 593-629.

[37] Anderson S, Bankier AT, Barrell BG, de-Bruijn MH, Coulson AR, Drouin J, Eperon IC, Nierlich DP, Roe BA, Sanger F, Schreier PH, Smith AJ, Staden R, Young IG. Sequence and organization of the human mitochondrial genome. Nature 1981;290(5806) 427-465.

[38] Andrews RM, Kubacka I, Chinnery PF, Lightowlers RN, Turnbull DM, Howell N. Reanalysis and revision of the Cambridge reference sequence for human mitochondrial DNA. Nature Genetics 1999;23(2) 147.

[39] Kasamatsu H, Vinograd J. Replication of circular DNA in eukaryotic cells. Annual Review of Biochemistry 1974;43(0) 695-719.

[40] Lutz S, Weisser HJ, Heizmann J, Pollak S. A third hypervariable region in the human mitochondrial D-loop. Human Genetics 1997;101(3) 384.

[41] Taanman JW. The mitochondrial genome: transcription, translation and replication. Biochimica et Biophysica Acta 1999;1410(2) 103-123.

[42] Monnat RJ, Reay DT. Nucleotide sequence identity of mitochondrial DNA from different human tissues. Gene 1986;43(3) 205-211.

[43] Tzagoloff A, Myers AM. Biogenesis of mitochondrial genetics. Annual Review of Biochemistry 1986; 55: 249-285.

[44] Gadaleta G, Pepe G, DeCandia G, Quagliariello C, Sbissá E, Saccone C. The complete
      nucleotide sequence of the Rattus norvegicus mitochondrial genome: cryptic signals
      revealed by comparative analysis between vertebrates. Journal of Molecular Evolu-
      tion 1989;28(6) 497-516.

[45] Lightowlers RN, Chinnery PF, Turnbull DM, Howell N. Mammalian mitochondrial
      genetics: heredity, heteroplasmy and disease. Trends in Genetics 1997;13(11) 450-455.

[46] Warburg O. On the origin of cancer cells. Science 1956;123(3191) 309-314.

[47] Pedersen PL. Tumor mitochondria and the bioenergetics of cancer cells. Progress in
      Experimental Tumor Research 1978; 22 190-274.

[48] Cuezva JM, Krajewska M, de Heredia ML, Krajewski S, Santamaría G, Kim H, Zapa-
      ta JM, Marusawa H, Chamorro M, Reed JC. The bioenergetic signature of cancer: a
      marker of tumor progression. Cancer Research 2002;62(22) 6674-6681.

[49] Arnould T, Vankoningsloo S, Renard P, Houbion A, Ninane N, Demazy C, Remacle
      J, Raes M. CREB activation induced by mitochondrial dysfunction is a new signaling
      pathway that impairs cell proliferation. The EMBO Journal 2002;21(1-2) 53-63.

[50] Rustin P. Mitochondria from cell death to proliferation. Nature Genetics 2002;30(4)
      352-353.

[51] Pelicano H, Xu RH, Du M, Feng L, Sasaki R, Carew JS, Hu Y, Ramdas L, Hu L, Keat-
      ing MJ, Zhang W, Plunkett W, Huang P. Mitochondrial respiration defects in cancer
      cells cause activation of Akt survival pathway through a redox-mediated mecha-
      nism. Journal of Cell Biology 2006;175(6) 913-923.

[52] Elstrom RL, Bauer DE, Buzzai M, Karnauskas R, Harris MH, Plas DR, Zhuang H, Ci-
      nalli RM, Alavi A, Rudin CM, Thompson CB. Akt stimulates aerobic glycolysis in
      cancer cells. Cancer Research 2004;64(11) 3892-3899.

[53] Plas DR, Thompson CB. Akt-dependent transformation: there is more to growth than
      just surviving. Oncogene 2005; 24(50) 7435-7442.

[54] López-Ríos F, Sánchez-Aragó M, García-García E, Ortega AD, Berrendero JR, Pozo-
      Rodríguez F, López-Encuentra A, Ballestín C, Cuezva JM. Loss of the mitochondrial
      bioenergetic capacity underlies the glucose avidity of carcinomas. Cancer Research
      2007;67(19) 9013-9017.

[55] Wu M, Neilson A, Swift AL, Moran R, Tamagnine J, Parslow D, Armistead S, Lemire
      K, Orrell J, Teich J, Chomicz S, Ferrick DA. Multiparameter metabolic analysis re-
      veals a close link between attenuated mitochondrial bioenergetic function and en-
      hanced glycolysis dependency in human tumor cells. American Journal of
      Physiology-Cell Physiology 2007;292(1) C125-136.

[56] Chance B, Sies H, Boveris A. Hydroperoxide metabolism in mammalian organs.
      Physiological Reviews 1979;59(3) 527-605.

[57] Burdon RH. Superoxide and hydrogen peroxide in relation to mammalian cell prolif-eration. Free Radical Biology and Medicine 1995;18(4) 775-794.

[58] Nose K, Shibanuma M, Kikuchi K, Kageyama H, Sakiyama S, Kuroki T. Transcrip-tional activation of early-response genes by hydrogen peroxide in a mouse osteoblas-tic cell line. European Journal of Biochemistry 1991;201(1) 99-106.

[59] Amstad PA, Krupitza G, Cerutti PA. Mechanism of c-fos induction by active oxygen. Cancer Research 1992;52(14) 3952-3960.

[60] Nose K, Ohba M. Functional activation of the Egr-1 (early growth response-1) gene by hydrogen peroxide. Biochemical Journal 1996;316 (Pt 2) 381-383.

[61] Sundaresan M, Yu ZX, Ferrans VJ, Sulciner DJ, Gutkind JS, Irani K, Goldschmidt-Clermont PJ, Finkel T. Regulation of reactive-oxygen-species generation in fibro-blasts by Rac1. Biochemical Journal 1996;318 (Pt 2) 379-382.

[62] Ha HC, Thiagalingam A, Nelkin BD, Casero RA Jr. Reactive oxygen species are criti-cal for the growth and differentiation of medullary thyroid carcinoma cells. Clinical Cancer Research 2000;6(9) 3783-3787.

[63] Harman D. Free radicals in aging. Molecular and Cellular Biochemistry 1988;84(2) 155-161.

[64] Ames BN, Shigenaga MK. Oxidants are a major contributor to aging. Annals of the New York Academy of Sciences 1992;663 85-96.

[65] Poulsen HE, Prieme H, Loft S. Role of oxidative DNA damage in cancer initiation and promotion. European Journal of Cancer Prevention 1998;7(1) 9-16.

[66] Zanssen S, Schon EA. Mitochondrial DNA mutations in cancer. PLoS Medicine 2005;2(11) e401.

[67] Grzybowska-Szatkowska L, Slaska B. Mitochondrial DNA and carcinogenesis (re-view). Molecular Medicine Reports 2012;6(5) 923-930.

[68] Kang D, Hamasaki N. Mitochondrial transcription factor A in the maintenance of mi-tochondrial DNA: overview of its multiple roles. Annals of the New York Academy of Sciences 2005;1042: 101-108.

[69] Chandra D, Singh KK. Genetic insights into OXPHOS defect and its role in cancer. Biochimica et Biophysica Acta 2011;1807(6) 620-625.

[70] Richter C. Pro-oxidants and mitochondrial Ca^{2+}: their relationship to apoptosis and oncogenesis. FEBS Letters 1993;325(1-2) 104-107.

[71] Orrenius S. Mitochondrial regulation of apoptotic cell death. Toxicology Letters 2004;149(1-3) 19-23.

[72] Nelson DA, Tan TT, Rabson AB, Anderson D, Degenhardt K, White E. Hypoxia and defective apoptosis drive genomic instability and tumorigenesis. Genes & Development 2004;18(17) 2095-2107.

[73] Kwong JQ, Henning MS, Starkov AA, Manfredi G. The mitochondrial respiratory chain is a modulator of apoptosis. Journal of Cell Biology 2007;179(6) 1163-1177.

[74] Raha S, Robinson BH. Mitochondria, oxygen free radicals, and apoptosis. American Journal of Medical Genetics 2001;106(1) 62-70.

[75] Kang BH, Plescia J, Dohi T, Rosa J, Doxsey SJ, Altieri DC. Regulation of tumor cell mitochondrial homeostasis by an organelle-specific Hsp90 chaperone network. Cell 2007;131(2) 257-270.

[76] Ghosh JC, Dohi T, Kang BH, Altieri DC. Hsp60 regulation of tumor cell apoptosis. Journal of Biological Chemistry 2008;283(8) 5188-5194.

[77] Holt IJ, Harding AE, Morgan-Hughes JA. Deletions of muscle mitochondrial DNA in patients with mitochondrial myopathies. Nature 1988;331(6158) 717-719.

[78] Wallace DC, Singh G, Lott MT, Hodge JA, Schurr TG, Lezza AM, Elsas LJ 2nd, Ni-koskelainen EK. Mitochondrial DNA mutation associated with Leber's hereditary optic neuropathy. Science 1988;242(4884) 1427-1430.

[79] Zeviani M, Moraes CT, DiMauro S, Nakase H, Bonilla E, Schon EA, Rowland LP. Deletions of mitochondrial DNA in Kearns-Sayre syndrome. Neurology 1988;38(9) 1339-1346.

[80] Penta JS, Johnson FM, Wachsman JT, Copeland WC. Mitochondrial DNA in human malignancy. Mutation Research 2001;488(2) 119-133.

[81] Chinnery PF, Schon EA. Mitochondria. Journal of Neurology, Neurosurgery, and Psychiatry 2003;74(9) 1188-1199.

[82] DiMauro S, Davidzon G. Mitochondrial DNA and disease. Annals of Medicine 2005;37(3) 222-232.

[83] Schapira AH. Mitochondrial diseases. Lancet. 2012;379(9828) 1825-1834. doi: 10.1016/S0140-6736(11)61305-6.

[84] DiMauro S, Schon EA. Mitochondrial respiratory-chain diseases. New England Journal of Medicine 2003;348(26) 2656-2668.

[85] Chatterjee A, Dasgupta S, Sidransky D. Mitochondrial subversion in cancer. Cancer Prevention Research 2011;4(5) 638-654.

[86] Salas A, Yao YG, Macaulay V, Vega A, Carracedo A, Bandelt HJ. A critical reassessment of the role of mitochondria in tumorigenesis. PLOS Medicine 2005;2(11) e296.

[87] Nie H, Shu H, Vartak R, Milstein AC, Mo Y, Hu X, Fang H, Shen L, Ding Z, Lu J, Bai Y. Mitochondrial common deletion, a potential biomarker for cancer occurrence, is

selected against in cancer background: a meta-analysis of 38 studies. PLoS One 2013;8(7) e67953.

[88] Brandon M, Baldi P, Wallace DC. Mitochondrial mutations in cancer. Oncogene 2006;25(34) 4647-4662.

[89] Chatterjee A, Mambo E, Sidransky D. Mitochondrial DNA mutations in human cancer. Oncogene 2006;25(34) 4663-4674.

[90] Yu M. Somatic mitochondrial DNA mutations in human cancers. Advances in Clinical Chemistry 2012;57 99-138.

[91] Polyak K, Li Y, Zhu H, Lengauer C, Willson JK, Markowitz SD, Trush MA, Kinzler KW, Vogelstein B. Somatic mutations of the mitochondrial genome in human colorectal tumours. Nature Genetics 1998;20(3) 291-293.

[92] Fliss MS, Usadel H, Caballero OL, Wu L, Buta MR, Eleff SM, Jen J, Sidransky D. Facile detection of mitochondrial DNA mutations in tumors and bodily fluids. Science 2000;287(5460) 2017-2019.

[93] Tan DJ, Bai RK, Wong LJC. Comprehensive scanning of somatic mitochondrial DNA mutations in breast cancer. Cancer Research 2002;62(4) 972-976.

[94] Zhu W, Qin W, Bradley P, Wessel A, Puckett CL, Sauter ER. Mitochondrial DNA mutations in breast cancer tissue and in matched nipple aspirate fluid. Carcinogenesis 2005;26(1) 145-152.

[95] Tseng LM, Yin PH, Yang CW, Tsai YF, Hsu CY, Chi CW, Lee HC. Somatic mutations of the mitochondrial genome in human breast cancers. Genes Chromosomes Cancer 2011;50(10) 800-811.

[96] Xu C, Tran-Thanh D, Ma C, May K, Jung J, Vecchiarelli J, Done SJ. Mitochondrial D310 mutations in the early development of breast cancer. British Journal of Cancer 2012;106(9) 1506-1511.

[97] Kumimoto H, Yamane Y, Nishimoto Y, Fukami H, Shinoda M, Hatooka S, Ishizaki K. Frequent somatic mutations of mitochondrial DNA in esophageal squamous cell carcinoma. International Journal of Cancer 2004;108(2) 228-231.

[98] Tan DJ, Chang J, Liu LL, Bai RK, Wang YF, Yeh KT, Wong LJ. Significance of somatic mutations and content alteration of mitochondrial DNA in esophageal cancer. BMC Cancer 2006;6:93.

[99] Lin CS, Chang SC, Wang LS, Chou TY, Hsu WH, Wu YC, Wei YH. The role of mitochondrial DNA alterations in esophageal squamous cell carcinomas. Journal of Thoracic and Cardiovascular Surgery 2010;139(1) 189-197.

[100] Lievre A, Blons H, Houllier AM, Laccourreye O, Brasnu D, Beaune P, Laurent-Puig P. Clinicopathological significance of mitochondrial D-Loop mutations in head and neck carcinoma. British Journal of Cancer 2006;94(5) 692-697.

[101] Lee HC, Li SH, Lin JC, Wu CC, Yeh DC, Wei YH. Somatic mutations in the D-loop and decrease in the copy number of mitochondrial DNA in human hepatocellular carcinoma. Mutation Research 2004;547(1-2) 71-78.

[102] Tamori A, Nishiguchi S, Nishikawa M, Kubo S, Koh N, Hirohashi K, Shiomi S, Inoue M. Correlation between clinical characteristics and mitochondrial D-loop DNA mutations in hepatocellular carcinoma. Journal of Gastroenterology 2004;39(11) 1063-1068.

[103] Yin PH, Wu CC, Lin JC, Chi CW, Wei YH, Lee HC. Somatic mutations of mitochondrial genome in hepatocellular carcinoma. Mitochondrion 2010;10(2) 174-182.

[104] Suzuki M, Toyooka S, Miyajima K, Iizasa T, Fujisawa T, Bekele NB, Gazdar AF. Alterations in the mitochondrial displacement loop in lung cancers. Clinical Cancer Research 2003;9(15) 5636-5641.

[105] Jin X, Zhang J, Gao Y, Ding K, Wang N, Zhou D, Jen J, Cheng S. Relationship between mitochondrial DNA mutations and clinical characteristics in human lung cancer. Mitochondrion 2007;7(5) 347-353.

[106] Choi SJ, Kim SH, Kang HY, Lee J, Bhak JH, Sohn I, Jung SH, Choi YS, Kim HK, Han J, Huh N, Lee G, Kim BC, Kim J. Mutational hotspots in the mitochondrial genome of lung cancer. Biochemical and Biophysical Research Communications 2011;407(1) 23-27.

[107] Liu VW, Shi HH, Cheung AN, Chiu PM, Leung TW, Nagley P, Wong LC, Ngan HY (2001) High incidence of somatic mitochondrial DNA mutations in human ovarian carcinomas. Cancer Research 2001; 61(16) 5998-6001.

[108] Van Trappen PO, Cullup T, Troke R, Swann D, Shepherd JH, Jacobs IJ, Gayther SA, Mein CA. Somatic mitochondrial DNA mutations in primary and metastatic ovarian cancer. Gynecologic Oncology 2007;104(1) 129-133.

[109] Jerónimo C, Nomoto S, Caballero OL, Usadel H, Henrique R, Varzim G, Oliveira J, Lopes C, Fliss MS, Sidransky D. Mitochondrial mutations in early stage prostate cancer and bodily fluids. Oncogene 2001;20(37) 5195-5198.

[110] Gomez-Zaera M, Abril J, Gonzalez L, Aguilo F, Condom E, Nadal M, Nunes V (2006) Identification of somatic and germline mitochondrial DNA sequence variants in prostate cancer patients. Mutation Research 2006;595(1-2) 42-51.

[111] Kloss-Brandstätter A, Schäfer G, Erhart G, Hüttenhofer A, Coassin S, Seifarth C, Summerer M, Bektic J, Klocker H, Kronenberg F. Somatic mutations throughout the entire mitochondrial genome are associated with elevated PSA levels in prostate cancer patients. American Journal of Human Genetics 2010;87(6) 802-812.

[112] Nagy A, Wilhelm M, Sukosd F, Ljungberg B, Kovacs G. Somatic mitochondrial DNA mutations in human chromophobe renal cell carcinomas. Genes Chromosomes Cancer 2002;35(3) 256-260.

[113] Tong BC, Ha PK, Dhir K, Xing M, Westra WH, Sidransky D, Califano JA. Mitochondrial DNA alterations in thyroid cancer. Journal Surgical Oncology 2003;82(3) 170-173.

[114] Carew JS, Zhou Y, Albitar M, Carew JD, Keating MJ, Huang P. Mitochondrial DNA mutations in primary leukemia cells after chemotherapy: clinical significance and therapeutic implications. Leukemia 2003;17(8) 1437-1447.

[115] Grist SA, Lu XJ, Morley AA. Mitochondrial mutations in acute leukemia. Leukemia 2004;18(7) 1313-1316.

[116] Schon EA, DiMauro S, Hirano M. Human mitochondrial DNA: roles of inherited and somatic mutations. Nature Review Genetics 2012;13(12) 878-890.

[117] Kirches E, Michael M, Woy C, Schneider T, Warich M-Kirches, Schneider-Stock R, Winkler K, Wittig H, Dietzmann K. Loss of heteroplasmy in the displacement loop of brain mitochondrial DNA in astrocytic tumors. Genes Chromosomes Cancer 1999;26(1) 80-83.

[118] Kirches E, Mawrin C, Schneider-Stock R, Krause G, Scherlach C, Dietzmann K. Mitochondrial DNA as a clonal tumor cell marker: gliomatosis cerebri. Journal of Neuro-Oncology 2003;61(1) 1-5.

[119] Kurtz A, Lueth M, Kluwe L, Zhang T, Foster R, Mautner VF, Hartmann M, Tan DJ, Martuza RL, Friedrich RE, Driever PH, Wong LJ. Somatic mitochondrial DNA mutations in neurofibromatosis type 1-associated tumors. Molecular Cancer Research 2004;2(8) 433-441.

[120] Vega A, Salas A, Gamborino E, Sobrido MJ, Macaulay V, Carracedo A. mtDNA mutations in tumors of the central nervous system reflect the neutral evolution of mtDNA in populations. Oncogene 2004;23(6) 1314-1320.

[121] Montanini L, Regna-Gladin C, Eoli M, Albarosa R, Carrara F, Zeviani M, Bruzzone MG, Broggi G, Boiardi A, Finocchiaro G. Instability of mitochondrial DNA and MRI and clinical correlations in malignant gliomas. Journal of Neuro-Oncology 2005;74(1) 87-89.

[122] Barthelemy C, de Baulny HO, Lombes A. D-loop mutations in mitochondrial DNA: link with mitochondrial DNA depletion? Human Genetics 2002;110(5) 479-487.

[123] Wong L, Tan D, Bai R, Yeh K, and Chang J. Molecular alterations in mitochondrial DNA of hepatocellular carcinomas: is there a correlation with clinicopathological profile? Journal of Medical Genetics 2004;41(5) e65.

[124] Maximo V, Soares P, Lima J, Cameselle-Teijeiro J, Sobrinho-Simoes M. Mitochondrial DNA somatic mutations (point mutations and large deletions) and mitochondrial DNA variants in human thyroid pathology: A study with emphasis on Hurthle cell tumors. American Journal of Pathology 2002;160(5) 1857-1865.

[125] Abnet CC, Huppi K, Carrera A, Armistead D, McKenney K, Hu N, Tang ZZ, Taylor
       PR, Dawsey SM. Control region mutations and the 'common deletion' are frequent in
       the mitochondrial DNA of patients with esophageal squamous cell carcinoma. BMC
       Cancer 2004;4: 30.

[126] Yin PH, Lee HC, Chau GY, Wu YT, Li SH, Lui WY, Wei YH, Liu TY, Chi CW. Altera-
       tion of the copy number and deletion of mitochondrial DNA in human hepatocellu-
       lar carcinoma. British Journal of Cancer 2004;90(12) 2390-2396.

[127] Wu CW, Yin PH, Hung WY, Li AF, Li SH, Chi CW, Wei YH, Lee HC. Mitochondrial
       DNA mutations and mitochondrial DNA depletion in gastric cancer. Genes Chromo-
       somes Cancer 2005;44(1) 19-28.

[128] Ye C, Shu XO, Wen W, Pierce L, Courtney R, Gao YT, Zheng W, Cai Q. Quantitative
       analysis of mitochondrial DNA 4977-bp deletion in sporadic breast cancer and be-
       nign breast diseases. Breast Cancer Research and Treatment 2008;108(3) 427-434.

[129] Peng TI, Yu PR, Chen JY, Wang HL, Wu HY, Wei YH, Jou MJ. Visualizing common
       deletion of mitochondrial DNA-augmented mitochondrial reactive oxygen species
       generation and apoptosis upon oxidative stress. Biochimica et Biophysica Acta
       2006;1762(2) 241-255.

[130] Corral-Debrinski M, Horton T, Lott MT, Shoffner JM, Beal MF, Wallace DC. Mito-
       chondrial DNA deletions in human brain: regional variability and increase with ad-
       vanced age. Nature Genetics 1992;2(4) 324-329.

[131] Kato T, Stine OC, McMahon FJ, Crowe RR. Increased levels of a mitochondrial DNA
       deletion in the brain of patients with bipolar disorder. Biological Psychiatry
       1997;42(10) 871-875.

[132] Yeung KY, Dickinson A, Donoghue JF, Polekhina G, White SJ, Grammatopoulos DK,
       McKenzie M, Johns TG, John JC. The identification of mitochondrial DNA variants in
       glioblastoma multiforme. Acta Neuropathologica Communications 2014;2(1): 1. doi:
       10.1186/2051-5960-2-1.

[133] Liang BC. Evidence for association of mitochondrial DNA sequence amplification
       and nuclear localization in human low-grade gliomas. Mutation Research 1996;354(1)
       27-33.

[134] Liang BC, Hays L. Mitochondrial DNA copy number changes in human gliomas.
       Cancer Letters 1996;105(2)167-173.

[135] Dmitrenko V, Shostak K, Boyko O, Khomenko O, Rozumenko V, Malisheva T, Sha-
       mayev M, Zozulya Y, Kavsan V. Reduction of the transcription level of the mitochon-
       drial genome in human glioblastoma. Cancer Letters 2005;218(1) 99-107.

[136] Salas A, Yao YG, Macaulay V, Vega A, Carracedo A, Bandelt HJ. A critical reassess-
       ment of the role of mitochondria in tumorigenesis. PLoS Medicine 2005;2:e296.

[137] Fang H, Lu J, Wei J, Shen LJ, Ding Z, Li H, Bai Y. Mitochondrial DNA mutations in the D-loop region may not be frequent in cervical cancer: a discussion on pitfalls in mitochondrial DNA studies. Journal of Cancer Research and Clinical Oncology 2009;135(4) 649-651.

7

Seizures in Children with Brain Tumours — Epidemiology, Significance, Management and Outcomes

Adrianna Ranger and David Diosy

1. Introduction

Cancer is the most frequently diagnosed disease-related cause of death among children and adolescents [1], and malignancies involving the brain are collectively the most common solid tumour [2, 3]. They are also either first or second in incidence overall (second only to leukaemia) in the United States (USA) [1, 4,7], Canada [8], and Mexico [9]. The *American Brain Tumour Association* has estimated that approximately 4,200 American children younger than age 20 would be diagnosed with a primary brain tumour in the year 2012, of whom three in four would be under the age of 15 years [10]. However, the overall prognosis for brain malignancies is much better in children than in adults, with up to half of paediatric brain cancer patients surviving long-term [11]. The reason for this enhanced survival in youths is that children and adolescents are much more likely than adults to have low-grade astrocytomas, in particular pilocytic astrocytomas and other low-grade gliomas that are almost never fatal and often cured, depending upon their location and surgical accessibility, rather than the grade III and IV astrocytomas that account for the majority of tumours among adults [12-14].

Long-term survival, even in the setting of cure, is not without problems, however, with empirical evidence accumulating that paediatric brain cancer survivors continue to suffer from significant morbidity [15-20] and, sometimes, early death [15]. Among the more common long-term sequelae of brain cancer and brain cancer treatment in children are seizures, which can be quite disabling and, at times, life-threatening in themselves [15, 21-30]. In one study, seizures were the number one predictor of disability in long-term brain cancer survivors [24, 25]. Seizures even increase a paediatric survivor's risk of suicide into adulthood [31]. In addition, there is a subset of children, up to 50% [32], whose low-grade brain cancer presents as seizures [26, 32-42]. Though the vast majority of epileptogenic tumours are supratentorial, some are not, especially among children in whom infratentorial tumours generally comprise the majority [43, 44], and in less typical locations like the thalamus and hypothalamus [38, 45-47]. Among thalamic tumours, for example, up to one third of paediatric patients present with seizures [38]. As such, and because even low-grade gliomas can nonetheless be infiltrative into high-function brain tissue [19, 48-50], while some of these lesions are totally resectable, others are not [51-54]. This creates dilemmas as to how aggressive to be, and therefore how much risk to take in their resection [55]. As well, the return of seizures at some distant time post-operatively may indicate tumour growth or relapse [28, 30, 56-66], transformation into a more aggressive lesion [28, 60, 65, 67, 68], or even the emergence of a secondary (e.g., radiation-induced) tumour [64].

Why seizures occur in patients with brain tumours is not entirely clear [27, 69-71], and several conjectures have been made, including alterations in regional metabolism and pH, immuno-logic activity, disordered neuronal function, altered vascular supply and permeability, the release of altered tumoral amino acids, proteins and enzymes, and abnormal protein transport and binding to receptors [27, 44, 69, 71-74]. Even genetic predispositions for tumour-related seizures have been postulated [71, 75]. A recent excellent review of current theories and empirical evidence on the pathogenesis of tumour-related epilepsy has been published by You et al. [74] Discussing the relative merits of each theory is a paper in itself, and beyond the scope of the current review.

Interestingly, tumour size has a somewhat paradoxical relationship with seizure occurrence, in that, though the opposite is true of low-grade lesions, high-grade gliomas that present with seizures tend to be smaller than those that present with other symptoms [76]. Moreover, high-grade lesions that present with seizures tend to have a better prognosis than lesions of the same size that present otherwise [77]. What this suggests is that the aggressiveness of the tumour might have an effect upon seizure development. This being said, low-grade lesions comprise the majority of epileptogenic tumours, both in children and adults [78]; and some tumour types — like gangliogliomas and dysembryoplastic neuroepithelial tumours (DNET) — are more likely to induce seizures than others [28].

In this chapter, we will thoroughly review the literature on seizures in paediatric brain cancer patients, looking at them (1) as a presenting symptom; (2) in the early tumour management/peri-operative period; and (3) long-term. Specific questions to be addressed in each of these sections are: How common are they? What is their history? How do they impact patients' lives, both short-and long-term, and in terms of management and prognosis? How do they effect management of the underlying tumour? How are seizures managed themselves? As much as possible, these questions will be answered by examining empirical evidence across a number of studies to provide, if not definitive answers, at least conclusions that are supported by published research.

2. Seizures as a presenting symptom of a brain tumour

2.1. How seizures present

A brain tumour is ultimately discovered in between one and three percent of children who present with new-onset seizures [40, 42], though a slightly higher percentage has been reported in children presenting with partial versus generalized seizures [79], and percentages as high as 20% have been reported in children undergoing epilepsy surgery [80]. From the reverse perspective, somewhere between 10 and 50% of brain tumours present with seizures as a symptom [69, 74, 81-83], and sometimes as the only symptom [32, 41, 84-86], with supratentorial and especially temporal lesions the most likely to be epileptogenic [44, 66, 78, 86-88]. In one study that compared children with supra-and infratentorial tumours, for example, among those with supratentorial lesions, 42% experienced vomiting as their first symptom, followed by seizures in 37%, and headache in 31% [43]. Meanwhile, 62% of children with an infratentorial lesion experienced headaches as their first symptom, with vomiting and ataxia accounting for most of the remainder, and seizures not observed in a single case.

Because children are more likely than adults to have infra-versus supratentorial lesions, the percentage of children presenting with seizures may be somewhat less than among adults, closer to the 10-20% than the 30-50% range [51, 89, 90], though 50% or more has been reported in some series [32, 35]. As in adults, of these epileptic tumours, the vast majority are supratentorial. For example, in their series of 157 children presenting to the hospital with brain tumour-related seizures, of mean age 3.3 years, Khan et al. found that 81% of the tumours were supratentorial and just 19% within the posterior fossa [82]. Meanwhile, Ianelli et al. reported that 80% of their 37 paediatric patients presenting with a temporal lobe malignancy had seizures as a presenting symptom [86]. Another excellent study on new-onset seizures presenting in children with brain cancers was published by Shady et al. [32] who analyzed 98 paediatric brain tumour patients and found that 50% percent of the children had seizures as part of their presentation, and 30% as their only presenting phenomenon; complex (55%) and simple (28%) partial seizures were the most common types, accounting for more than three quarters of all cases. Pre-operative electroencephalography (EEG) accurately lateralized to the tumour side in 88% of the cases and to the correct lobe in 56%. In addition, tumours involving cerebral cortex were much more likely than non-cortical lesions to present with seizures (59% vs. 15% of patients, respectively), with temporal and frontal lobe lesions exhibiting the highest incidence of seizures. Moreover, whereas 88% of gangliogliomas and 86% of oligoastrocytomas were associated with seizures, seizures were noted in just 21% of the patients with an anaplastic astrocytoma. Finally, as described elsewhere [32, 77], patients with seizures at presentation had a better prognosis than those without (p=0.02) [32].

Virtually every possible tumour type has been reported presenting as seizures, especially low-grade gliomas [27, 30, 32, 34, 37, 39, 70-72, 75, 76, 78, 91-93] and glioneuronal tumours like ganglioglioma and dysembryoplastic neuroepithelial tumour [28, 44, 62, 73, 88, 89, 91, 94, 95]; but including oligodendroglioma [77, 96, 97], cortical ependymoma [98], medulloblastoma

[47], subependymal giant cell astrocytoma (SEGA) [99], meningioma [10]⁰, thalamic and cerebellar glioma [38, 46], and a variety of atypical, systemic and metastatic tumours, like primary meningeal osteosarcoma [84], acute lymphoblastic leukemia [101], anaplastic large cell lymphoma [102], neuroblastoma [103], melanoma [104], various sarcomas [105, 106], Ewing's sarcoma [107], malignant germ cell tumours [108], and others [16, 109].

There is no stereotypical seizure presenting as an early symptom of a brain tumour. Early seizures may be generalized, simple partial, complex partial, or mixed, depending upon the tumour's size, location, level of aggressiveness, and other factors [24, 26, 27, 33, 34, 37, 70, 74, 77, 82, 87, 110-115]. This being said, among children, seizures as a presenting symptom of brain tumour are most commonly complex or simple partial, versus generalized, with complex partial seizures generally accounting for from 50% to as high as 85% of all new-onset seizures [32, 63, 69, 86, 115-117]. The lone series in which this was not true was that reported by Hirsch et al., in which complex and simple partial seizures together only accounted for half of all cases [118]. The percentages generally reported for children and adolescents are somewhat different than for adults, in whom tumour-associated seizures tend to be more evenly distributed across the four most typical seizure types [58]. Other atypical and, therefore, less well recognized forms of seizure have been described in children as well, including gelastic seizures, characterized by uncontrolled fits of inappropriate laughter [45], tics and Tourrette-like symptoms [119], and sympathetic storms in a 7-year old with a midbrain glioma [120]. In addition, especially in the paediatric population, tumors may arise in the setting of a variety of familial syndromes such as neurofibromatosis types 1 [121] and 2 [122], and tuberous sclerosis [123]. Seizures in these conditions are often blong-standing, frequent, and intractable because of the numerous non-neoplastic lesions that can involve the CNS [55, 124, 125]. In such patients, the diagnosis of a new neoplastic lesion can be especially challenging [124, 126].

The diagnosis of brain tumour does not always quickly follow the onset of seizures. In one study reported by Ibrahim et al., for example, the time from seizure onset to tumour diagnosis among ten children presenting with seizures ranged from two weeks to two years, averaging six months [37]. A wide range of opinions and practices exist regarding how aggressive to pursue diagnostic imaging in children presenting with seizures [36, 41, 51, 79, 80, 100, 127-133]. For example, in one series of eighteen patients between the ages of 1 month and 13 years who presented with seizures and were discovered to have DNETs between January 1992 and December 2004, the preoperative evaluation included magnetic resonance (MR) imaging and interictal scalp electro-encephalography (EEG) in all patients, but functional MR imaging also was performed in eight patients, video monitoring with scalp EEG during seizures in 12 patients, interictal single-photon emission computerized tomography (SPECT) scanning in one patient, and ictal SPECT scanning in two patients [132]. Meanwhile, in their 2010 review of eleven clinical trials for anti-epileptic drugs (AEDs) conducted over the preceding two years, Jansky et al. noted that none of the trials required MRI as part of the patient enrollment protocol [128]. Increasingly, with advances in imaging and the recognition that the resection of epileptogenic lesions is both safe and effective for many patients, there seems to be growing opinion that the initial work-up of new-onset non-febrile seizures in children should include both an EEG and MRI, despite the likelihood that the majority of imaging studies will be either normal or inconclusive [134, 135]. As discussed in the next section, mounting evidence suggests that new-onset seizures in the setting of a tumour, and conversely, tumours in the setting of new-onset seizures both have therapeutic and prognostic implications.

2.2. Implications of brain-tumour induced seizures

Having a child's brain tumour present as seizures adds therapeutic complexity with respect to how the patient is initially managed, since peri-operative control of seizures is obviously considered of extreme clinical importance. The type of seizure a patient has also may have prognostic significance, both in terms of patient survival [65, 136] and how easily the seizures are controlled with anti-epilepsy drugs (AED), both peri-operatively and long-term. How well AEDs work, in turn, may have implications relating to how aggressive surgical resection should be.

Although no reliable data have been published for children, adults who present with seizures as their sole symptom tend to have less aggressive or advanced lesions than those who present with symptoms or signs of increased intracranial pressure like papilloedema, headaches [65], neurological or cognitive deficits [65, 136]. Although this intrinsically makes sense — the fewer the symptoms, the less aggressive or advanced the disease — extrapolating these findings to children must be done with caution, because a disproportionate number of paediatric lesions tend to be brainstem tumours that, though usually low-grade and non-epileptogenic, often are non-resectable because of their location and proximity to function-rich neural tissue [2, 3, 137-139]. Nonetheless, especially among supratentorial lesions, it makes sense that having seizures present before all other symptoms develop is a hopeful prognostic sign, given that low-grade gliomas and other so-called benign lesions tend to be associated with much higher seizure rates than high-grade lesions [32, 87, 91, 113, 140, 141].

Having seizures in the presence of a tumour has implications with respect to management of the seizures as well, in that studies have shown that such seizures tend to be more resistant to AEDs than idiopathic seizures [133, 142]. This appears to be especially true for patients who present with a history of numerous seizures [142]. This likelihood of *drug resistance*, which has been formally defined as *"the failure of adequate trials of two tolerated, appropriately-chosen and used antiepileptic drug schedules (whether as monotherapies or in combination) to achieve sustained seizure freedom"* [143], may play a role in determining the aggressiveness of surgery for tumour resection. For example, given the clear superiority of epilepsy surgery over medical management alone, in terms of achieving freedom from seizures in patients with intractable seizures (65% vs. 8% in one relatively recent meta-analysis [144]), a decision might be made to pursue more aggressive resection in a patient with repeated new-onset seizures upon initial work-up of seizures and diagnosis of their brain tumour, versus the patient who presents with a single seizure prior to tumour detection. Moreover, for many epileptogenic lesions, surgical resection often leads to either complete resolution of seizures, sometimes without the need for continued AEDs, or to a marked reduction in their frequency, as will be elaborated upon next.

2.3. General principles of management

How tumor-induced seizures are managed largely depends upon the aggressiveness and location, and therefore, the prognosis of the underlying tumour. In patients with invariably terminal forms of cancer, including primary brain neoplasms like glioblastoma multiforme (GBM), and metastatic spread to brain, the goal usually is to prolong life over months to, at most, a few years, while preserving as high a quality of life as possible. In both adult and paediatric patients with high-grade astrocytomas like GBM, even partial resection of terminal lesions has been shown both to prolong life and reduce the frequency and severity of seizures [145-147]. Clearly, such surgery needs to be performed as soon after diagnosis of the lesion as possible to have any effect upon outcome. Such is not the case in many patients with low-grade tumours like stage I and II gliomas and gangliogliomas, in whom progression of the tumour may be so slow as to be virtually undetectable, and patients can live for years without apparent disease progression, so that any decision to surgically remove the offending lesion may be delayed for years [58, 93, 148, 149]. This being said, there has been increasing emphasis on surgically resecting low-grade tumours early in the course of disease [131] for a multiplicity of reasons. Among these reasons are that anywhere from 20% to roughly one third of low-grade gliomas (LGG) fail to respond to anti-epileptic medications [72, 150], and many that do respond require more than a single AED [150], placing patients, and especially children, at risk for long-term drug toxicities [23, 24, 59, 71, 151-153]. Among the various documented toxicities of AEDs are wide-ranging adverse effects on cognitive function [23, 153], which already may be impaired because of the tumour itself and the radiation therapy sometimes administered to treat it [18, 20, 154-156]. Moreover, surgical resection of LGG has been shown to enhance long-term survival [19] and to significantly improve the likelihood of seizure control [27, 70].

Though the data are not definitive, there is some evidence suggesting that, among the various seizure types, partial seizures, either simple or complex, may be less likely to respond to anti-epileptic drugs than generalized or mixed seizures [93, 157, 158]. This resistance may be noted initially, so that seizure control is never achieved; but it also may develop over time, so that seizure control is lost and never regained [158, 159]. In such patients, therefore, there may even be an increased incentive to pursue surgical resection of the tumour+/-any adjacent epileptogenic foci, if the lesion can be accessed with no undue risk.

Several studies have shown that radical removal of an epileptogenic brain tumour is a strong, and likely the strongest, predictor of seizure freedom [127]. However, additional predictors include the type of seizure, the histopathology of the tumour, the age of the patient at the time of surgery, and the duration of epilepsy [127]. Among the various tumour histologies, tumours that are non-resectable due to infiltration, like high-grade astrocytomas, can be problematic over the patient's relatively brief period of survival [160]. However, as stated earlier, such high-grade lesions tend to be less often epileptogenic than their low-grade counterparts [32, 87, 91, 113, 140, 141]. In long-term brain cancer survivors, glioneuronal tumours, and particularly low-grade gliomas, gangliogliomas and dysembryoplastic neuroepithelial tumours (DNETs), often produce quite drug-resistant epilepsy in children, so that complete surgical resection of the tumour is typically considered the primary focus of treatment [28, 61-63, 88, 94, 116, 132].

In such patients, post-operative seizure-freedom rates often approach or exceed 80% [35, 48, 51, 58, 66, 86, 88, 90, 93, 115, 157, 161-169].

Traditionally, there has been some concern about being too aggressive with younger children with brain tumours, because of the risk of long-term adverse effects on neurological develop-ment, the risk of secondary neoplasms, and other neurological sequelae [155]. That such risks exist is certainly true of radiation therapy [18, 20, 64, 153-156], but it also is true of surgery [170]. However, recent studies have shown that surgery to resect epileptogenic brain tumours is both effective and safe for the vast majority of infants and toddlers [35, 55, 171]. In one large survey, for example, data were collected retrospectively on 116 patients less than 3-years old from eight centers across Canada from January 1987 to September 2005 who had undergone epilepsy surgery [171]. Among the various seizure aetiologies were malformations of cortical develop-ment (n=57), tumours (22), Sturge-Weber syndrome (19), and infarcts (8), with 10 cases either of unknown or some other cause. Seizure onset was in the first year of life in 82%, and the mean age at the time of the initial surgery was 15.8 months (range: 1-35 months). Second surgeries were performed in 27 patients, with six patients requiring a third surgical procedure. Among the initial 116 procedures performed were 40 hemispheric operations, 33 cortical resections, 35 lesionectomies, 7 temporal lobectomies, and one callosotomy. Of the 151 operations, including the 27 second and six third procedures, only one resulted in a surgery-related death. The most common surgical complications were infection, in 17 patients, and aseptic meningitis in 13. Of 107 patients assessed more than one year postoperatively, 72 (67.3%) were seizure free (Engel I), 15(14%) had experienced at least a 90% reduction in seizures (Engel II), and 12 had at least a 50% reduction (Engel III), with only eight exhibiting no benefit (Engel IV). Moreover, 55.3% of the children exhibited signs of improved development post-operatively [171].

Consequently, regardless of patient age, the focus for most patients with low-grade lesions has become, whenever possible without the undue risk of peri-operative death or long-term adverse neurological sequelae, to attempt total or at least subtotal tumor resection earlier rather than later in the course of disease. Debate rages, however, as to how aggressive to be achieving this goal, whether or not resecting the lesion alone is enough, and what intra-operative technologies to use to aid in identifying tumour margins and other epileptogenic foci. Moreover, not all patients will be eligible for surgery and will have to rely on non-neurosur-gical treatments alone, most notably anti-epileptic drugs (AEDs) and radiation therapy. The next section briefly discusses the benefits, risks and utilization of AEDs both prior to and in lieu of surgery.

3. Anti-Epileptic Drugs (AEDs)

An extensive review paper could be written discussing the various advantages and disadvan-tages, indications and contra-indications, and drug-drug interactions that exist for the extensive list of anti-epileptic drugs that now are available for use in patients with brain tumour-induced epilepsy, all of which is beyond the scope of the current review. Here, we briefly describe the roles of AEDs, both in prophylaxis against and control of tumour-induced seizures, some of the risks of prolonged use, and at least the theoretical advantages of the new class of non-enzyme inducing drugs.

3.1. AEDs for seizure prophylaxis

In three recent surveys of neurosurgeons, including one survey specifically of members of the *American Association of Neurologic Surgeons* (AANS), the majority (up to 70%) of respondents reported prophylactically initiating AEDs in brain tumour patients who had not yet experienced a seizure [172-174]. This practice of prescribing AEDs prophylactically in brain tumour patients with no seizure history persists, even though empirical evidence addressing this practice is inconclusive at best [78, 81, 127, 140, 172]. Moreover, many authors and the most current *American Association of Neurology* practice parameters argue against it [113, 140, 172, 175, 176]. The argument of AED detractors is that both meta-analyses published since 2000 to address this issue failed to provide sufficient evidence to promote their prophylactic use in brain-tumour patients without seizures [173, 177]. The first meta-analysis, published in 2000 by Glantz et al. [173], analyzed 12 studies, of which four were randomized controlled trials and eight were considered to be "well-designed observational studies with concurrent controls", sufficient to be classified as class II evidence. Not one of these twelve studies demonstrated a statistical advantage of the AED being studied (phenytoin, depakote, or phenobarbital) over placebo [173]. The second, somewhat more stringent meta-analysis, published in 2004 by Sirven et al [177], only included five RCTs, assessing the prophylactic use of either phenobarbital, phenytoin, or valproic acid. Of the five trials, four identified no statistical benefit of AED use for peri-operative seizure prophylaxis. The one exception was a 1983 study published by North et al [178], in which not only patients with brain tumours, but patients who had undergone craniotomies for aneurisms and head injuries were included. A closer, empirical look at these data reveals no advantage at all when brain tumours are considered alone: seizures occurred in 9/42 on phenytoin, and in 5/39 on placebo (OR=1.11, 95% CI=0.58, 2.12). Further considering just those patients with glial tumours (versus meningiomas, sellar tumours, and metastases), seizures occurred in three of 16 on phenytoin versus just one of 16 on placebo (1.15; 0.42, 3.19) [178]. Overall meta-analysis across the five RCT confirmed the lack of any AED benefit at both one week (OR, 0.91; 95% confidence interval [CI], 0.45-1.83) and six months (OR, 1.01; 95% CI, 0.51-1.98) of follow-up. The AEDs also exhibited no effect on seizure prevention for specific tumours, including primary glial tumors (OR, 3.46; 95% CI, 0.32-37.47), cerebral metastases (OR, 2.50; 95% CI, 0.25-24.72), and meningiomas (OR, 0.62; 95% CI, 0.10-3.85) [177].

More recently, in a review published in 2011, Kargiotis et al. non-statistically examined published evidence on more currently-used AED, including the newer non-enzyme inducing drugs, and concluded that, among patients with either brain metastases or primary brain tumors who have never experienced seizures, prophylactic anticonvulsant treatment might be justified, but only for up to six months postoperatively after surgical excision of the cerebral tumour, since most of these patients will never experience seizures, and the anti-epileptic drugs may cause toxicity and adverse interactions with chemotherapeutic treatments administered to control the neoplasm itself [109]. For such prophylaxis, the authors argued that newer antiepileptic drugs like levetiracetam and oxcarbazepine are preferable to older agents like phenytoin and carbamazepine [109]. To date, however, no hard evidence supports any of these recommendations, and certainly not in children.

In a study by Hardesty et al., only 7.4% of 223 paediatric patients with brain tumours but no history of seizures experienced even a single seizure during their surgical admission, even though only 4.4% of patients had been started on a prophylactic AED [179]. This percentage is similar to the 8.0% observed among those on placebo in a controlled study in which 127 patients awaiting brain tumour surgery, ranging in age from 16 to 84 years, were randomized to receive either phenytoin 15mg/kg intravenously in the operating room, followed by 100 mg three times daily, either by mouth or intravenously, for seven days or placebo [180]. Thereafter, the dose of each was tapered. The 30-day incidence of seizures actually was higher in the phenytoin group (10.0%) than in controls (8.0%), albeit not statistically so. Moreover, the rate of complications was 18.0% versus 0% in the treatment versus placebo group, respectively (p < 0.001).

In the Hardesty study on youths [179], dependent factors associated with peri-operative seizures included a supratentorial tumour, patient age less than two years, and the presence of post-operative hyponatraemia due to either the syndrome of inappropriate antidiuretic hormone (SIADH) or cerebral salt wasting. No other factor was independently predictive of incident seizures, including tumour type, the lobe of the brain affected, the amount of operative blood loss, and the length of surgery [179]. Consequently, though children and adolescents who are awaiting brain-tumour resection and have recurrent seizures might warrant the initiation of an AED pre-operatively, and perhaps also children under age two years with a supratentorial tumour and those with highly-epileptogenic tumours like DNETs, even in the absence of seizures, the prophylactic use of these drugs is far from empirically justified. What is more prudent is to monitor all patients carefully throughout the peri-operative period to identify clinical factors that might place the child at risk, like electrolyte imbalances and fever.

3.2. AEDs for seizure control

Although in some small series of patients, seizures have been found to occur in up to 50% of paediatric patients with a brain tumour [170], in most populations, the overall inci-dence of seizures in this patient population is considerably lower, in the 10-20% range [51, 89, 90]. This is largely due to the infratentorial location of the majority of paediatric tumours, where very few are epileptogenic [37]. As such, only a small minority of children and adolescents with a brain tumour will likely ever require an AED, and almost all will have a supratentorial lesion. For example, from a database of 334 patients up to 21-years old, Sogawa et al. only identified 32 (10%) who had been started on an AED [83]; 94% of these 32 tumours were supratentorial, and 78% were glial [83]. Similarly, in their series of 280 patients between the ages of two months and 18 years of age, Khan et al. identified only 55 (20%) patients who had required an AED, among whom 49 (89%) had a supratentorial lesion [90]. This being said, over a 20-year period at a single institution, Khan et al. followed 157 patients who had presented with seizures and a brain tumour during childhood or adolescence, all of whom had been on at least one AED at some point [82]. Of these patients, phenytoin was the first AED used for 52 patients, carbamazepine for 38 patients, gabapentin for 31, and phenobarbitol for 14. Sixty-two of these patients ultimately were taken off all AEDs; but 17 of these 62 (27%) suffered seizure recurrence [181].

DNETs and gangliogliomas, which typically become manifest during childhood, adolescence or young adulthood, represent only a small percentage of CNS tumours in either youths or adults [6]. However, these tumours are almost always associated with seizures. Consequently, they comprise a disproportionate percentage of tumour-associated epilepsy cases [28, 44, 62, 73, 88, 89, 91, 94, 95]. Moreover, DNETs tend to be extremely resistant to AED therapy [62, 182-186]. Consequently, though AEDs generally are initiated in such patients, the majority ultimately will require surgical resection.

There is virtually no debate that AEDs are of use in treating brain tumour patients with seizures, in patients with repeated seizures awaiting surgery, in patients in whom tumour resection is infeasible, and in those whose seizures remain refractory despite surgery. However, there is concern about the risks of their long-term use, especially in patients who require on-going chemotherapy for their brain malignancy due to drug interactions and mutually-shared toxicities [81, 83, 127, 140, 151, 159, 172, 176], 187]; and significant debate regarding when and how AEDs should be discontinued post-operatively.

One of the biggest issues relating to AEDs is their potential interactions with anti-neoplastic drugs administered to control tumours and prolong survival. In a paper reviewing anti-epileptic drugs, Kargiotis et al. [109] listed 25 chemotherapeutic medications that interact with AEDs, most commonly carbamazepine, phenobarbitol, phenytoin and primidone, but also valproic acid. Common interactions are the AED accelerating metabolism of the chemotherapeutic drug, and the chemotherapeutic drug reducing serum levels of the AED [109], two results that potentially accentuate each other — when AED levels fall, AED doses must be increased to achieve seizure control, which will further increase metabolism of the chemotherapeutic drug, resulting in its doses needing to be increased, and so on. Included on their list of 25 drugs were 13 drugs often selected for the treatment of brain metastases, as well as nine drugs currently used to treat glioblastomas, six drugs to treat medulloblastomas, and five to treat malignant meningiomas.

In the current paper, Table 1 lists these interactions in reverse, indicating those anti-neoplastic drugs used for CNS malignancies that have had documented interactions with each of the five AEDs listed above. What is clear from this table is that all but valproic acid interacts with almost all of the chemo-therapeutic drugs typically used for CNS cancers.

The only drug on the list published by Kargiotis et al. [109] this is not considered to interact with AEDs is temozolomide (TMZ), a less toxic and more-easily tolerated orally-administered drug that effectively crosses the blood-brain barrier [188] and is now commonly used for both high-grade [189] and low-grade [190, 191] gliomas, as well as for brain metastases [192] and melanomas, often in combination with radiation therapy. There also is evidence that TMZ itself reduces the frequency of seizures, independent of AED dose. In one study in which 39 patients receiving TMZ (mean age 46.0 years) were followed for a mean 39 months and compared with 30 patients not on TMZ (mean age 41.5 years), patients on TMZ experienced a 59% reduction in seizure frequency versus just 13% in controls (p < 0.001) [150]. However, for reasons that are not entirely understood, TMZ appears to be less effective in children [193]. For this reason, other anti-neoplastic drugs typically are prescribed in children and adolescents, particularly multiple-drug regimens that include carboplatin and vincristine [193-195], two drugs both documented to interact with the older, cytochrome P450-inducing anti-eptiletics [109] (Table 1).

Meanwhile, evidence continues to mount documenting both the effectiveness and safety of newer-generation AEDS, like levetiracetam, oxcarbazepine and pregabalin [152, 196-204]. Though direct comparisons against the older drugs are generally lacking, theoretical advantages include the lack of any effect on cytochrome P450, and the fact that these drugs generally target specific risk factors for tumour-induced seizures [81]. Recently, in a survey of 32 paediatric brain-tumour patients requiring AEDs for seizure control, Sogawa et al. found that patients who had been started on any the newer–generation drugs (levetiracetam, oxcarbaze-pine and lamotrigine) were three times as likely to remain on these drugs than those started on one of the older drugs like valproic acid, phenytoin, and phenobarbitol (73% vs. 28%, respectively, p=0.04) [83]. Although the sample was small, there also was evidence of increased toxicity with the older drugs, with five versus just two adverse events resulting in drug discontinuation [83].

Of course, the treatment of brain tumours is anything but a static field. In attempts to reduce tumour progression and prolong survival, newer chemotherapeutic drugs are continuously being tested. Some, like nimotuzumab [205]and bevacizumab [206], both of them antibodies against epithelial growth factor receptors (EGFR), have been demonstrating considerable promise, and this may have implications for which AEDs are best tolerated as interactions and mutual toxicities become clearer. What is evident is that AEDs, in themselves, are usually inadequate to control seizures in most patients with epileptogenic brain tumours. And while novel treatments like stereotactic radiosurgery [154], vagus nerve stimulation [207], and ionizing radiation [208] are emerging, at this time optimal management of a child or adolescent with epilepsy caused by a brain tumour almost always necessitates resection of the lesion itself.

4. Surgical resection of epileptogenic brain tumours

4.1. The benefits and risks of surgery

In recent years, there has been a trend towards earlier surgical intervention in young patients with low-grade epileptogenic tumours; but is this justified? One potential justification is the risk of malignant transformation of low-grade tumours which, even though uncommon, has been described for virtually all tumour types and often is catastrophic [60, 64, 65, 67, 68, 97, 112, 131, 209-213]. A second justification pertains to improved seizure control and the decreased reliance on AEDs, with some patients potentially able to discontinue anti-epileptic medications altogether[59], [61, 181, 185]. But how successful is tumour resection in terms of controlling or eliminating seizures?

Table 2 lists 26 studies [35, 51, [61-63, 86, 90, 94, 96, 132, 148, 149, 168, 182, 184, 185, 214-223] published over the past two decades in which seizure outcomes in children and adolescents undergoing surgery to remove epileptogenic brain neoplasms were examined. Across these 26 studies are 741 patients, ranging in age from one month to 21 years of age, with a mean age of 9.1 years and a mean duration of post-operative follow-up of more than four years (overall mean=52 months, with individual study means ranging from 12 to 148 months). Though one study [86] included six paediatric patients with high-grade gliomas (either GBM or grade III astrocytoma), and another indicated 11 patients with either grade III or grade IV lesions [35], almost all of the remaining 724 patients had low-grade (grade I or II) lesions, including various low-grade gliomas and glioneuronal tumours, and less typically epileptogenic tumours like craniopharyngiomas and a dysplastic cyst. Spanning these studies, surgical approaches clearly differed, with some surgeons either largely or exclusively performing lesionectomies alone, others performing further procedures like partial lobectomies [86, 148] and amygdylohypo-campectomies [182], and still others using various intra-operative mapping technologies like electrocortography (ECoG) [63, 132, 184, 214] to identify and ultimately resect extra-tumoral epileptogenic tissue. However, the ubiquitous goal was total tumour resection, whenever possible, an objective that was achieved in roughly two-thirds of cases.

Overall, the series with the lowest total resection rates were those that included a number of oligodendrogliomas (ODG), with resection rates ranging from 30% in a study exclusively of ODG and ODG-mixed lesions [96] and 40% in an older study in which half the patients had ODG [219], to 58% and 61% in studies in which the proportion of ODG was considerably lower [90, 220]. This discovery is not unexpected, given the highly infiltrative nature of these tumours [77, 96, 97, 191].

The outcomes of surgery otherwise were impressive, with almost four out of every five patients (77.7%) seizure free at the time of the final follow-up assessment, and 92.6% experiencing a significant improvement in their seizures from baseline, to Engel class 1, 2 or 3. Examining these data further reveals moderately strong, borderline statistically-significant correlations between the percentage of total resections achieved within any given series and the rate of seizure freedom (r=0.37, p=0.08), and between the percentage of total resections and the percentage of patients whose seizures were improved post-operatively (r=0.36, p=0.09). However, no correlation is apparent between the duration of follow-up and either outcome (r=0.06, p=0.78 and r=0.26, p=0.22, respectively), suggesting that it was the surgical procedure, rather than post-operative management, that influenced seizure outcomes.

There also were no peri-operative deaths among the 741 patients, some of whom even underwent second procedures to resect residual tumour detected by imaging after the first procedure. The overall operative complication rate, adjusted for missing data, was 11.7%, with the vast majority of complications and new neurological deficits transient and completely resolved within weeks to months of the procedure. As stated above, a small number of patients required repeat surgeries to achieve seizure control, sometimes associated with total tumour resection. For example, in one series a second surgery was required in three of 29 paediatric patients with supratentorial gangliogliomas, and all became seizure free after the second operation [216].

The studies by Jo et al. [223] and Gaggero et al. [35] are of special note because all the patients were infants, under the age of 5 and 3 years, respectively. In the first small series of 14 patients of mean age 2.7 years (32 months) [223], total resection of the epileptogenic lesion was achieved in 71%, as was total seizure freedom an average of 35 months post-operatively. In addition, all 14 infants experienced a significant reduction in seizure frequency, either being totally seizure free or having seizures limited to auras alone [223]. There also were no deaths and no reported operative complications. In the second study, which included 20 infants under age 3 years (mean age 1.5 years), eleven of the 20 children had either a grade III or grade IV neoplasm, including four choroid plexus carcinomas, one anaplastic oligodendroglioma, one anaplastic ependymoma, one immature teratoma, two glioblastoma multiforme, one PNET and one neuroblastoma [35]. Despite this, total resection was achieved in 70% of the children, seizure freedom beyond four years in 55%, and seizure improvement in 90%. Interestingly, all 20 patients lived beyond four years, and 17 remained alive at eight years of follow-up [35]. These two studies that imply both the effectiveness and safety of aggressive brain tumour resection in infants is counter to another study on 18 infants under one year of age who had a variety of grade I through IV lesions [170]. In this series, there was only one peri-operative death, due to massive brain haemorrhage in an 8-month old child with a deep, right parieto-occipital ganglioglioma. However, three patients had new-onset seizures following surgery, and an additional three had worsened neurological deficits. Of the nine patients who had pre-operative seizures, three improved, five did not improve, and one died. Overall, as of the paper's publication, only eight of the twenty patients had survived beyond infancy, with five now into adulthood (ages 18 – 26) [170]; two of the adult survivors were severely disabled at the time of the report, both having a Karnofsky score [224] of just 40%.

Also worth noting from Table 2 are the six studies in which only patients with dysembryoplastic neuroepithelial tumours (DNETs) were included (Table 3) [61, 62, 94, 132, 182, 184]. These six studies encompass 132 patients, of mean age 9.7 years, amongst whom total tumour resection was achieved in almost 82%, seizure freedom in 87%, and seizure improvement in all but a single patient (99%). However, the adjusted surgical complication rate was slightly higher than that noted across all 26 studies.

Table 4 lists four additional studies of note. Among these four additional studies, three were excluded from the previous table and its summation totals because vascular and other non-neoplastic lesions were intermingled with non-vascular lesions, with no data provided to distinguish between them; and the fourth was excluded because all the patients had tuberous sclerosis, in which brain tubors often cause uncontrolled seizures [225, 226]. The fifteen patients in this fourth study all had subependymal giant cell astrocytomas (SEGA), a tumour that is found in between five and fifteen percent of TS patients [123], typically developing in the region of the foramen of Monro, where it frequently causes obstructive hydrocephalus. Seizures primarily result from a broad array of intra-cerebral tumors, which include the cortical tubers mentioned above, and subependymal nodules, in addition to SEGA [225, 226]. The long-term prognosis therefore is poor, with death primarily resulting from intractable seizures or SEGA-induced obstructive hydrocephalus [225, 226]. As such, it is not unexpected that Cuccia et al. [99] failed to achieve either seizure freedom or any meaningful clinical improvement in seizure frequency in any of their patients. The inherent complexities of SEGA removal, given the relative inaccessibility of these tumours, also could account for the high complication rate (6 of 15, 40%).

The three remaining studies [117, 227, 228] involved a high proportion of non-neoplastic lesions that were not analyzed distinctly from neoplastic cases. Mean seizure free rates across the three studies ranged from a low of 56% to a high of 81%, with seizure improvement noted in 81.3% and 92.4% in the two studies in which this outcome was reported [117, 227]. Although no deaths were reported, almost one in four patients (73 of 320, 22.8%) had a significant post-operative complication, likely due to the highly vascular nature of many of the lesions and the increased risk of intracranial bleeding.

4.2. Post-operative management

According to the 30 studies (26+4) analysed above, the rate of post-operative complications among patients with epileptogenic brain tumours is low, likely somewhere between 10 and 20 percent, depending upon the nature of the tumour resected, its location, and perhaps other factors as well. The risk of peri-operative mortality also appears to be exceedingly low, with not a single surgery-related death reported among those 873 patients.

Few papers have been published on the post-operative management of paediatric brain tumour patients. What has been reported is that youths tend to experience different intra-operative and post-operative complications than adults, and that these complications affect both short and long-term outcomes, including disability, mortality and hospital and PICU lengths of stay and, hence, direct health care costs [229, 230]. Among the various risk factors for complications are fluid and electrolyte imbalances, which may be especially significant in children. One also must consider that volume of blood loss is all relative to the age and size of the child, given that a human's total blood volume varies dramatically relative to their age and size: falling from roughly 85 to 90 ml per kg in term neonates, to roughly 85 ml/kg in infants, 80 ml/kg in children under age 10, 70-75 ml in children > 10 and adolescents, and 70ml/kg in adults [231, 232]. Clearly then, 100 ml of blood loss may mean nothing to an adult, but may represent 25% or more of the total blood volume of a newborn.

In general, the most common fluid and electrolyte abnormalities observed after brain surgery in children relate to serum sodium levels, with hyponatraemia secondary to either the syndrome of inappropriate diuretic hormone (SIADH) secretion or cerebral salt wasting syndrome, and hypernatraemia caused by diabetes insipidis (DI) [233-236]. In one series of 79 children, for example, water and sodium disorders were noted in 36 (46%): 23 (29%) with DI, 12 (15%) with SIADH, and a single patient with cerebral salt wasting [236]. Why this is especially important in the paediatric patient in whom an epileptogenic brain tumour has been resected is that sodium disturbances are a significant risk factor for seizures. In one study involving 223 paediatric patients with epileptic brain tumours undergoing 229 surgical procedures, post-operative hyponatraemia — due to either SIADH or cerebral salt wasting — was one of just three independent factors associated with peri-operative seizures, the other two being a supratentorial tumour and patient age less than two years [179].

In another study of 105 paediatric patients post brain tumor resection admitted to the PICU, patients required an average of 0.7 unexpected intensive care unit interventions, mostly secondary to sodium abnormalities, followed by new neurologic deficits, paresis, and seizures

[237]. Interestingly, however, 68% of the patients were stable enough to be transferred out of the PICI within 24 hours of surgery.

With respect to anti-epileptic drugs, the same applies post-operatively as pre-operatively, in that there is generally no need to initiate AEDs in patients who have not yet experienced seizures, given the lack of evidence documenting any benefit of prophylaxis [180, 238]. This being said, there are no clear guidelines as to when and how to discontinue AEDs if they have been initiated pre-operatively, and there is always the potential risk of withdrawal-induced seizures [59]. In one study of 332 mostly adult patients, but including some as young as age 16, among those with AEDs that had been initiated to treat seizures pre-operatively, patients with a longer history of seizures (p<0.001) and those with simple partial seizures (p=0.004) were found to be especially likely to continue to have seizures in the immediate post-operative period, as well as poorer control long-term [58]. If AEDs are started post-operatively to reduce the risk of seizures following the trauma of surgery in a patient who otherwise has not had seizures, they generally should be administered short-term [239].

5. When seizures persist or recur

In virtually every series we have reviewed, patients were described who underwent resection of their epileptogenic brain tumour, with apparently successful removal of the tumour, yet no achieved control of seizures. Additional patients were noted to suffer from the post-operative onset of new seizures [170]. And still others had complete control of their seizures, only to relapse later, either while still on an anti-epileptic drug or after all AEDs had been withdrawn. Each of these three scenarios has implications with respect to patient prognosis and management.

5.1. Implications of post-operative seizures

The clinical implications of seizures that either start or re-start months or years after the initial resection of tumour are somewhat different than seizures that start immediately post-operatively or that started pre-operatively and failed to resolve with surgery. The major concern with the latter two scenarios is that tumour resection either was incomplete, or that extra-tumoral epileptogenic tissue was not removed. Over the years, attempts have been made to optimize the resection of epileptogenic lesions by both better delineating their margins and identifying extra-tumoral epileptogenic tissue, using intra-operative tools like electrocorticography (ECoG) to identify potential seizure-inducing tissue irregularities like cortical dysplasia [63, 77, 93, 132, [1] [6][3], 184, 214, 216, 240, 241]. This has led to debate regarding the relative benefits and safety of performing epilepsy surgery rather than just lesionectomies in patients with tumour-triggered seizures [242]; though, in fact, many surgeons have been utilizing additional surgical steps like lobectomies, amygdylohypocampectomies and, in extreme cases, hemispherectomies for decades [63, 86, 94, 117, 132, 148, 149, 168, 182, 185, 214, 217, 218, 222, 227, 243]. To date, almost no direct empirical comparisons have been undertaken. In perhaps the most methodologically sound study, Gelinas et al. retrospectively compared

34 patients who underwent ECoG-aided epilepsy surgery and 33 patients who had undergone simple lesionectomies without ECoG, all between the ages of 3 months and 16 years, in Vancouver, Canada [214]. One year post-operatively, the two treatment arms were virtually identical, with roughly 80% of patients in each group seizure free. However, at a mean follow-up of 5.8 years, there was a trend towards improved seizure freedom in patients in the ECoG group, with 79% versus 61% patients still seizure free (p=0.08). The investigators also noted no increase in neurological morbidity among patients who had undergone the more extensive ECoG-guided cortical resection, and that these patients were less likely to require repeat epilepsy surgery [214]. Why this has implications post-operatively relates to the potential need for re-operation, as discussed in the next section.

If the major concern of continued seizures is residual tumour or other epileptogenic tissue, the major concerns with later tumour recurrence are multiple. They include the possibility: (1) that the tumour itself is re-growing, having never been fully resected; (2) that the tumour has undergone malignant transformation; or (3) that some secondary tumour has started to develop, perhaps as a consequence of brain irradiation, chemotherapy, or some other cause. The risk of second brain malignancies is especially high in patients with CNS tumour-associated familial syndromes like neurofibromatosis types 1 [121] and 2 [122], tuberous sclerosis [123], von Hippel Lindau disease [244, 245], and basal cell nevus syndrome [246], with some of these tumours originating within the brain and others the result of metastatic spread from some extra-cranial site. All of the above-mentioned scenarios warrant investigation, which will include diagnostic imaging, due to their potentially dire consequences

Re-growth of tumour is anticipated among children with high-grade lesions, especially glioblastomas [81, 146, 247]. However, although long-term prognoses remain dismal, small improvements in survival times are being reported even among patients with GBMs, relating to advanced surgical techniques, the introduction of real-time, intra-operative imaging and brain mapping, and combining TMZ with radiation therapy [147, 189, 247-250]. Recall that in one study in which eleven of the 20 children had either a grade III or grade IV lesion, including two GBMs, a grade IV PNET, and a grade IV neuroblastoma, all 20 patients lived beyond four years [35]. Nonetheless, when the return of seizures leads to the discovery of grade IV tumour progression, surgery is almost never indicated. Instead, radiation therapy, chemotherapy, or both can be used and may be effective at reducing seizures [81, 208]. The recurrence of seizures does not necessarily indicate tumour progression, however. Sometimes, intrinsic changes within the tumour itself render AEDs less effective, so that switching or combining drugs may be beneficial [72]. As mentioned in Section 3, in such cases, care must be taken to avoid interactions between chemotherapeutic and anti-epileptic drugs [109].

Tumour re-growth also in anticipated in many low-grade gliomas and other neuroglial tumours when total resection is not achieved, and this can be manifested by the recurrence or worsening of seizures. This being said, malignant transformation has been documented with virtually every form of low-grade brain tumour, especially low-grade gliomas [65, 68, 112, 131], but also traditionally-benign lesions like DNETS [64, 67, 209-211], gangliogliomas [209, 212], meningiomas [251, 252], vestibular schwannomas [251], pituitary adenomas [251], and haemangioblastomas [251], among others. Glioblastomas have even been documented to arise at the site of previously totally-resected tumours [253]. Previously-controlled seizures generally are harder to control once malignant-transformation has occurred, even independent of tumour size or rate of progression [78]. Identification of such transformation therefore has implications in terms of patient prognosis, and management of both the tumour and the seizures.

Finally, the late recurrence of seizures can represent the formation of a secondary tumour, perhaps induced by brain irradiation or chemotherapy [251].

5.2. Surgical management of persistent and recurrent seizures

Whether seizures start immediately after surgery, later along in follow-up, or never fully remit, in all three scenarios, some patients will have seizures that remain uncontrolled despite the use of AEDs. In our review of the 26 studies listed in Table 2, as well as in various other case series and case studies, we found that, occasionally, patients undergo second or even third resections to remove either residual tumour that is now identified on post-operative imaging, or a residual or newly-identified epileptogenic focus. Though sometimes prolonged attempts are made to control the seizures with medication prior to the second surgery, in some cases, surgery is almost immediate, even within a few days of the initial procedure [254]. In one multi-centre survey that involved 116 children under age 3 undergoing epilepsy surgery for a variety of causes, 27 children were brought into the operating room for a second procedure, and six of these for a third procedure to control seizures [171]. Both the approaches and results of these second operations are mixed. In terms of the former, attempts are usually made to resect any residual or newly-discovered tumour, as well as to identify and resect other epileptogenic foci. Approaches range from simple lesionectomies to lobectomies and, in the most severe cases, hemispherectomies [243].

Table 5 summarizes ten studies we identified, published over the past two decades, in which second operative procedures were performed [46, 77, 157, [1] [6][2], 171, 216, 242, 254-256]. Half of these studies were exclusive to paediatric patients, while the other half included children, adolescents and adults. The study by Steinbok et al. was restricted to infants under the age of 3 years at the time of their initial surgery [171]. In this study, six of the patients required a third surgical procedure prior to achieving their final seizure outcome. Follow-up for most of these studies was approximately two years, but sometimes not reported. Overall, slightly less than half of the patients (46%) achieved seizure freedom, with roughly half the remainder (where reported) achieving at least a significant reduction in seizures. As with the first procedures, operative mortality was low, with only one death in 132 patients and 138 procedures.

6. Conclusions

A brain tumour is identified in one to three percent of non-febrile seizures that occur in a child. Meanwhile, seizures occur in between one in ten and one in five paediatric patients with a brain tumour, often as a presenting symptom. Most are associated with low-grade gliomas, like pilocytic astrocytoma, or with neuroglial tumours like ganglioglioma or dysembryoplastic neuroectodermal tumour (DNET). There is no empirical justification for initiating an anti-epileptic drug in a brain tumour patient without seizures, and some would restrict their use to those patients who experience at least two ictal episodes.

The cornerstone of management in most patients with a low-grade lesion is surgical resection, both because doing so often prolongs survival and reduces or eliminates seizures. Overall, almost 80% of children who undergo surgery to for resection of an epileptogenic brain tumour will attain prolonged seizure-freedom, and more than 90% will experience at least some meaningful clinical improvement, associated with a negligible risk of death in experienced surgical hands. Risks may be greater and results poorer in very small infants (under one year of age), but most-preschool children can undergo epilepsy-lesion resections safely and with benefit. Significant surgical complications occur in 10-20% of patients and include fluid and electrolyte imbalances, as well as typically short-lived neurological deficits in most patients, so that vigilant post-operative monitoring is essential.

Late post-operative seizure recurrence is an ominous sign that can be a harbinger of tumour recurrence, progression, or malignant transformation, as well as the appearance of new tumours, especially in patients with familial tumour syndromes like neurofibromatosis and tuberous sclerosis, and those who have received brain irradiation. When low-grade tumours recur and cause seizures, second resections may be effective at again controlling seizures.

These claims must be interpreted with caution, however, given that many essential questions remain unanswered — like whether more extensive epilepsy surgery is more effective or as safe as lesionectomy alone; and what factors best predict outcomes. In addition, with the emergence of new anti-epileptics, new anti-neoplastic treatments, and new surgical technologies, the management of epilepsy in children and adolescents with brain tumours appears to be rapidly changing.

AED	Interactions with
Phenytoin	carboplain, cisplatin, cyclophosphamide, dacarbazine, erlotinib, etoposide, fluorouracil, ifosfamide, imatanib, irinotecan, carmustine, lomustine, paclitaxel, procarbazine, tegafur, teniposide, thiotepa, topotecan, vincristine
Carbamazepine	cisplatin, cyclophosphamide, erlotinib, etoposide, ifosfamide, imatinib, irinotecan, carmustine, lomustine, palitaxel, procarbazine*, teniposide, thiotepa, topotecan, vincristine
Phenobarbitol	cyclophosphamide, erlotinib, etoposide, ifosfamide, imatinib, irinotecan, carmustine, lomustine, paclitaxel, procarbazine, teniposide, thiotepa, topotecan, vincristine
Primidone	cyclophosphamide, erlotinib, etoposide, ifosfamide, imatinib, irinotecan, carmustine, lomustine, paclitaxel, procarbazine, teniposide, thiotepa, topotecan, vincristine
Valproic Acid	cisplatin, cyclophosphamide, vorinostat

*Carbamazepine is contraindicated in patients on procarbazine

Table 1. Anti-epileptic drugs (AED) and their interactions with CNS anti-neoplastic drugs

* Some patients died before final seizure assessment; ** Three patients underwent a second reaction; *** These 16 patients part of a larger series with other seizure aetiologies included

GG=ganglioglioma; DNET=dysembryoplastic neuroepithelial tumor; PGNT=papillary glioneuronal tumor; LGG=low-grade glioma; ODG=oligodendroglioma; AC=astrocytoma; CPP=choroid plexus papilloma; CP=craniopharyngioma; L=lesionectomy; L+E=lesionectomy+additional resection of adjacent epileptogenic tissue; L+A=lesionectomy+amygdylohypocampectomy; L+L=lesionectomy+lobectomy; TL=temporal lobectomy; L+L+A=lesionectomy+lobectomy+amygdylohypocampectomy; AHC=amygdylohypocampectomy; (T)=all temporal lesions

Table 2. Seizure response to surgical resection of epileptogenic tumor

Table 3. Seizure response to surgical resection of dysembroplastic neuroectodermal tumors

Vasc=vascular lesions; SEGA=subependymal cell astrocytoma; TS=tuberous sclerosis; FU=follow-up

Table 4. Seizure response to surgical resection of epileptogenic tumor – studies including vascular lesions

First Author	Year Published	# Subjects	Mean Age (y)*	# Seizure Free
Benifla	2006	12	13.5	7
Chae	2001	1	0.3	1
Gonzalez-Martinez	2007	57	24.7	22
Im	2002	3	16.5	3
Jooma	1995	8	24.0	5
Lombardi	1997	1	?	1
Ojemann	2012	4	8.5	2
Steinbok	2009	24	1.5	12
Tian	2011	9	13.7	3
Whittle	1995	4	36.0	0
Totals		123		56
Mean			15.4	
Percentages				45.5%

Table 5. Seizure response to a second surgical resection

Author details

Adrianna Ranger[1*] and David Diosy[2]

*Address all correspondence to: aranger@uwo.ca

1 Department of Clinical Neurological Sciences, Division of Neurosurgery, Children's Hospital-London Health Sciences Center, Western University, London, Ontario, Canada

2 Department of Clinical Neurological Sciences, Division of Neurology, London Health Sciences Center, Western University, London, Ontario, Canada

References

[1] Centers for Disease Control and Prevention (CDC). Trends in childhood cancer mortality--United States, 1990-2004. *MMWR Morb Mortal Wkly Rep.* 2007;56:1257-1261.

[2] Centers for Disease Control and Prevention (CDC): Trends in childhood cancer mortality--United States, 1990-2004. *MMWR Morb Mortal Wkly Rep.* 2007;56:1257-1261.

[3] Ellison LF, De P, Mery LS, Grundy PE. Canadian Cancer Society's Steering Committee for Canadian Cancer Statistics.: Canadian cancer statistics at a glance: cancer in children. *CMAJ.* 2009;180:422-424.

[4] Linet MS, Ries LA, Smith MA, Tarone RE, Devesa SS. Cancer surveillance series: recent trends in childhood cancer incidence and mortality in the United States. *J Natl Cancer Inst.* 1999;91:1051-1058.

[5] Bunin GR, Feuer EJ, Witman PA, Meadows AT. Increasing incidence of childhood cancer: report of 20 years experience from the greater Delaware Valley Pediatric Tumor Registry. *Paediatr Perinat Epidemiol.* 1996;10:319-338.

[6] Gurney, J. G., Smith, M. A., and Bunin, G. R. CNS and miscellaneous intra-cranial and intraspinal neoplasms. SEER Pediatric Monograph, National Cancer Institute, 51-63. 2001. Ref Type: Serial (Book,Monograph)

[7] National Cancer Institute. A Snapshot of Pediatric Cancers: Incidence on Mortality Rate Trends. 2011. Ref Type: Report

[8] Ellison LF, De P, Mery LS, Grundy PE, Canadian Cancer Society's Steering Committee for Canadian Cancer Statistics. Canadian cancer statistics at a glance: cancer in children. *CMAJ 2009 Feb 17;180(4):422-4.* 2009;180:422-424.

[9] Rendón-Macías ME, Ramos-Becerril C, Bernardez-Zapata I, Iglesias-Leboreiro J. [Cancer epidemiology in children and adolescents at private health care (1995-2004)] [Article in Spanish]. *Rev Med Inst Mex Seguro Soc.* 2008;46:353-360.

[10] Brain Tumor Facts. American Brain Tumor Association. 2012. Ref Type: Electronic Citation

[11] Dolecek TA, Propp JM, Stroup NE, Kruchko C. CBTRUS statistical report: primary brain and central nervous system tumors diagnosed in the United States in 2005-2009. *Neuro Oncol.* 2012;14:1-49.

[12] Sievert AJ, Fisher MJ. Pediatric low-grade gliomas. *J Child Neurol.* 2009;24:1397-1408.

[13] Qaddoumi I, Sultan I, Gajjar A. Outcome and prognostic features in pediatric gliomas: a review of 6212 cases from the Surveillance, Epidemiology, and End Results database. *Cancer.* 2009;115:5761-5770.

[14] Taylor MD, Sanford RA, Boop FA. Cerebellar pilocytic astrocytomas. In: Albright AL, Pollack IF, Adelson PD, eds. *Principles and Practice of Pediatric Neurosurgery.* New York: Thieme Medical pUBLISHERS, iNC.; 2008:655-67.

[15] Sato I, Higuchi A, Yanagisawa T et al. Impact of Late Effects on Health-Related Quality of Life in Survivors of Pediatric Brain Tumors: Motility Disturbance of Limb(s), Seizure, Ocular/Visual Impairment, Endocrine Abnormality, and Higher Brain Dysfunction. *Cancer Nurs 2014 Mar 13 [Epub ahead of print].* 2014.

[16] Huang LT, Hsiao CC, Weng HH, Lui CC. Neurologic complications of pediatric systemic malignancies. *J Formos Med Assoc*. 1996;95:209-212.

[17] Lovely MP. Symptom management of brain tumor patients. *Semin Oncol Nurs*.
2004;20:273-283.

[18] Packer RJ, Gurney JG, Punyko JA et al. Long-term neurologic and neurosensory sequelae in adult survivors of a childhood brain tumor: childhood cancer survivor
study. *J Clin Oncol*. 2003;21:3255-3261.

[19] Shields LB, Choucair AK. Management of Low-Grade Gliomas: A Review of Patient-
Perceived Quality of Life and Neurocognitive Outcome. *World Neurosurg 2014 Feb 19
pii: S1878-8750(14)00164-8 doi: 10 1016/j wneu 2014 02 033 [Epub ahead of print]*. 2014.

[20] Vargo M. Brain tumor rehabilitation. *Am J Phys Med Rehabil*. 2011;90:S50-S62.

[21] Sato I, Higuchi A, Yanagisawa T et al. Impact of Late Effects on Health-Related Quality of Life in Survivors of Pediatric Brain Tumors: Motility Disturbance of Limb(s),
Seizure, Ocular/Visual Impairment, Endocrine Abnormality, and Higher Brain Dysfunction. *Cancer Nurs [Epub ahead of print]*. 2014.

[22] Armstrong GT. Long-term survivors of childhood central nervous system malignancies: the experience of the Childhood Cancer Survivor Study. *Eur J Paediatr Neurol*.
2010;14:298-303.

[23] Klein M, Engelberts NH, van der Ploeg HM et al. Epilepsy in low-grade gliomas: the
impact on cognitive function and quality of life. *Ann Neurol*. 2003;54:514-520.

[24] Maschio M, Dinapoli L. Patients with brain tumor-related epilepsy. *J Neurooncol*.
2012;109:1-6.

[25] Maschio M, Sperati F, Dinapoli L et al. Weight of epilepsy in brain tumor patients. *J
Neurooncol*. 2014;118:385-393.

[26] Riva M. Brain tumoral epilepsy: a review. *Neurol Sci*. 2005;26 Suppl 1:S42.

[27] Ruda R, Trevisan E, Soffietti R. Epilepsy and brain tumors. *Curr Opin Oncol*.
2010;22:611-620.

[28] Thom M, Blumcke I, Aronica E. Long-term epilepsy-associated tumors. *Brain Pathol*.
2012;22:350-379.

[29] Ullrich NJ. Neurologic sequelae of brain tumors in children. *J Child Neurol*.
2009;24:1446-1454.

[30] Wells EM, Gaillard WD, Packer RJ. Pediatric brain tumors and epilepsy. *Semin Pediatr Neurol*. 2012;19:3-8.

[31] Brinkman TM, Liptak CC, Delaney BL, Chordas CA, Muriel AC, Manley PE. Suicide
ideation in pediatric and adult survivors of childhood brain tumors. *J Neurooncol*.
2013;113:425-432.

[32] Shady JA, Black PM, Kupsky WJ et al. Seizures in children with supratentorial astro-glial neoplasms. *Pediatr Neurosurg.* 1994;21:23-30.

[33] Backus RE, Millichap JP. The seizure as a manifestation of intracranial tumor in childhood. *Pediatrics.* 1962;29:978-984.

[34] Blume WT, Girvin JP, Kaufmann JC. Childhood brain tumors presenting as chronic uncontrolled focal seizure disorders. *Ann Neurol.* 1982;12:538-541.

[35] Gaggero R, Consales A, Fazzini F et al. Epilepsy associated with supratentorial brain tumors under 3 years of life. *Epilepsy Res.* 2009;87:184-189.

[36] Gaillard WD, Chiron C, Cross JH et al. Guidelines for imaging infants and children with recent-onset epilepsy. *Epilepsia.* 2009;50:2147-2153.

[37] Ibrahim K, Appleton R. Seizures as the presenting symptom of brain tumours in children. *Seizure.* 2004;13:108-112.

[38] Martinez-Lage JF, Perez-Espejo MA, Esteban JA, Poza M. Thalamic tumors: clinical presentation. *Childs Nerv Syst.* 2002;18:405-411.

[39] Rutledge SL, Snead OC3, Morawetz R, Chandra-Sekar B. Brain tumors presenting as a seizure disorder in infants. *J Child Neurol.* 1987;2:214-219.

[40] Sjors K, Blennow G, Lantz G. Seizures as the presenting symptom of brain tumors in children. *Acta Paediatr.* 1993;82:66-70.

[41] Sun DC, Shen EY, Wong TT. Epilepsy as the sole manifestation of brain tumor--report of two cases. *Zhonghua Min Guo Xiao Er Ke Yi Xue Hui Za Zhi.* 1995;36:142-145.

[42] Williams BA, Abbott KJ, Manson JI. Cerebral tumors in children presenting with epilepsy. *J Child Neurol.* 1992;7:291-294.

[43] Klitbo DM, Nielsen R, Illum NO, Wehner PS, Carlsen N. Symptoms and time to diagnosis in children with brain tumours. *Dan Med Bull.* 2011;58:A4285.

[44] Shamji MF, Fric-Shamji EC, Benoit BG. Brain tumors and epilepsy: pathophysiology of peritumoral changes. *Neurosurg Rev.* 2009;32:275-284.

[45] Coppola G, Spagnoli D, Sciscio N, Russo F, Villani RM. Gelastic seizures and low-grade hypothalamic astrocytoma: a case report. *Brain Dev.* 2002;24:183-186.

[46] Chae JH, Kim SK, Wang KC, Kim KJ, Hwang YS, Cho BK. Hemifacial seizure of cerebellar ganglioglioma origin: seizure control by tumor resection. *Epilepsia.* 2001;42:1204-1247.

[47] Ho CH, Chen SJ, Juan CJ, Lee HS, Tsai SH, Fan HC. Sudden death due to medulloblastoma: a case report. *Acta Neurol Taiwan.* 2013;22:76-80.

[48] Berger MS, Ghatan S, Geyer JR, Keles GE, Ojemann GA. Seizure outcome in children with hemispheric tumors and associated intractable epilepsy: the role of tumor removal combined with seizure foci resection. *Pediatr Neurosurg.* 1991;17:185-191.

[49] Berger MS. Functional mapping-guided resection of low-grade gliomas. *Clin Neurosurg.* 1995;42:437-452.

[50] Chang EF, Clark A, Smith JS et al. Functional mapping-guided resection of low-grade gliomas in eloquent areas of the brain: improvement of long-term survival. Clinical article. *J Neurosurg.* 2011;114:566-573.

[51] Fattal-Valevski A, Nissan N, Kramer U, Constantini S. Seizures as the clinical presenting symptom in children with brain tumors. *J Child Neurol.* 2013;28:292-296.

[52] Consales A, Striano P, Nozza P et al. Glioneuronal tumors and epilepsy in children: seizure outcome related to lesionectomy. *Minerva Pediatr.* 2013;65:609-616.

[53] Gump WC, Skjei KL, Karkare SN. Seizure control after subtotal lesional resection. *Neurosurg Focus.* 2013;34:E1.

[54] Babini M, Giulioni M, Galassi E et al. Seizure outcome of surgical treatment of focal epilepsy associated with low-grade tumors in children. *J Neurosurg Pediatr.* 2013;11:214-223.

[55] Jo KI, Shin HJ, Hong SC. Seizure outcomes of lesionectomy in pediatric lesional epilepsy with brain tumor--single institute experience. *Brain Dev.* 2013;35:810-815.

[56] Kim YH, Park CK, Kim TH et al. Seizures during the management of high-grade gliomas: clinical relevance to disease progression. *J Neurooncol.* 2013;113:101-109.

[57] Chaichana KL, Parker SL, Oliva A, Quinones-Hinojosa A. Long-term seizure outcomes in adult patients undergoing primary resection of malignant brain astrocytomas. Clinical article. *J Neurosurg.* 2009;111:282-292.

[58] Chang EF, Potts MB, Keles GE et al. Seizure characteristics and control following resection in 332 patients with low-grade gliomas. *J Neurosurg.* 2008;108:227-235.

[59] Das RR, Artsy E, Hurwitz S et al. Outcomes after discontinuation of antiepileptic drugs after surgery in patients with low grade brain tumors and meningiomas. *J Neurooncol.* 2012;107:565-570.

[60] Luyken C, Blumcke I, Fimmers R et al. The spectrum of long-term epilepsy-associated tumors: long-term seizure and tumor outcome and neurosurgical aspects. *Epilepsia.* 2003;44:822-830.

[61] Minkin K, Klein O, Mancini J, Lena G. Surgical strategies and seizure control in pediatric patients with dysembryoplastic neuroepithelial tumors: a single-institution experience. *J Neurosurg Pediatr.* 2008;1:206-210.

[62] Nolan MA, Sakuta R, Chuang N et al. Dysembryoplastic neuroepithelial tumors in childhood: long-term outcome and prognostic features. *Neurology.* 2004;62:2270-2276.

[63] Ogiwara H, Nordi DR, DiPatri AJ, Alden TD, Bowman RM, Tomita T. Pediatric epileptogenic gangliogliomas: seizure outcome and surgical results. *J Neurosurg Pediatr.* 2010;5:271-276.

[64] Ray WZ, Blackburn SL, Casavilca-Zambrano S et al. Clinicopathologic features of recurrent dysembryoplastic neuroepithelial tumor and rare malignant transformation: a report of 5 cases and review of the literature. *J Neurooncol.* 2009;94:283-292.

[65] Smits A, Duffau H. Seizures and the natural history of World Health Organization Grade II gliomas: a review. *Neurosurgery.* 2011;68:1326-1333.

[66] Tandon N, Esquenazi Y. Resection strategies in tumoral epilepsy: is a lesionectomy enough? *Epilepsia.* 2013;54:72-78.

[67] Hammond RR, Duggal N, Woulfe JM, Girvin JP. Malignant transformation of a dysembryoplastic neuroepithelial tumor. Case report. *J Neurosurg.* 2000;92:722-725.

[68] Unal E, Koksal Y, Cimen O, Paksoy Y, Tavli L. Malignant glioblastomatous transformation of a low-grade glioma in a child. *Childs Nerv Syst.* 2008;24:1385-1389.

[69] Schaller B, Ruegg SJ. Brain tumor and seizures: pathophysiology and its implications for treatment revisited. *Epilepsia.* 2003;44:1223-1232.

[70] Ruda R, Bello L, Duffau H, Soffietti R. Seizures in low-grade gliomas: natural history, pathogenesis, and outcome after treatments. *Neuro Oncol.* 2012;14:iv55-iv64.

[71] van Breemen M, Wilms EB, Vecht CJ. Epilepsy in patients with brain tumours: epidemiology, mechanisms, and management. *Lancet Neurol.* 2007;6:421-430.

[72] Calatozzolo C, Pollo B, Botturi A et al. Multidrug resistance proteins expression in glioma patients with epilepsy. *J Neurooncol.* 2012;110:129-135.

[73] Alkonyi B, Mittal S, Zitron I et al. Increased tryptophan transport in epileptogenic dysembryoplastic neuroepithelial tumors. *J Neurooncol.* 2012;107:365-372.

[74] You G, Sha Z, Jiang T. The pathogenesis of tumor-related epilepsy and its implications for clinical treatment. *Seizure.* 2012;21:153-159.

[75] Berntsson SG, Malmer B, Bondy ML, Qu M, Smits A. Tumor-associated epilepsy and glioma: are there common genetic pathways? *Acta Oncol.* 2009;48:955-963.

[76] Lee JW, Wen PY, Hurwitz S et al. Morphological characteristics of brain tumors causing seizures. *Arch Neurol.* 2010;67:336-342.

[77] Whittle IR, Beaumont A. Seizures in patients with supratentorial oligodendroglial tumours. Clinicopathological features and management considerations. *Acta Neurochir (Wien).* 1995;135:19-24.

[78] Rosati A, Tomassini A, Pollo B et al. Epilepsy in cerebral glioma: timing of appearance and histological correlations. *J Neurooncol.* 2009;93:395-400.

[79] Kramer U, Nevo Y, Reider-Groswasser I et al. Neuroimaging of children with partial seizures. *Seizure.* 1998;7:115-118.

[80] Harvey AS, Cross JH, Shinnar S, Mathern GW, ILAE Pediatric Epilepsy Surgery Survey Taskforce. Defining the spectrum of international practice in pediatric epilepsy surgery patients. *Epilepsia.* 2008;49:146-155.

[81] Perucca E. Optimizing antiepileptic drug treatment in tumoral epilepsy. *Epilepsia.* 2013;54:97-104.

[82] Khan RB, Hunt DL, Boop FA et al. Seizures in children with primary brain tumors: incidence and long-term outcome. *Epilepsy Res.* 2005;64:85-91.

[83] Sogawa Y, Kan L, Levy AS, Maytal J, Shinnar S. The use of antiepileptic drugs in pediatric brain tumor patients. *Pediatr Neurol.* 2009;41:192-194.

[84] Dagcinar A, Bayrakli F, Yapicier O, Ozek M. Primary meningeal osteosarcoma of the brain during childhood. Case report. *J Neurosurg Pediatr.* 2008;1:325-329.

[85] Fulton SP, Clarke DF, Wheless JW, Ellison DW, Ogg R, Boop FA. Angiocentric glioma-induced seizures in a 2-year-old child. *J Child Neurol.* 2009;24:852-856.

[86] Iannelli A, Guzzetta F, Battaglia D, Iuvone L, Di Rocco C. Surgical treatment of temporal tumors associated with epilepsy in children. *Pediatr Neurosurg.* 2000;32:248-254.

[87] Bromfield EB. Epilepsy in patients with brain tumors and other cancers. *Rev Neurol Dis.* 2004;1:S27-S33.

[88] Wallace D, Ruban D, Kanner A et al. Temporal lobe gangliogliomas associated with chronic epilepsy: long-term surgical outcomes. *Clin Neurol Neurosurg.* 2013;115:472-476.

[89] Shamji MF, Vassilyada M, Lam CH, Montes JL, Farmer JP. Congenital tumors of the central nervous system: the MCH experience. *Pediatr Neurosurg.* 2009;45:368-374.

[90] Khan RB, Boop FA, Onar A, Sanford RA. Seizures in children with low-grade tumors: outcome after tumor resection and risk factors for uncontrolled seizures. *J Neurosurg.* 2006;104:377-382.

[91] Lynam LM, Lyons MK, Drazkowski JF et al. Frequency of seizures in patients with newly diagnosed brain tumors: a retrospective review. *Clin Neurol Neurosurg.* 2007;109:634-638.

[92] Ruda R, Trevisan E, Soffietti R. Low-grade gliomas. *Handb Clin Neurol.* 2012;105:437-450.

[93] Englot DJ, Berger MS, Barbaro NM, Chang EF. Predictors of seizure freedom after resection of supratentorial low-grade gliomas. A review. *J Neurosurg.* 2011;115:240-244.

[94] Spalice A, Ruggieri M, Grosso S et al. Dysembryoplastic neuroepithelial tumors: a prospective clinicopathologic and outcome study of 13 children. *Pediatr Neurol.* 2010;43:395-402.

[95] Karremann M, Pietsch T, Janssen G, Kramm CM, Wolff JE. Anaplastic ganglioglioma in children. *J Neurooncol.* 2009;92:157-163.

[96] Razack N, Baumgartner J, Bruner J. Pediatric oligodendrogliomas. *Pediatr Neurosurg.* 1998;28:121-129.

[97] Wang KC, Chi JG, Cho BK. Oligodendroglioma in childhood. *J Korean Med Sci.* 1993;8:110-116.

[98] Lehman NL, Jordan MA, Huhn SL et al. Cortical ependymoma. A case report and review. *Pediatr Neurosurg.* 2003;39:50-54.

[99] Cuccia V, Zuccaro G, Sosa F, Monges J, Lubienieky F, Taratuto AL. Subependymal giant cell astrocytoma in children with tuberous sclerosis. *Childs Nerv Syst.* 2003;19:232-243.

[100] Amirjamshidi A, Mehrazin M, Abbassioun K. Meningiomas of the central nervous system occurring below the age of 17: report of 24 cases not associated with neurofibromatosis and review of literature. *Childs Nerv Syst.* 2000;16:406-416.

[101] Goldsby RE, Liu Q, Nathan PC et al. Late-occurring neurologic sequelae in adult survivors of childhood acute lymphoblastic leukemia: a report from the Childhood Cancer Survivor Study. *J Clin Oncol.* 2010;28:324-331.

[102] Karikari O, Thomas KK, Lagoo A, Cummings TJ, George TM. Primary cerebral ALK-1-positive anaplastic large cell lymphoma in a child. Case report and literature review. *Pediatr Neurosurg.* 2007;43:516-521.

[103] Astigarraga I, Lejarretta R, Navajas A, Fernandez-Teijeiro A, Imaz I, Bezanilla JL. Secondary central nervous system metastases in children with neuroblastoma. *Med Pediatr Oncol.* 1996;27:529-533.

[104] Lopez-Castilla J, Diaz-Fernandez F, Soult JA, Munoz M, Barriga R. Primary leptomeningeal melanoma in a child. *Pediatr Neurol.* 2001;24:390-392.

[105] Postovsky S, Ash S, Ramu IN et al. Central nervous system involvement in children with sarcoma. *Oncology.* 2003;65:118-124.

[106] Postovsky S, Moaed B, Krivoy E, Ofir R, Ben Arush MW. Practice of palliative sedation in children with brain tumors and sarcomas at the end of life. *Pediatr Hematol Oncol.* 2007;24:409-415.

[107] Shuper A, Cohen IJ, Mor C, Ash S, Kornreich L, Zaizov R. Metastatic brain involvement in Ewing family of tumors in children. *Neurology.* 1998;51:1336-1338.

[108] Spunt SL, Walsh MF, Krasin MJ et al. Brain metastases of malignant germ cell tumors in children and adolescents. *Cancer.* 2004;101:620-626.

[109] Kargiotis O, Markoula S, Kyritsis AP. Epilepsy in the cancer patient. *Cancer Chemother Pharmacol.* 2011;67:489-501.

[110] Hughlings-Jackson J. Localised convulsions from tumour of the brain. *Brain.* 1882;5:364-374.

[111] Jackson JH. Localized convulsions from tumors of the brain. *Brain.* 1882;36:4-374.

[112] Loiacono G, Cirillo C, Chiarelli F, Verrotti A. Focal epilepsy associated with glioneuronal tumors. *ISRN Neurol 2011:867503 doi: 10 5402/2011/867503 Epub 2011 Jul 7.* 2011.

[113] Rossetti AO, Stupp R. Epilepsy in brain tumor patients. *Curr Opin Neurol.* 2010;23:603-609.

[114] White JC, Liu CT, Mixter WJ. Focal epilepsy; a statistical study of its causes and the results of surgical treatment; epilepsy secondary to intracranial tumors. *N Engl J Med.* 1948;238:891-899.

[115] Zaatreh MM, Firlik KS, Spencer DD, Spencer SS. Temporal lobe tumoral epilepsy: characteristics and predictors of surgical outcome. *Neurology.* 2003;61:636-641.

[116] Consales A, Striano P, Nozza P et al. Glioneuronal tumors and epilepsy inchildren:seizureoutcome related to lesionectomy. *Minerva Pediatr.* 2013;65:609-616.

[117] Kim SK, Wang KC, Hwang YS et al. Epilepsy surgery in children: outcomes and complications. *J Neurosurg Pediatr.* 2008;1:277-283.

[118] Hirsch JF, Sainte Rose C, Pierre-Kahn A, Pfister A, Hoppe-Hirsch E. Benign astrocytic and oligodendrocytic tumors of the cerebral hemispheres in children. *J Neurosurg.* 1989;70:568-572.

[119] Luat AF, Behen ME, Juhasz C, Sood S, Chugani HT. Secondary tics or tourettism associated with a brain tumor. *Pediatr Neurol.* 2009;41:457-460.

[120] Goh KY, Conway EJ, DaRosso RC, Muszynski CA, Epstein FJ. Sympathetic storms in a child with a midbrain glioma: a variant of diencephalic seizures. *Pediatr Neurol.* 1999;21:742-744.

[121] Hottinger AF, Khakoo Y. Neuro-oncology of Neurofibromatosis Type 1. *Curr Treat Options Neurol.* 2009;11:306-314.

[122] Lu-Emerson C, Plotkin SR. The neurofibromatoses. Part 2: NF2 and schwannomatosis. *Rev Neurol Dis.* 2009;6:E81-E86.

[123] Goh S, Butler W, Thiele EA. Subependymal giant cell tumors in tuberous sclerosis complex. *Neurology.* 2004;63:1457-1461.

[124] Ferner RE, Huson SM, Thomas N et al. Guidelines for the diagnosis and management of individuals with neurofibromatosis 1. *J Med Genet.* 2007;44:81-8.

[125] Hou JW, Wang PJ, Wang TR. Tuberous sclerosis in children. *Zhonghua Min Guo Xiao Er Ke Yi Xue Hui Za Zhi.* 1994;35:102-107.

[126] Roaches ES, Gomez MR, Northrup H. Tuberous sclerosis complex consensus conference: revised clinical diagnostic criteria. *J Child Neurol.* 1998;13:624-628.

[127] Guerrini R, Rosati A, Giordano F, Genitori L, Barba C. The medical and surgical treatment of tumoral seizures: current and future perspectives. *Epilepsia.* 2013;54:84-90.

[128] Jansky J, Kovacs N, Gyimesi C, Fogarasi A, Doczi T, Wiebe S. Epilepsy surgery, antiepileptic drug trials, and the role of evidence. *Epilepsia.* 2010;51:1004-1009.

[129] Kumar A, Juhasz C, Asano E, Sood S, Muzik O, Chugani HT. Objective detection of epileptic foci by 18F-FDG PET in children undergoing epilepsy surgery. *J Nucl Med.* 2010;51:1901-1907.

[130] Maytal J, Krauss JM, Novak G, Nagelberg J, Patel M. The role of brain computed tomography in evaluating children with new onset of seizures in the emergency department. *Epilepsia.* 2000;41:950-954.

[131] Prabhu VC, Khaldi A, Barton KP et al. Management of diffuse low-grade cerebral gliomas. *Neurol Clin.* 2010;28:1037-1059.

[132] Sandberg DI, Ragheb J, Dunoyer C, Bhatia S, Olavarria G, Morrison G. Surgical outcomes and seizure control rates after resection of dysembryoplastic neuroepithelial tumors. *Neurosurg Focus.* 2005;18:E5.

[133] Spooner CG, Berkovic SF, Mitchell LA, Wrennal JA, Harvey AS. New-onset temporal lobe epilepsy in children: lesion on MRI predicts poor seizure outcome. *Neurology.* 2006;67:2147-2153.

[134] Taheri MR, Krauthamer A, Otjen J, Khanna PC, Ishak GE. Neuroimaging of migrational disorders in pediatric epilepsy. *Curr Probl Diagn Radiol.* 2012;41:11-19.

[135] Hardasmalani MD, Saber M. Yield of diagnostic studies in children presenting with complex febrile seizures. *Pediatr Emerg Care.* 2012;28:789-791.

[136] Lote K, Egeland T, Hager B et al. Survival, prognostic factors, and therapeutic efficacy in low-grade glioma: a retrospective study in 379 patients. *J Clin Oncol.* 1997;15:3129-3140.

[137] Recinos PF, Sciubba DM, Jallo GI. Brainstem tumors: where are we today? *Pediatr Neurosurg.* 2007;43:192-201.

[138] Shuper A, Kornreich L, Loven D, Michowitz S, Schwartz S, Cohen IJ. Diffuse brain stem gliomas. Are we improving outcome? *Childs Nerv Syst.* 1998;14:578-581.

[139] Freeman CR, Farmer JP. Pediatric brain stem gliomas: a review. *Int J Radiat Oncol Biol Phys*. 1998;40:265-271.

[140] van Breeman MS, Vecht CJ. Optimal seizure management in brain tumor patients. *Curr Neurol Neurosci Rep*. 2005;5:207-213.

[141] Vecht CJ, Wilms EB. Seizures in low-and high-grade gliomas: current management and future outlook. *Expert Rev Anticancer Ther*. 2010;10:663-669.

[142] Kwan P, Brodie MJ. Early identification of refractory epilepsy. *N Engl J Med*. 2000;342:314-319.

[143] Kwan P, Arzimanoglou A, Berg AT et al. Definition of drug resistant epilepsy: consensus proposal by the ad hoc Task Force of the ILAE Commission on Therapeutic Strategies. *Epilepsia*. 2010;51:1069-1077.

[144] Wiebe S. Effectiveness and safety of epilepsy surgery: what is the evidence? *CNS Spectr*. 2004;9:120-122.

[145] Kim YH, Park CK, Kim TM et al. Seizures during the management of high-grade gliomas: clinical relevance to disease progression. *J Neurooncol*. 2013;113:101-109.

[146] Verla T, Babu R, Agarwal V, Halvorson KG, Adamson DC. Treatment outcomes and prognostic factors of pediatric glioblastoma multiforme. *Neurosurgery*. 2014;61:217-218.

[147] Napolitino M, Vaz G, Lawson TM et al. Glioblastoma surgery with and without intraoperative MRI at 3.0T. *Neurochirurgie 2014 Jun 26 pii: S0028-3770(14)00064-2 doi: 10 1016/j neuchi 2014 03 010 [Epub ahead of print]*. 2014.

[148] Cataltepe O, Turanli G, Yalnizoglu D, Topcu M, Akalan N. Surgical management of temporal lobe tumor-related epilepsy in children. *J Neurosurg*. 2005;102:280-287.

[149] Uliel-Sibony S, Kramer U, Fried I, Fattal-Valevski A, Constantini S. Pediatric temporal low-grade glial tumors: epilepsy outcome following resection in 48 children. *Childs Nerv Syst*. 2011;27:1413-1418.

[150] Sherman JH, Moldovan K, Yeoh HK et al. Impact of temozolomide chemotherapy on seizure frequency in patients with low-grade gliomas. *J Neurosurg*. 2011;114:1617-1621.

[151] Cramer JA, Mintzer S, Wheless J, Mattson RH. Adverse effects of antiepileptic drugs: a brief overview of important issues. *Expert Rev Neurother*. 2010;10:885-891.

[152] Maschio M, Dinapoli L. Lecture: profile of risks and benefits of new antiepileptic drugs in brain tumor-related epilepsy. *Neurol Sci*. 2011;32:S259-S262.

[153] Taphoorm MJ. Neurocognitive sequelae in the treatment of low-grade gliomas. *Semin Oncol*. 2003;30:45-48.

[154] Chang EF, Quigg M, Oh DC et al. Predictors of efficacy after stereotactic radiosurgery for medial temporal lobe epilepsy. *Neurology.* 2010;74:165-172.

[155] Grenier Y, Tomita T, Marymont MH, Byrd S, Burrowes DM. Late postirradiation occlusive vasculopathy in childhood medulloblastoma. Report of two cases. *J Neurosurg.* 1998;89:460-464.

[156] Shuper A, Yaniv Y, Michowitz S et al. Epilepsy associated with pediatric brain tumors: the neuro-oncologic perspective. *Pediatr Neurol.* 2003;29:232-235.

[157] Jooma R, Yeh HS, Privitera MD, Gartner M. Lesionectomy versus electrophysiologically guided resection for temporal lobe tumors manifesting with complex partial seizures. *J Neurosurg.* 1995;83:231-236.

[158] Siegel AM. Presurgical evaluation and surgical treatment of medically refractory epilepsy. *Neurosurg Rev.* 2004;27:1-18.

[159] Pati S, Alexopoulos AV. Pharmacoresistant epilepsy: from pathogenesis to current and emerging therapies. *Cleve Clin J Med.* 2010;77:457-467.

[160] Riva M, Salmaggi A, Marchioni E et al. Tumour-associated epilepsy: clinical impact and the role of referring centres in a cohort of glioblastoma patients. A multicentre study from the Lombardia Neurooncology Group. *Neurol Sci.* 2006;27:345-351.

[161] Alexiou GA, Varela M, Sfakianos G, Prodromou N. Benign lesions accompanied by intractable epilepsy in children. *J Child Neurol.* 2009;24:697-700.

[162] Benifla M, Otsubo H, Ochi A et al. Temporal lobe surgery for intractable epilepsy in children: an analysis of outcomes in 126 children. *Neurosurgery.* 2006;59:1203-1213.

[163] Berger MS, Ghatan S, Haglund MM, Dobbins J, Ojemann GA. Low-grade gliomas associated with intractable epilepsy: seizure outcome utilizing electrocorticography during tumor resection. *J Neurosurg.* 1993;79:62-69.

[164] Chang EF, Christis C, Sullivan JE et al. Seizure control outcomes after resection of dysembryoplastic neuroepithelial tumor in 50 patients. *J Neurosurg Pediatr.* 2010;5:123-130.

[165] Duffau H, Capelle L, Lopes M, Bitar.A., Sichez JP, van Effenterre R. Medically intractable epilepsy from insular low-grade gliomas: improvement after an extended lesionectomy. *Acta Neurochir (Wien).* 2002;144:563-572.

[166] Fried I, Kim JH, Spencer DD. Limbic and neocortical gliomas associated with intractable seizures: a distinct clinicopathological group. *Neurosurgery.* 1994;34:815-823.

[167] Giuloni M, Rubboli G, Marucci G et al. Seizure outcome of epilepsy surgery in focal epilepsies associated with temporomesial glioneuronal tumors: lesionectomy compared with tailored resection. *J Neurosurg.* 2009;111:1275-1282.

[168] Packer RJ, Sutton LN, Patel KM et al. Seizure control following tumor surgery for childhood cortical low-grade gliomas. *J Neurosurg.* 1994;80:998-1003.

[169] Zentner J, Hufnagel A, Wolf HK et al. Surgical treatment of neoplasms associated with medically intractable epilepsy. *Neurosurgery.* 1997;41:378-386.

[170] Mehrotra N, Shamji MF, Vassilyada M, Ventureyra EC. Intracranial tumors in first year of life: the CHEO experience. *Childs Nerv Syst.* 2009;25:1563-1569.

[171] Steinbok P, Gan PY, Connolly MB et al. Epilepsy surgery in the first 3 years of life: a Canadian survey. *Epilepsia.* 2009;50:1442-1449.

[172] Stevens GH. Antiepileptic therapy in patients with central nervous system malignancies. *Curr Neurol Neurosci Rep.* 2006;6:311-318.

[173] Glantz MJ, Cole BF, Forsyth PA et al. Practice parameter: anticonvulsant prophylaxis in patients with newly diagnosed brain tumors. Report of the Quality Standards Subcommittee of the American Academy of Neurology. *Neurology.* 2000;54:1886-1893.

[174] Siomin V, Angelov L, Li L, Vogelbaum MA. Results of a survey of neurosurgical practice patterns regarding the prophylactic use of anti-epilepsy drugs in patients with brain tumors. *J Neurooncol.* 2005;74:211-215.

[175] van Breeman M, Wilms EB, Vecht CJ. Epilepsy in patients with brain tumours: epidemiology, mechanisms, and management. *Lancet Neurol.* 2007;6:421-430.

[176] Vecht CJ, van Breeman M. Optimizing therapy of seizures in patients with brain tumors. *Neurology.* 2006;67:S10-S13.

[177] Sirven JI, Wingerchuk DM, Drazkowski JF, Lyons MK, Zimmerman RS. Seizure prophylaxis in patients with brain tumors: a meta-analysis. *Mayo Clin Proc.* 2004;79:1489-1494.

[178] North JB, Penhall RK, Hanieh A, Frewin DB, Taylor WB. Phenytoin and postoperative epilepsy. A double-blind study. *J Neurosurg.* 1983;58:672-677.

[179] Hardesty DA, Sanborn MR, Parker WE, Storm PB. Perioperative seizure incidence and risk factors in 223 pediatric brain tumor patients without prior seizures. *J Neurosurg Pediatr.* 2011;7:609-615.

[180] Wu AS, Trinh VT, Suki D et al. A prospective randomized trial of perioperative seizure prophylaxis in patients with intraparenchymal brain tumors. *J Neurosurg.* 2013;118:873-883.

[181] Khan RB, Onar A. Seizure recurrence and risk factors after antiepilepsy drug withdrawal in children with brain tumors. *Epilepsia.* 2006;47:375-379.

[182] Bilginer B, Yalnizoglu D, Soylemezoglu F et al. Surgery for epilepsy in children with dysembryoplastic neuroepithelial tumor: clinical spectrum, seizure outcome, neuroradiology, and pathology. *Childs Nerv Syst.* 2009;25:485-491.

[183] Chan CH, Bittar RG, Davis GA, Kalnins RM, Fabinyi GC. Long-term seizure outcome following surgery for dysembryoplastic neuroepithelial tumor. *J Neurosurg.* 2006;104:62-69.

[184] Lee J, Lee BL, Joo EY et al. Dysembryoplastic neuroepithelial tumors in pediatric patients. *Brain Dev.* 2009;31:671-681.

[185] Ramantani G, Kadish NE, Anastasopoulos C et al. Epilepsy surgery for glioneuronal tumors in childhood: avoid loss of time. *Neurosurgery.* 2014;74:648-657.

[186] Chassoux F, Daumas-Duport C. Dysembryoplastic neuroepithelial tumors: where are we now?Chassoux F1, Daumas-Duport C. *Epilepsia.* 2013;54:129-134.

[187] Ruggiero A, Rizzo D, Mastrangelo S, Battaglia D, Attina G, Riccardi R. Interactions between antiepileptic and chemotherapeutic drugs in children with brain tumors: is it time to change treatment? *Pediatr Blood Cancer.* 2010;54:193-198.

[188] Baker SD, Wirth M, Statkevich P et al. Absorption, metabolism, and excretion of 14C-temozolomide following oral administration to patients with advanced cancer. *Clin Cancer Res.* 1999;5:309-317.

[189] Yang LJ, Zhou CF, Lin ZX. Temozolomide and radiotherapy for newly diagnosed glioblastoma multiforme: a systematic review. *Cancer Invest.* 2014;32:31-36.

[190] Pouratian N, Schiff D. Management of low-grade glioma. *Curr Neurol Neurosci Rep.* 2010;10:224-231.

[191] van den Bent MJ, Snijders TJ, Bromberg JE. Current treatment of low grade gliomas. *Memo.* 2012;5:223-227.

[192] Zhu W, Zhou L, Qian JQ, Qiu TZ, Shu YQ, Liu P. Temozolomide for treatment of brain metastases: A review of 21 clinical trials. *World J Clin Oncol.* 2014;5:19-27.

[193] Hummel TR, Chow LM, Fouladi M, Franz D. Pharmacotherapeutic management of pediatric gliomas : current and upcoming strategies. *Paediatr Drugs.* 2013;15:29-42.

[194] Packer RJ, Lange B, Ater J et al. Carboplatin and vincristine for recurrent and newly diagnosed low-grade gliomas of childhood. *J Clin Oncol.* 1993;11:850-856.

[195] Packer RJ, Ater J, Allen J et al. Carboplatin and vincristine chemotherapy for children with newly diagnosed progressive low-grade gliomas. *J Neurosurg.* 1997;86:747-754.

[196] Maschio M, Dinapoli L, Saveriano F et al. Efficacy and tolerability of zonisamide as add-on in brain tumor-related epilepsy: preliminary report. *Acta Neurol Scand.* 2009;120:210-212.

[197] Maschio M, Dinapoli L, Mingoia M et al. Lacosamide as add-on in brain tumor-related epilepsy: preliminary report on efficacy and tolerability. *J Neurol.* 2011;258:2100-2104.

[198]   Maschio M, Dinapoli L, Sperati F et al. Levetiracetam monotherapy in patients with brain tumor-related epilepsy: seizure control, safety, and quality of life. *J Neurooncol.* 2011;104:205-214.

[199]   Maschio M, Dinapoli L, Sperati F et al. Effect of pregabalin add-on treatment on seizure control, quality of life, and anxiety in patients with brain tumour-related epilepsy: a pilot study. *Epileptic Disord.* 2012;14:388-397.

[200]   Maschio M, Dinapoli L, Sperati F et al. Oxcarbazepine monotherapy in patients with brain tumor-related epilepsy: open-label pilot study for assessing the efficacy, tolerability and impact on quality of life. *J Neurooncol.* 2012;106:651-656.

[201]   Newton HB, Goldlust SA, Pearl D. Retrospective analysis of the efficacy and tolerability of levetiracetam in brain tumor patients. *J Neurooncol.* 2006;78:99-102.

[202]   Newton HB, Dalton J, Goldlust SA, Pearl D. Retrospective analysis of the efficacy and tolerability of levetiracetam in patients with metastatic brain tumors. *J Neurooncol.* 2007;84:293-296.

[203]   Novy.J., Stupp R, Rossetti AO. Pregabalin in patients with primary brain tumors and seizures: a preliminary observation. *Clin Neurol Neurosurg.* 2009;111:171-173.

[204]   Rossetti AO, Jeckelmann S, Novy.J., Roth P, Weller M, Stupp R. Levetiracetam and pregabalin for antiepileptic monotherapy in patients with primary brain tumors. A phase II randomized study. *Neuro Oncol.* 2014;16:584-588.

[205]   Cabanas R, Saurez G, Alert J et al. Prolonged use of nimotuzumab in children with central nervous system tumors: safety and feasibility. *Cancer Biother Radiopharm.* 2014;29:173-178.

[206]   Narayana A, Kunnakkat S, Chacko-Mathew J et al. Bevacizumab in recurrent high-grade pediatric gliomas. *Neuro Oncol.* 2010;12:985-990.

[207]   Boon P, Raedt R, de Herdt V, Wyckhuys T, Vonck K. Electrical stimulation for the treatment of epilepsy. *Neurotherapeutics.* 2009;6:218-227.

[208]   Chalifoux R, Elisevich K. Effect of ionizing radiation on partial seizures attributable to malignant cerebral tumors. *Stereotact Funct Neurosurg.* 1996;67:169-182.

[209]   Aronica E, Leenstra S, van Veelen CW et al. Glioneuronal tumors and medically intractable epilepsy: a clinical study with long-term follow-up of seizure outcome after surgery. *Epilepsy Res.* 2001;43:179-191.

[210]   Chuang NA, Yoon JM, Newbury RO, Crawford JR. Glioblastoma Multiforme Arising From Dysembryoplastic Neuroepithelial Tumor in a Child in the Absence of Therapy. *J Pediatr Hematol Oncol 2013 Dec 4 [Epub ahead of print].* 2013.

[211]   Moazzam AA, Wagle N, Shiroishi MS. Malignant transformation of DNETs: a case report and literature review. *Neuroreport.* 2014;25:894-899.

[212]   Moreno A, de Felipe J, Garcia Sola R, Navarro A, Ramon y Cajal S. Neuronal and mixed neuronal glial tumors associated to epilepsy. A heterogeneous and related group of tumours. *Histol Histopathol.* 2001;16:613-622.

[213]   Yang T, Pruthi S, Geyer JR, Ojemann JG. MRI changes associated with vigabatrin treatment mimicking tumor progression. *Pediatr Blood Cancer.* 2010;55:1221-1223.

[214]   Gelinas JN, Battison AW, Smith S, Connolly MB, Steinbok P. Electrocorticography and seizure outcomes in children with lesional epilepsy. *Childs Nerv Syst.* 2011;27:381-390.

[215]   Giulioni M, Galassi E, Zucchelli M, Volpi L. Seizure outcome of lesionectomy in glioneuronal tumors associated with epilepsy in children. *J Neurosurg Ped.* 2005;102:288-293.

[216]   Im SH, Chung CK, Cho BK, Lee SK. Supratentorial ganglioglioma and epilepsy: postoperative seizure outcome. *J Neurooncol.* 2002;57:59-66.

[217]   Kan P, Van Orman C, Kestle JR. Outcomes after surgery for focal epilepsy in children. *Childs Nerv Syst.* 2008;24:587-591.

[218]   Khajavi K, Comair YG, Wyllie E, Palmer J, Morris HH, Hahn JF. Surgical management of pediatric tumor-associated epilepsy. *J Child Neurol.* 1999;14:15-25.

[219]   Kim SK, Wang KC, Cho BK. Intractable seizures associated with brain tumor in childhood: lesionectomy and seizure outcome. *Childs Nerv Syst.* 1995;11:634-638.

[220]   Kim SK, Wang KC, Hwang YS, Kim KJ, Cho BK. Intractable epilepsy associated with brain tumors in children: surgical modality and outcome. *Childs Nerv Syst.* 2001;17:445-452.

[221]   Consales A, Striano P, Nozza P et al. Glioneuronal tumors and epilepsy inchildren:seizureoutcome related to lesionectomy. *Minerva Pediatr.* 2013;65:609-616.

[222]   Babini M, Giulioni M, Galassi E et al. Seizure outcome of surgical treatment of focal epilepsy associated with low-grade tumors in children. *J Neurosurg Pediatr.* 2013;11:214-223.

[223]   Jo KI, Chung SB, Jo KW, Kong DS, Seol HJ, Shin HJ. Microsurgical resection of deep-seated lesions using transparent tubular retractor: pediatric case series. *Childs Nerv Syst.* 2011;27:1989-1994.

[224]   Karnofsky DA, Burchenal JH. The Clinical Evaluation of Chemotherapeutic Agents in Cancer. In: MacLeod CM, ed. *Evaluation of Chemotherapeutic Agents.* New York, NY: Columbia University Press; 1949:196.

[225]   Grajkowska W, Kotulska K, Jurkiewicz E, Matyja E. Brain lesions in tuberous sclerosis complex. Review. *Folia Neuropathol.* 2010;48:139-149.

[226] Orlova KA, Crino PB. The tuberous sclerosis complex. *Ann N Y Acad Sci.* 2010;1184:87-105.

[227] Bourgeois M, Sainte-Rose C, Lellouch-Tubiana A et al. Surgery of epilepsy associated with focal lesions in childhood. *J Neurosurg.* 1999;90:833-842.

[228] Sonderkaer S, Schmiegelow M, Carstensen H, Nielsen LB, Muller J, Schmiegelow K. Long-term neurological outcome of childhood brain tumors treated by surgery only. *J Clin Oncol.* 2003;21:1347-1351.

[229] Mekitarian Filho E, Brunow de Carvalho W, Cavalheiro S, Horigoshi NK, Freddi NA. Perioperative factors associated with prolonged intensive care unit and hospital length of stay after pediatric neurosurgery. *Pediatr Neurosurg.* 2011;47:423-429.

[230] Drake JM, Riva-Cambrin J, Jea A, Auguste K, Tamber M, Lamberti-Pasculli M. Prospective surveillance of complications in a pediatric neurosurgery unit. *J Neurosurg Pediatr.* 2010;5:544-548.

[231] Graham GR. Blood volume in children. *Ann R Coll Surg Engl.* 1963;33:149-158.

[232] Guidance: Blood Draw Guidelines. University of Michigan Medical School. 2013. Ref Type: Electronic Citation

[233] Lobel DA. Pediatric Intensive Care Unit Management of Neurosurgical Diseases. In: Lobel DA, Lee MR, Duhaime A-C, eds. *The Central Nervous System in Pediatric Critical Illness and Injury.* London: Springer; 2009:1-10.

[234] Hammer GB, Krane EJ. Perioperative care of the child with acute neurological disease. In: Hammer GB, Andrews BT, eds. *Pediatric Neurosurgical Intensive Care.* Park Ridge, IL: American Association of Neurological Surgeons (AANS); 1997:25-36.

[235] Segura Matute S, Balaguer Gargallo M, Cambra Lasaosa FJ, Zambudio Sert S, Martin Rodrigo JM, Palomeque Rico A. [Fluid and electrolyte disorders following surgery for brain tumors]. [Article in Spanish]. *An Pediatr (Barc).* 2007;67:225-230.

[236] Hiranrat P, Katavetin P, Supornsilchai V, Wacharasindhu S, Srivuthana S. Water and sodium disorders in children undergoing surgical treatment of brain tumors. *J Med Assoc Thai.* 2003;86:S152-S159.

[237] Spentzas T, Escue JE, Patters AB, Varelas PN. Brain tumor resection in children: neurointensive care unit course and resource utilization. *Pediatr Crit Care Med.* 2010;11:718-722.

[238] Pruitt AA. Treatment of Medical Complications in Patients with Brain Tumors. *Curr Treat Options Neurol.* 2005;7:323-336.

[239] Michelucci R. Optimizing therapy of seizures in neurosurgery. *Neurology.* 2006;67:S14-S18.

[240] Asano E, Benedek K, Shah A et al. Is intraoperative electrocorticography reliable in children with intractable neocortical epilepsy? *Epilepsia.* 2004;45:1091-1099.

[241] Wennberg R, Quesney LF, Lozano A, Olivier A, Rasmussen T. Role of electrocorticography at surgery for lesion-related frontal lobe epilepsy. *Can J Neurol Sci.* 1999;26:33-39.

[242] Lombardi D, Marsh R, de Tribolet N. Low grade glioma in intractable epilepsy: lesionectomy versus epilepsy surgery. *Acta Neurochir Suppl.* 1997;68:70-74.

[243] Terra-Bustamante VC, Inuzuka LM, Fernandes RM et al. Outcome of hemispheric surgeries for refractory epilepsy in pediatric patients. *Childs Nerv Syst.* 2007;23:321-326.

[244] Butman JA, Linehan WM, Lonser RR. Neurologic manifestations of von Hippel-Lindau disease. *JAMA.* 2008;300:1334-1342.

[245] Richard S, Campello C, Taillandier L, Parker F, Resche F. Haemangioblastoma of the central nervous system in von Hippel-Lindau disease. French VHL Study Group. *J Intern Med.* 1998;243:547-553.

[246] Shanley S, Ratcliffe J, Hockey A, et al. Nevoid basal cell carcinoma syndrome: review of 118 affected individuals. *Am J MedGenet.* 1994;50:282-290.

[247] Yang T, Temkin N, Barber J et al. Gross total resection correlates with long-term survival in pediatric patients with glioblastoma. *World Neurosurg.* 2013;79:537-544.

[248] Hart MG, Garside R, Rogers G, Stein K, Grant R. Temozolomide for high grade glioma. *Cochrane Database Syst Rev 2013 Apr 30;4:CD007415 doi: 10 1002/14651858 CD007415 pub2.* 2013.

[249] Ho RHVK, Reijneveld JC, Enting et al. Changing incidence and improved survival of gliomas. *Eur J Cancer 2014 Jun 24 pii: S0959-8049(14)00718-7 doi: 10 1016/j ejca 2014 05 019 [Epub ahead of print].* 2014.

[250] Weller M, Gorlia T, Cairncross JG et al. Prolonged survival with valproic acid use in the EORTC/NCIC temozolomide trial for glioblastoma. *Neurology.* 2011;77:1156-1164.

[251] Evans DG, Birch JM, Ramsden RT, Sharif S, Baser ME. Malignant transformation and new primary tumours after therapeutic radiation for benign disease: substantial risks in certain tumour prone syndromes. *J Med Genet.* 2006;43:289-294.

[252] Osipov V, Ho KC, Krouwer HG, Meyer G, Shidham VB. Post-radiation dedifferentiation of meningioma into osteosarcoma. *BMC Cancer.* 2002;2:34.

[253] Pereira EA, Dabbous B, Qureshi HU, Ansorge O, Bojanic S. Rapid development of glioblastoma at the site of atypical meningioma resection. *Br J Neurosurg.* 2010;24:471-473.

[254] Gonzalez-Martinez JA, Srikijvilaikul T, Nair D, Bingaman WE. Long-term seizure outcome in reoperation after failure of epilepsy surgery. Neurosurgery. 2007;60:873-880.

[255] Ojemann JG, Hersonskey TY, Abeshaus S et al. Epilepsy surgery after treatment of pediatric malignant brain tumors. Seizure. 2012;21:624-630.

[256] Tian AG, Edwards MS, Williams AJ, Olson DM. Epilepsy surgery following brain tumor resection in children. J Neurosurg Pediatr. 2011;7:229-234.

8

Radiation-Induced Glioma

Ryuya Yamanaka and Azusa Hayano

1. Introduction

Radiation therapy is widely used for patients with intracranial tumors. However, there are many complications, including cerebral atrophy, calcifying microangiopathy, radiation necrosis, leukoencephalopathy and development of radiation-induced tumors [1-5]. Radiation-induced central nervous system (CNS) neoplasms are recognized in patients who have had therapeutic radiotherapy to the head or face [6]. Radiation-induced CNS neoplasms are rare, but the cumulative risk of brain tumor after therapeutic cranial irradiation is reported as 0.5-2.7% at 15 years [7]. Among radiation-induced CNS neoplasms, meningiomas are about 70%, gliomas about 20% and sarcomas less than 10% [4,6,8]. In children, high-grade gliomas are the most common radiation-induced tumor [9]. Type of post-radiation gliomas are glioblastoma (GBM) in 75% and anaplastic astrocytoma in 25% [7]. Brada et al. [6] described a relative risk of secondary glioma of 7.92 times higher than that of the normal non-irradiated population, with an average latency period to glioma diagnosis of 7 years, in 334 patients with pituitary lesions, irradiated to a median dose of 45 Gy for the sellar region. Cahan et al. [10] established criteria to diagnose a radiotherapy induced brain tumor. These criteria were modified in 1972 by Schrantz and Araoz [11] as follows:(1) the tumor must appear within the irradiated field; (2) the tumor was not present prior to the radiotherapy; (3) a sufficient latency period must elapse between irradiation and appearance of the tumor (usually>5 years); (4) the radiation induced tumor must be histologically proven and a different histological type from the original neoplasm treated by the radiation therapy.

2. Radiation-induced gliomas in the literature

In a review of the literature, 191 cases of radiation-induced glioma that analyzed in detail were identified in the period 1960-2014 [9,12-120]. The latency period from the irradiation to the onset of the secondary glioma ranged from 6 months to 50 years, with an average of 11.1 years. More than 40 Gy irradiation was delivered in 50% of cases, with an average of 37.2 Gy. As shown in Table 1, 29 grade II, 37 grade III and 97 grade IV gliomas had been reported, and no specific grade had been shown in other 28 cases. Grade II gliomas developed after 10.7 years, and grade IV gliomas developed after 10.6 years from the time of irradiation. The radiation dose of grade II gliomas for primary lesion is 29.7 Gy, grade III 37.4 Gy and grade IV 37.3 Gy, respectively. There was a significant difference of radiation dose between grade II and grade IV glioma (p<0.05). In Table 2 and 3, the relation of primary lesion and radiation dose, latency to radiation induced glioma occurrence, glioma grade are shown. The latency in acute lymphoblastic leukemia (ALL) / acute myeloblastic leukemia (AML), Hodgkin/non-Hodgkin lymphoma and cancer patients is short compared to that of intracranial and scalp lesion. And, the irradiated dose in ALL/AML patients is rather small compared to that of intracranial lesion. Patients with ALL/AML and Hodgkin/non-Hodgkin lymphoma are usually intensively treated with anticancer agents with carcinogenic effects, so the patients may suffer from glioma by the synergistic effects of prophylactic irradiation and chemotherapy.

WHO grade	Number of cases	Irradiated dose (Gy)	Latency (years)
Grade II	29	29.7±18.4	10.7±7.7
Grade III	37	37.4±15.9	12.6±8.6
Grade IV	97	37.3±17.5	10.7±6.6

Table 1. Radiation induced glioma

	Number of cases	Irradiated dose (Gy)	Latency (years)	Radiation induced glioma
Pituitary adenoma	20	52.2±12.7	13.5±7.5	Grade III/IV 16, II 3
Craniopharyngioma	15	63.9±7.0	11.7±7.0	Grade III/IV 13, II 1
Medulloblastoma	16	44.9±9.5	15.8±12.2	Grade III/IV 12, II 4
Germ cell tumor	10	44.9±8.5	15.2±13.4	Grade III/IV 9, II 1
Optic glioma/ Retinoblastoma	6	46.5±10.9	7.2±2.4	Grade IV 6
Menigioma/Neurinoma	6	38.4±14.2	10±5.7	Grade III/IV 5, II 1
Low grade glioma	12	47.0±7.8	13.5±10.1	Grade III/IV 11, II 1

Table 2. Radiation induced glioma of intracranial primary lesion

	Number of cases	Irradiated dose (Gy)	Latency (years)	Radiation induced glioma
ALL/AML	64	23.6±7.6	8.6±3.9	Grade III/IV 52, II 10
Hodgkin/non-Hodgkin Lymphoma	6	35.6±10.7	8±5.7	Grade III/IV 6
Cancer	6	60.5±15.4	8±3.2	Grade III/IV 6
Scalp lesion (non-cancer)	14	12.2±12.1	15.5±9.2	Grade III/IV 9, II 5

ALL: acute lymphoblastic leukemia, AML: acute myeloblastic leukemia

Table 3. Radiation induced glioma of extracranial primary lesion

3. Genetic characteristics of radiation-induced glioma

In a patient reported by Gessi [36], the genetic alterations were p53 mutation (C to G transition at codon 176 of Exon 5), loss of heterozygosity (LOH) of 17p and 19q, O(6)-methylguanine DNA methyltransferase (MGMT) promoter methylation, and no amplification of epidermal growth factor receptor (EGFR). In Yang's case [115], p53 mutation (deletion at codon 233 of Exon 7 and a C to G transition at codon 278 of Exon 8) and no amplification of EGFR were reported. In Tada's case [104], 3-bp homozygous deletion in exon 7 of the p53 gene was described. In Kon's case [58], although LOH and amplification of EGFR, phosphatase and tensin analog (PTEN) was not observed, LOH of 1p, K-ras, p16, p53 were observed. In Alexous's two cases, LOH of 1p was found in both cases [15]. Nine radiation-induced high-grade gliomas were studied for possible molecular alterations in p53, PTEN, K-ras, EGFR, and p16 by Brat [121]. Exon 8 of p53 gene mutation (G to A substitution in codon 285) is detected in one case, EGFR amplification in 2 cases and p16/ methylthioadenosine phosphorylase (MTAP) gene deletion in 2 cases [121]. However, genetic alterations similar to those described in spontaneous, sporadic primary GBM, except the absence of PTEN mutations in the radia-tion-induced group were found. Radiation-induced GBMs have a lower percent of EGFR and p16 alterations than primary GBM [121]. Donson et al. [122] demonstrated by gene expression analysis genetic homogenity relative to de-novo gliomas, suggesting a common precursor cell for radiation-induced gliomas. It is not well known about the molecular alteration of radiation-induced gliomas, due to the limited number of cases and limited genes were analyzed.

4. Therapeutic implications

Radiation-induced glioma is difficult to treat; radiotherapy is not always a therapeutic option because the patient has already been exposed to radiation. However there are several patients reported who had a sustained remission following chemotherapy alone or radiochemothera-py. About the reports of treatment of radiation-induced glioma, a dramatic response and prolonged survival by carmustine, nimustine hydrochloride and temozolomide were reported [52, 58, 71, 75]. These tumors have a poor prognosis due to their intrinsic resistance to treatment and the difficulty using aggressive therapies in previously irradiated patients. However, vigorous chemotherapeutic approaches may yield prolonged disease control in some patients with radiation-induced glioma. The relationship of 1p LOH and chemosensitivity in oligo-dendroglial tumors is well known [123]. 1p LOH may account for the marked response to chemotherapy [52,58], although the reason of the chemosensitivity is not discussed in other case. In Fukui's case [32], 40 Gy of local radiotherapy and chemotherapy with nimustine hydrochloride and Interferone-β yielded dramatic response. The patient received 15 Gy of whole brain radiotherapy 7 years prior to the onset of radiation-induced glioma. Although the tolerable radiation dose is not well known after initial radiation therapy, additional radio-therapeutic approaches may yield prolonged disease control in some patients with radiation-induced glioma. The marked chemo and radiosensitivity should be further investigated for the development of glioma therapy.

5. Conclusion

In case that intracranial and extracranial lesions are treated by standard fractionated radiation or stereotatic radiosurgery, radiation-induced gliomas should be considered as possible long-term side effect. And the patients should be followed for a long term, even long after the period of risk for relapse of the primary site has passed.

Author details

Ryuya Yamanaka* and Azusa Hayano

*Address all correspondence to: ryaman@koto.kpu-m.ac.jp

Graduate School for Health Care Science, Kyoto Prefectural University of Medicine, Kyoto, Japan

References

[1] Mikhael MA. Radiation necrosis of the brain: correlation between patterns on com-puted tomography and dose of radiation. J Comput Assist Tomogr 1979;3(2):241-9.

[2] Jacoby CG, Tewfik HH, Blackwelder JT. Cerebellar atrophy developing after cranial irradiation. J Comput Assist Tomogr 1982;6(1):159-62.

[3]   Dooms GC, Hecht S, Brant-Zawadzki M, Berthiaume Y, Norman D, Newton TH. Brain radiation lesions. MR imaging. Radiology 1986;158(1):149-55.

[4]   Ron E, Modan B, Boice JD Jr, Alfandary E, Stovall M, Chetrit A, Katz L. Tumors of the brain and nervous system after radiotherapy in childhood. N Engl J Med 1988; 319(16):1033-9.

[5]   Devivo DC, Malas D, Nelson JS, Land VJ. Leukoencephaly in childhood leukemia. Neurology 1997;27(7):609-13.

[6]   Brada M, Ford D, Ashley S, Bliss JM, Crowley S, Mason M, Rajan B, Traish D. Risk of second brain tumour after conservative surgery and radiotherapy for pituitary adenoma. Br Med J 1992;304(6838):1343-6.

[7]   Paulino AC, Mai WY, Chintagumpala M, Taher A, Teh BS. Radiation-induced malignant gliomas: is there a role for reirradiation? Int J Radiat Oncol Biol Phys 2008;71:1381-7.

[8]   Musa BS, Pople IK, Cummins BH. Intracranial meningiomas following irradiation--a growing problem? Br J Neurosurg 1995;9(5):629-37.

[9]   Pettorini BL, Park YS, Caldarelli M, Massimi L, Tamburrini G, Di Rocco C. Radiation-induced brain tumours after central nervous system irradiation in childhood: a review. Childs Nerv Syst 2008; 24: 793–805.

[10] Cahan WG, Woodard HQ, Higinbotham NL, Stewart FW, Coley EL. Sarcoma arising in irradiated bone; report of 11 cases. Cancer1948; 1(1):3-29.

[11] Schrantz JL, Araoz CA. Radiation induced meningeal fibrosarcoma. Arch Pathol 1972;93(1):26-31.

[12] Ahn SJ, Kim IO. Spinal cord glioblastoma induced by radiation therapy of nasopharyngeal rhabdomyosarcoma with MRI findings: case report. Korean J Radiol 2012;13(5):652-7.

[13] Albert RE, Omran AR, Brauer EW, Freed R. Follow-up study of patients treated by X-ray for tinea capitis. Am J Public Health 1966; 56:2114–20.

[14] Alexander MJ, DeSalles AA, Tomiyasu U. Multiple radiation-induced intracranial lesions after treatment for pituitary adenoma. Case report. J Neurosurg 1998;88(1): 111-5.

[15] Alexiou GA, Moschovi M, Georgoulis G, Neroutsou R, Stefanaki K, Sfakianos G, Prodromou N. Anaplastic oligodendrogliomas after treatment of acute lymphoblastic leukemia in children: report of 2 cases. J Neurosurg Pediatr 2010;5(2):179-83.

[16] Anderson JR, Treip CS. Radiation-induced intracranial neoplasms: a report of three possible cases. Cancer 1984; 53:426–9.

[17] Bachman DS, Ostrow PT. Fatal long-term sequela following radiation "cure" for ependymoma. Ann Neurol 1978; 4:319–21.

[18] Balasubramaniam A, Shannon P, Hodaie M, Laperriere N, Michaels H, Guha A. Glioblastoma multiforme after stereotactic radiotherapy for acoustic neuroma: case report and review of the literature. Neuro Oncol 2007;9(4):447-53.

[19] Barnes ARE, Liwnicz BH, Schellhas HE, Altshuller G, Aron BS, Lippert WR. Successful treatment of placental choriocarcinoma metastatic to brain followed by primary brain glioblastoma. Gynecol Oncol 1982;13:108–14.

[20] Bazan C, New PZ, Kaghan-Hallet KS. MRI of radiation-induced spinal cord glioma. Neuroradiology 1990;32:331–3.

[21] Berman EL, Eade TN, Brown D, Weaver M, Glass J, Zorman G, Feigenberg SJ. Radiation-induced tumor after stereotactic radiosurgery for an arteriovenous malformation: case report. Neurosurgery 2007;61(5):E1099.

[22] Beute BJ, Fobben ES, Hubschmann O, Zablow A, Eanelli T, Solitare G. Cerebellar gliosarcoma: report of a probable radiation-induced neoplasm. AJNR 1991;12:554–6.

[23] Bonilha L, Borges G, Fernandes YB, Ramina R, Carelli EF, Alvarenga M. Pilocytic astrocytoma following radiotherapy for craniopharyngioma: case report. Arq Neuropsiquiatr 2000;58(3A):731-5.

[24] Chung CK, Stryker JA, Cruse R, Vanucci R, Towfighi J. Glioblastoma multiforme following prophylactic cranial irradiation and intrathecal methotrexate in a child with acute lymphoblastic leukaemia. Cancer 1980; 47:2563–6.

[25] Clifton MD, Amromin GD, Perry MC, Abadir R, Watts C, Levy N. Spinal cord glioma following irradiation for Hodgkin's disease. Cancer 1980; 45:2051–5.

[26] Cohen MS, Kushner MJ, Dell S. Frontal lobe astrocytoma following radiotherapy for medulloblastoma. Neurology 1988; 31:616–9.

[27] Diersse G, Alvarez G, Figols J. Anaplastic astrocytoma associated with previous radiotherapy: report of three cases. Neurosurgery 1988; 6:1095–7.

[28] Doskaliyev A, Yamasaki F, Kenjo M, Shrestha P, Saito T, Hanaya R, Sugiyama K, Kurisu K. Secondary anaplastic oligodendroglioma after cranial irradiation: a case report. J Neurooncol 2008;88(3):299-303.

[29] Edwards MK, Terry JG, Montebello JF, Hornback NB, Kuharik MA. Gliomas in children following radiation therapy for lymphoblastic leukemia. Acta Radiol Suppl 1986;369:651-3.

[30] Enchev Y, Ferdinandov D, Kounin G, Encheva E, Bussarsky V. Radiation-induced gliomas following radiotherapy for craniopharyngiomas: a case report and review of the literature. Clin Neurol Neurosurg 2009;111(7):591-6.

[31]   Fontana M, Stanton C, Pompili A, Amadori S, Mandelli F, Meloni G, Riccio A, Rubin-
       stein LJ. Late multifocal gliomas in adolescents previously treated for lymphoblastic
       leukaemia. Cancer 1987; 60:1510–8.

[32]   Fukui K, Inamura T, Nakamizo A, Ikezaki K, Inoha S, Nakamura K, Matsuzaki A,
       Fukui M. A case showing effective radiotherapy for a radiation-induced glioblasto-
       ma. No Shinkei Geka 2001;29(7):673-7.

[33]   Fuller GN, Kaba SE, Ginsberg LE, McCutcheon IE, Langford LA. Late sequelae of
       treated pleomorphic xanthoastrocytoma: malignant brain stem astrocytoma occur-
       ring 15 years after radiation therapy. J Neurooncol 1997;32(1):57-61.

[34]   Furuta T, Sugiu K, Tamiya T, Matsumoto K, Ohmoto T. Malignant cerebellar astrocy-
       toma developing 15 years after radiation therapy for a medulloblastoma. Clin Neurol
       Neurosurg 1998;100(1):56-9.

[35]   García-Navarro V, Tena-Suck ML, Celis MA, Vega R, Rembao D, Salinas C. Anaplas-
       tic astrocytoma post radiotherapy of pineal germinoma. Arq Neuropsiquiatr
       2009;67(3A):707-9.

[36]   Gessi M, Maderna E, Guzzetti S, Cefalo G, Massimino M, Solero CL, Finocchiaro G,
       Pollo B. Radiation-induced glioblastoma in a medulloblastoma patient: a case report
       with molecular features. Neuropathology 2008;28(6):633-9.

[37]   Grabb PA, Kelly DR, Fulmer BB, Palmer C. Radiation-induced glioma of the spinal
       cord. Pediatr Neurosurg 1996;25:214–9.

[38]   Guthjahr P, Dietrich E. Risiko zweiter maligner neoplasien nach erfolgreicher Tu-
       morbehadlung in Kindersalter. Deutch Med Wochenshr 1979; 104:969–72.

[39]   Hamasaki K, Nakamura H, Ueda Y, Makino K, Kuratsu J. Radiation-induced glio-
       blastoma occurring 35 years after radiation therapy for medulloblastoma: case report.
       Brain Tumor Pathol 2010;27(1):39-43.

[40]   Haselow RE, Nesbit M, Dehner LP, Knam FM, McHugh R, Lewitt SH. Second neo-
       plasm following megavoltage radiation in a pediatric population. Cancer 1978;
       42:1185–91.

[41]   Hill MD, Mackenzie I, Mason WP. Radiation-induced glioma presenting as diffuse
       leptomeningeal gliomatosis: a case report. J Neurooncol 2001;55(2):113-6.

[42]   Huang CI, Chiou WH, Ho DM. Oligodendroglioma occurring after radiation therapy
       for pituitary adenoma. J Neurol Neurosurg Psychiatry 1987;50(12):1619-24.

[43]   Hufnagel TJ, Kim JH, Lesser R, Miller JM, Abrahams JJ, Piepmeier J, Manuelidis EE.
       Malignant glioma of optic chiasm eight years after radiotherapy for prolactinoma.
       Arch Ophtalmol 1988;106:1701–5.

[44]   Jones A. Supervoltage X-ray therapy after of intracranial tumors. Ann R Soc Surg
       Eng1960;27:310–54.

[45] Judge MR, Eden OB, O'Neill P. Cerebral glioma after cranial prophylaxis for acute lymphoblastic leukaemia. Br Med J (Clin Res Ed) 1984; 289:1038-9.

[46] Kaido T, Hoshida T, Uranishi R, Akita N, Kotani A, Nishi N, Sakaki T. Radiosurgery-induced brain tumor: case report. J Neurosurg 2001;95:710-3.

[47] Kamide T, Nakada M, Hayashi Y, Suzuki T, Hayashi Y, Uchiyama N, Kijima T, Hamada J. Radiation-induced cerebellar high-grade glioma accompanied by meningioma and cavernoma 29 years after the treatment of medulloblastoma: a case report. J Neurooncol 2010;100(2):299-303.

[48] Kaschten B, Flandroy P, Reznik M, Hainaut H, Stevenaert A. Radiation-induced gliosarcoma: case report and review of the literature. J Neurosurg 1995;83:154-62.

[49] Kato N, Kayama T, Sakurada K, Saino M, Kuroki A. Radiation-induced glioblastoma: a case report. No To Shinkei 2000;52:413-8.

[50] Kawaguchi S, Kashiwaba T, Koiwa M, Shimoyama M, Kobayashi N, Fukushi Y, Tokuda K. Two autopsied cases of radiation-induced gliosarcoma. No Shinkei Geka 1991;19(3):285-90.

[51] Kawanabe Y, Sawada M, Yukawa H, Ueda S, Sasaki N, Koizumi T, Kihara S, Hoshimaru M. Radiation-induced spinal cord anaplastic astrocytoma subsequent to radiotherapy for testicular seminoma. Neurol Med Chir (Tokyo) 2012;52(9):675-8.

[52] Khoo HM, Kishima H, Kinoshita M, Goto Y, Kagawa N, Hashimoto N, Maruno M, Yoshimine T. Radiation-induced anaplastic ependymoma with a remarkable clinical response to temozolomide: a case report. Br J Neurosurg 2013;27(2):259-61.

[53] Kikkawa Y, Suzuki SO, Nakamizo A, Tsuchimochi R, Murakami N, Yoshitake T, Aishima S, Okubo F, Hata N, Amano T, Yoshimoto K, Mizoguchi M, Iwaki T, Sasaki T. Radiation-induced spinal cord glioblastoma with cerebrospinal fluid dissemination subsequent to treatment of lymphoblastic lymphoma. Surg Neurol Int. 2013;4:27.

[54] Kitanaka C, Shitara N, Nakagomi T, Nakamura H, Genka S, Nakagawa K, Akanuma A, Aoyama H, Takakura K. Postradiation astrocytoma: report of two cases. J Neurosurg 1989;70:469-74.

[55] Kleriga E, Sher JH, Nallainathan SK, Stein SC, Sacher M. Development of cerebellar malignant astrocytoma at site of medulloblastoma treated 11 years earlier. J Neurosurg 1979;49:445-9.

[56] Komaki S, Komaki R, Chol H, Correa-Paz F. Radiation and drug-induced intracranial neoplasm with angiographic demonstration. Neurol Med Chir (Tokio) 1977;17:55-62.

[57] Komatsu F, Kawaguchi H, Tsugu H, Oshiro S, Komatsu M, Fukushima T, Nabeshima K, Inoue T. Radiation-induced astrocytoma with rapid malignant transformation: case report. Neurol Med Chir (Tokyo) 2011;51(3):243-6.

[58] Kon T, Natsumeda M, Taki T, Takahashi H, Fujii Y, Yamanaka R. Radiation-induced glioblastoma following radiotherapy for pituitary adenomas: marked response to chemotherapy. J Neurol Neurophysiol 2013;4:155.

[59] Lach M, Wallace CJ, Krcek J, Curry B. Radiation-associated gliosarcoma. Can Assoc Radiol J 1996;47(3):209-12.

[60] Leung J, Guiney M. Secondary tumours after prophylactic cranial irradiation. Australas Radiol 1996;40(1):43-4.

[61] Liwnicz BH, Berger TS, Liwnicz RG. Radiation associated gliomas. A report of four cases and analysis of postradiation tumors of the central nervous system. Neurosurgery 1985;17:436–45.

[62] Loeffler JS, Niemierko A, Chapman P. Second tumors after radiosurgery: tip of the iceberg or a bump in the road? Neurosurgery 2003; 52:1436–42.

[63] Maat-Schieman MLC, Bots GTAM, Thomeer RTWM. Malignant astrocytoma following radiotherapy for craniopharyngioma. Br J Radiol 1985; 58:480–2.

[64] Malde R, Jalali R, Muzumdar D, Shet T, Kurkure P. Gliosarcoma occurring 8 years after treatment for a medulloblastoma. Childs Nerv Syst 2004;20(4):243-6.

[65] Malone M, Lumley H, Erdohazi M. Astrocytoma as a second malignancy in patients with acute lymphoblastic leukaemia. Cancer 1986;57:1979–85.

[66] Marus G, Levin V, Rutherford GS. Malignant glioma following radiotherapy for unrelated primary tumors. Cancer 1986; 58:886–94.

[67] Matsumura H, Takimoto H, Shirata M, Hirata M, Ohnishi T, Hayakawa T. Glioblastoma following radiotherapy in a patient with tuberous sclerosis. Neurol Med Chir (Tokio) 1998; 38:287–91.

[68] McWhirter WR, Pearn JH, Smith H, O'Regan P. Cerebral astrocytoma as a complication of acute lymphoblastic leukaemia. Med J Aust 1986;45:96–7.

[69] Menon G, Nair S, Rajesh BJ, Rao BR, Radhakrishnan VV.Malignant astrocytoma following radiotherapy for craniopharyngioma. J Cancer Res Ther 2007;3(1):50-2.

[70] Miyazawa T, Aida S, Shima K. Hemorrhagic cerebellar anaplastic glioma appearing 12 years after prophylactic cranial radiotherapy for acute lymphocytic leukemia. Neurol Med Chir (Tokyo) 2008;48(3):126-30.

[71] Monje ML, Ramakrishna NR, Young G, Drappatz J, Doherty LM, Wen PY, Kesari S. Durable response of a radiation-induced, high-grade cerebellar glioma to temozolomide. J Neurooncol 2007;84(2):179-83.

[72] Myong NH, Park BJ. Malignant glioma arising at the site of an excised cerebellar hemangioblastoma after irradiation in a von Hippel-Lindau disease patient. Yonsei Med J 2009;50(4):576-81.

[73] Muzumdar DP, Desai K, Goel A. Glioblastoma multiforme following prophylactic cranial irradiation and intrathecal methotrexate on a child with acute lymphoblastic leukaemia: a case report. Neurol India 1999; 47:142–4.

[74] Ng C, Fairhall J, Rathmalgoda C, Stening W, Smee R. Spinal cord glioblastoma multiforme induced by radiation after treatment for Hodgkin disease. Case report. J Neurosurg Spine 2007;6(4):364-7.

[75] Nicolardi L, DeAngelis LM. Response to chemotherapy of a radiation-induced glioblastoma multiforme. J Neurooncol 2006;78(1):55-7.

[76] Nishio S, Morioka T, Inamura T, Takeshita I, Fukui M, Sasaki M, Nakamura K, Wakisaka S. Radiation-induced brain tumors: potential late complications of radiation therapy for brain tumors. Acta Neurochir 1998;140:763–70.

[77] Okamoto S, Handa H, Yamashita J. Post-irradiation brain tumors. Neurol Med Chir (Tokyo) 1985;25:528–33.

[78] Osumi AK, Mclendon RE, Tien RD, Friedman HS, Graham M, Hockenberger B, Halperin EC, Oakes WJ. Well differentiated astrocytoma occurring nine years after radiation therapy for medulloblastoma. Clin Neuropathol 1994;13(5):281-5.

[79] Palma L, Vagnozzi R, Annino L, Ciappetta P, Maleci A, Cantore GP. Post-radiation glioma in a child. Case report and review of the literature. Child's Nervous System 1988;4:296–301.

[80] Pearl GS, Mirra SS, Miles ML. Glioblastoma multiforme occurring 13 years after treatment of a medulloblastoma. Neurosurgery 1980;6:546–51.

[81] Platt JH, Blue JM, Schold SC, Burger PC. Glioblastoma multiforme after radiotherapy for acromegaly. Neurosurgery 1983;13:85–9.

[82] Preissig SH, Bohmfalk GL, Reichel GW, Smith M. Anaplastic astrocytoma following radiation for a glomus jugulare tumor. Cancer 1979;43:2243–7.

[83] Raffel C, Edwards MSB, Davis RL, Albin AR. Postirradiation cerebellar glioma: case report. J Neurosurg 1985;63:300–3.

[84] Rappaport ZH, Loren D, Ben-Ahron A. Radiation-induced cerebellar glioblastoma multiforme subsequent to treatment of an astrocytoma of the cervical spinal cord. Neurosurgery 1991;4:606–8.

[85] Riffaud L, Bernard M, Lesimple T, Morandi X. Radiation-induced spinal cord glioma subsequent to treatment of Hodgkin's disease: case report and review. J Neurooncol 2006;76(2):207-11.

[86] Rimm IL, Li FC, Tarbell NJ, Winston KR, Sallan SE. Brain tumors after cranial irradiation for childhood acute lymphoblastic leukaemia: a 13-years experience from Dana-Farber Cancer Institute and The Children's Hospital. Cancer 1987;59:1506–8.

[87]   Rittinger O, Kranzinger M, Jones R, Jones N. Malignant astrocytoma arising 10 years
       after combined treatment of craniopharyngioma. J Pediatr Endocrinol Metab 2003;
       16: 97–101.

[88]   Robinson RG. A second brain tumor and irradiation. J Neurol Neurosurg Psychiatry
       1978;41:1005–12.

[89]   Saenger EL, Silverman FN, Sterling FT, Turner ME. Neoplasia following therapeutic
       irradiation for benign conditions in childhood. Radiology 1960;74:889–904.

[90]   Saiki S, Kinouchi T, Usami M, Nakagawa H, Kotake T. Glioblastoma multiforme af-
       ter radiotherapy for metastatic brain tumor of testicular cancer. Int J Urol 1997;4(5):
       527-9.

[91]   Salvati M, D'Elia A, Melone GA, Brogna C, Frati A, Raco A, Delfini R. Radio-induced
       gliomas: 20-year experience and critical review of the pathology. J Neurooncol
       2008;89(2):169-77.

[92]   Sanders J, Sale GE, Ramberg R, Clift R, Buckner CD, Thomas ED. Glioblastoma mul-
       tiforme in a patient with acute lymphoblastic leukaemia who received a marrow
       transplant. Transplant Proc 1982;14:770–4.

[93]   Schmidbauer M, Budka H, Bruckner CD, Vorkapic P. Glioblastoma developing at the
       site of a cerebellar medulloblastoma treated six years earlier. J Neurosurg 1987;71:77–
       82.

[94]   Shamisa A, Bance M, Nag S, Tator C, Wong S, Noren G, Guha A. Glioblastoma multi-
       forme occurring in a patient treated with gamma knife surgery: case report and re-
       view of the literature. J Neurosurg 2001;94:816–21.

[95]   Shapiro S, Mcaly JJ. Late anaplastic glioma in children previously treated for acute
       lymphoblastic leukaemia. Pediatr Neurosci 1989;15:176–89.

[96]   Shapiro S, Mcaly JJ, Sartorius C. Radiation-induced intracranial malignant gliomas. J
       Neurosurg 1989;71:77–82.

[97]   Shore RE, Albert RE, Pasternack BS. Follow-up study of patients treated by X-ray ep-
       ilation for tinea capitis. Arch Environ Health 1976;31:21–8.

[98]   Simmons NE, Laws ER Jr. Glioma occurrence after sellar irradiation: case report and
       review. Neurosurgery 1998;42(1):172-8.

[99]   Snead OC, Acker JD, Morawetz RW, Benton JW. High resolution computerized to-
       mography with coronal and sagittal reconstruction in the diagnosis of brain tumors
       in children. Childs Brain 1982; 9:1–9.

[100] Soffer D, Gomori JM, Pomeranz S, Siegal T. Gliomas following low dose irradiation
       to the head: report of three cases. J Neurooncol 1998;6:67–72.

[101] Sogg RL, Donaldson SS, Yorke CH. Malignant astrocytoma following radiotherapy for craniopharyngioma. J Neurosurg 1978;48:622–7.

[102] Suda Y, Mineura K, Kowada M, Ohishi H. Malignant astrocytoma following radiotherapy in pituitary adenoma: case report. No Shinkei Geka 1989;17(8):783-8.

[103] Tada M, Sawamura Y, Abe H, Iggo R. Homozygous p53 gene mutation in a radiation-induced glioblastoma 10 years after treatment for an intracranial germ cell tumor: a case report. Neurosurgery 1997;40:393–6.

[104] Tamura M, Misumi S, Kurosaki S, Shibasaki T, Ohye C. Anaplastic astrocytoma 14 years after radiotherapy for pituitary adenoma. No Shinkei Geka 1992;20(4):493-7.

[105] Tanriover N, Ulu MO, Sar M, Uzan M. Anaplastic oligoastrocytoma: previous treatment as a possible cause in a child with acute lymphoblastic leukemia. Childs Nerv Syst 2007;23(4):469-73.

[106] Tolnay M, Kaim A, Probst A, Ulrich J. Subependymoma of the third ventricle after partial resection of a craniopharyngioma and repeated postoperative irradiation. Clin Neuropathol 1996;15(2):63-6.

[107] Tomita H, Nogaki H, Shibata Y, Tamaki N. Brain stem glioma induced by radiotherapy: report of a case. No Shinkei Geka 1995;23:151–5.

[108] Tsang RW, Lapierre NJ, Simpson WJ, Brierley MB, Panzarella T, Smyth S. Glioma arising after radiation therapy for pituitary adenoma: a report of four patients and estimation of risk. Cancer 1993;72:2227–33.

[109] Tsutsumi S, Yasumoto Y, Ito M. Pediatric multicentric glioma occurring after cranial irradiation. J Clin Neurosci 2009;16(8):1086-8.

[110] Ushio Y, Anta N, Yoshimine T, Nagatami N, Mogami H. Glioblastoma after radiotherapy for craniopharyngioma: case report. Neurosurgery 1987;21:33–8.

[111] Utsunomiya A, Uenohara H, Suzuki S, Nishimura S, Nishino A, Arai H, Sakurai Y, Suzuki H. A case of anaplastic astrocytoma arising 8 years after initial treatment by partial resection and irradiation for central neurocytoma. No To Shinkei 2001;53(8): 747-51.

[112] Walter AW, Hancock ML, Pui C-H, Hudson MM, Ochs J, Rivera G, Pratt C, Boyett J, Kun L. Secondary brain tumors in children treated for acute lymphoblastic leukaemia at St. Jude Children's Research Hospital. J Clin Oncol 1998;16(12):3761-7.

[113] Walters TR. Childhood acute lymphocytic leukemia with a second neoplasm. Am J Pediatr Hematol Oncol 1979;1:285–7.

[114] Yang SY, Wang KC, Cho BK, Kim YY, Lim SY, Park SH, Kim IH, Kim SK. Radiation-induced cerebellar glioblastoma at the site of a treated medulloblastoma: case report. J Neurosurg 2005;102(4 Suppl):417-22.

[115] Yeung YF, Wong GK, Zhu XL, Ma BB, Hk NG, Poon WS. Radiation-induced spinal glioblastoma multiforme. Acta Oncol 2006;45(1):87-90.

[116] Yu J, Yong WH, Wilson D, Black KL. Glioblastoma induction after radiosurgery for meningioma. Lancet 2000;356:1576–7.

[117] Zagzag D, Miller DC, Cangiarella J, Allen JC, Greco MA. Brainstem glioma after radiation therapy for acute myeloblastic leukemia in a child with Down syndrome. Possible pathogenetic mechanisms. Cancer 1992;70(5):1188-93.

[118] Zampieri P, Zorat PL, Mingrino S, Soattin GB. Radiation-associated cerebral gliomas. Report of two cases and review of the literature. J Neurosurg Sci 1989;3:271–9.

[119] Zochodne DW, Cairncross JG, Arce FP, MacDonald JC, Blume WT, Girvin JP, Kaufmann JC. Astrocytoma following scalp radiotherapy in infancy. Can J Neurol Sci 1984;11:475–8.

[120] Zuccarello M, Sawaya R, DeCourten-Myers G. Glioblastoma after radiation therapy for meningioma: case report and review of the literature. Neurosurgery 1986;19:114–9.

[121] Brat DJ, James CD, Jedlicka AE, Connolly DC, Chang E, Castellani RJ, Schmid M, Schiller M, Carson DA, Burger PC. Molecular genetic alterations in radiation-induced astrocytomas. Am J Pathol1999; 154:1431–8.

[122] Donson AM, Erwin NS, Kleinschmidt-DeMasters BK, Madden JR, Addo-Yobo SO, Foreman NK. Unique molecular characteristics of radiation-induced glioblastoma. J Neuropathol Exp Neurol 2007;66(8):740-9.

[123] Thiessen B, Maguire JA, McNeil K, Huntsman D, Martin MA, Horsman D. Loss of heterozygosity for loci on chromosome arms 1p and 10q in oligodendroglial tumors: relationship to outcome and chemosensitivity. J Neurooncol 2003;64(3):271-8.

9

Tumor Microenvironment — Perivascular and Perinecrotic Niches

Davide Schiffer, Marta Mellai, Laura Annovazzi,
Cristina Casalone and Paola Cassoni

1. Introduction

Tumor microenvironment is a dynamic concept that includes, beside tumor cells, everything is not tumor cells. It consists of cells, soluble factors, signaling molecules, extracellular matrix (ECM), and mechanical cues that can promote neoplastic transformation, support tumor growth and invasion, protect the tumor from host immunity and foster therapeutic resistance [1]. It is organ-specific and in the brain it is not yet fully understood. In addition to cancer cells, it contains different stromal cells mainly represented by endothelial cells, microglia/macrophages, and reactive astrocytes [2], but other cell types should be considered such as fibroblasts, pericytes, immune cells, *etc.* (Figure 1). These cells are heterogeneously distributed in the tumor, according to its different phenotypes and relevant biological significances.

2. Microenvironment cell components

2.1. Microglia/macrophages

Malignant gliomas are rich in microglia/macrophages that are classified as ramified or resident microglia, ameboid or activated microglia, macrophages and perivascular microglia [3]. They are called tumor-associated macrophages (TAM) and lack apparent phagocytic activity [4].They are considered as both intrinsic to the central nervous system (CNS) and blood-borne arrived, subjected to the local production of chemoattractant factors [5]; they share surface markers [6], but it has been demonstrated that microglia are chemokine (C-X3-C motif) receptor 1 (CX3CR1)+/chemokine (C-C motif) receptor 2 (CCR2)– and monocytes are CCR2+/

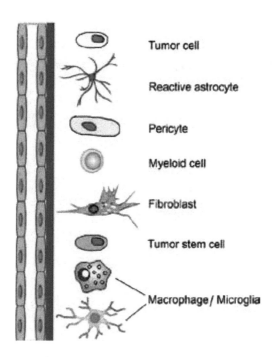

Figure 1. Scheme of the relationship between vessels/endothelium and microenvironment cells.

CX3CR1– [7]. In acute conditions microglia is blood-derived, from adult haematopoietic stem cells (HSCs), even though macrophages in adult renew independently from HSCs. Their majority derives from Tie2+ pathway generating eritro-myeloid progenitors, distinct from HSCs, from the yolk sac they migrate in the various organs [8].

It is still debated whether they are included in or they are distinct from pro-inflammatory cells. They increase both in the center and at the periphery of the tumors [9] and it has been calculated that up to one third of the cells in glioma biopsies are represented by macrophages [9,10] (Figure 2A,B). In the tissue, microglia/macrophages are found as small or large clusters around vessels or necroses, whereas at the periphery or around the tumor they are more regularly distributed. Undoubtedly, they proliferate in response to tumor growth and they have a cytotoxic defense function [11], as well as the capacity for antigen presentation [12], but they can also promote tumor infiltration and proliferation [13,14]. An inverse correlation between TAM infiltration and glioblastoma multiforme (GBM) prognosis [15] and promotion of tumor progression have been found [16].

Together with fibroblasts, pericytes, neutrophils, mast cells, lymphocytes, dendritic and endothelial cells, macrophages belong to the category of stromal cells that interact with the tumor, as discussed before, *via* cell-cell or by cytokine or chemokine-mediated signaling. Tumor cells may influence stromal cells to produce growth factors such as vascular endothelial growth factor (VEGF), tumor necrosis factor alpha (TNF-α), transforming growth factor beta (TGF-β), interleukin 1 (IL-1) or CXC ligand 2 (CXCL2), CXCL8, CXCL12 that promote angiogenesis and tumor growth. Conversely, tumor cells are stimulated to produce chemokines that influence angiogenesis [16] and growth. There is both an autocrine and a paracrine tumor growth stimulation [17]. The enrichment in stromal cells, especially microglia/macrophages, in the brain adjacent to tumor (BAT) strongly influences immunoregulation and tumor growth on the one side, and it represents a defense from the tumor on the other side.

The existence of a positive relationship between microglia/macrophages and tumor-initiating cells (TICs) in the two opposite directions is relevant to the problem [18]. The vessels can be associated or not with macrophages (Figure 2C,D) even with only one (Figure 2E). They occur obviously in circumscribed necroses (Figure 2F). Basically, any glioma-associated monocytic cell with macrophage characteristics has been called "tumor associated microglia". It shows a functional phenotype different from the inflammatory one and promotes glioma cell migration and tumor growth [19]. Migration promotion is accomplished through matrix metalloprotei-nases (MMPs) released by microglia [20,21] and CX3CL1 with its receptor (CX3CR1) [22]. The demonstration that microglia/macrophages promote glioma progression means that their inhibition can be a useful therapeutic tool [23]. Macrophages have long been recognized as critical components of immunity against tumors, because, when appropriately stimulated, they can attack tumor cells by contact interaction or by secreting cytotoxic and cytostatic factors [24]. However, they can also contribute to tumor development, by secretion of growth factors such as angiogenic factors, proteinases, which degrade the matrix, and immunosuppressor factors [25]. Their dual function is mainly exerted through TNF that demonstrates both an anticancer [26] and a tumorigenic activity [27]. However, it has also been shown that TNF can reduce glioma growth and prolong patient survival [28].

One specific question is the role of immune cells in the tumor microenvironment. These cells through cytokines, growth factors, chemokines and cerebrospinal fluid (CSF) interfere with tumor initiation, angiogenesis, proliferation and invasion [29]. IL-1β is the primary factor of microglia that enhances TGF-β, that, in turn, inhibits lymphocyte proliferation by suppressing antiglioma responses [30]. IL-1β also stimulates VEGF, epidermal growth factor receptor (EGFR) and MMP9 for angiogenesis, proliferation and invasion [31].

Macrophages can be subdivided into M1 and M2 subtypes, according their polarization status, supporting tumor suppression or progression, respectively [32]. As shown by the marker MHCII [33], they are strongly M2 in GBM [34]. In summary, it can be stated that macrophages support tumor progression and that tumor recruit macrophages [35]. There is an interrela-tionship between glioma stem cells (GSCs) and TAMs in GBM and it was shown that the former express Periostin, a member of the Fasciclin family (POSTN) [36] that has a supportive role in various tumors. TAM density correlates with POSTN in GBM and disrupting it TAM density is reduced so that GSCs secrete POSTN to recruit M2 that support tumor growth [37]. It was then showed that POSTN is highly expressed in high grade in comparison with low grade tumors [38]. How POSTN acts in potentiating tumor progression in niches has been widely discussed [39].

2.2. Reactive astrocytes

Reactive astrocytes can be sometimes confused with tumor cells, mainly because their phenotype changes over time until their complete maturation. There are analogies between glial reaction and physiological maturation of astrocytes during embryogenesis. In the initial phases, the fine processes originate directly from the cell soma and then from the thick and long processes [40]. Nestin and Vimentin would be the main markers of immature astrocytes whereas glial fibrillary acidic protein (GFAP) is the main marker of mature astrocytes [41,42].

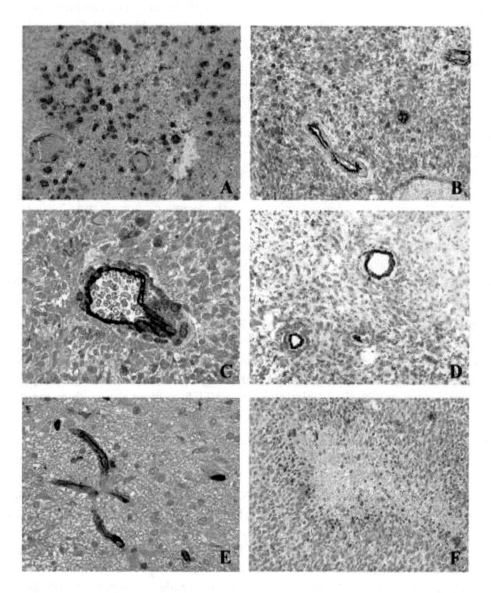

Figure 2. Glioblastoma. Macrophages/microglia. A – Cluster of macrophages in a proliferating area, not in relation with vessels; x200. B – Regular distribution of macrophages/microglia in a proliferating area not in relation with vessels; x200. C – Cluster of macrophages around a middle size vessel; x400. D – One vessel is surrounded by a crowd of macrophages, the other has none; x200. E – Capillaries with a macrophage adherent to the wall; x200. F – Macrophages in a perinecrotic palisade; x400. All double staining CD68-CD34, Alkaline Phosphatase Red and DAB, respectively.

It is still a debated question whether tumor infiltration can be recognized by magnetic resonance imaging (MRI), not only when adjacent to tumor, but also at distance. It has been observed, for example, that low grade gliomas, which preferentially locate in the *insula* and in the supplementary motor area, spread along distinct subcortical *fasciculi* [43]. By analyzing different peritumor areas with different MRI methods, it has been shown that fractional anisotropy and not apparent diffusion coefficient can be used to evaluate glioma cell invasion. An attempt to classify different peritumoral tissues by a voxel-wise analytical solution using serial diffusion MRI has been made [44].

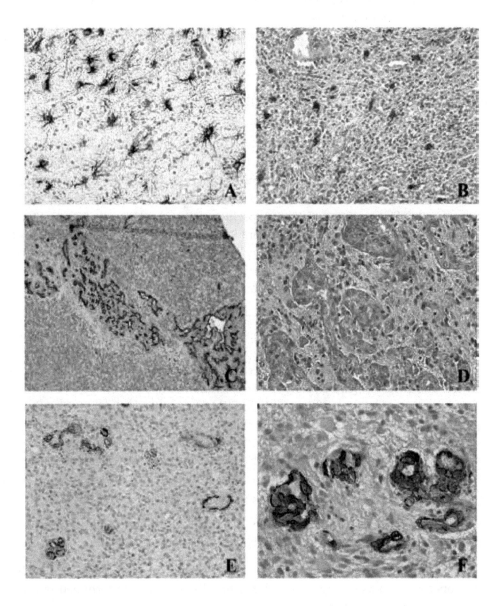

Figure 3. Glioblastoma. Reactive astrocytes. A – Regular distribution of reactive astrocytes in a cortex with mild infiltration. Some adhere to small vessels; GFAP, x200, DAB. B – Proliferating area with reactive astrocytes entrapped; almost only the large cytoplasm is visible; GFAP, x200, DAB. C – *Glomeruli*: multi-channel formations; double staining CD68-CD34, x100, DAB and Alkaline Phosphatase Red, respectively; D – Microvascular proliferations; x200, H&E. E – Pericytes; α-SMA, x200, DAB. F – *Id.* x400.

Peritumoral reactive gliosis (Figure 3A) has a particular importance because of three main characteristics: reactive astrocytes divide by mitosis as tumor cells do, they progressively lose Nestin and increase GFAP expression, as during development, and they may regionally exert a series of metabolic and molecular influences [45]. The most important point is that reactive astrocytes may be included in the advancing tumor (Figure 3B), in which they progressively become no more recognizable from tumor cells. The question is whether they disappear suffocated by the high tumor cell density, or if they remain, unrecognizable from tumor cells, to contribute to the pleomorphic aspect of gliomas, or if they even can be transformed into tumor cells [46]. There are evidences that reactive astrocytes support tumor progression [2].

3. The glioma origin and the stem cell theory

The existence of a similarity between cancer cells and embryonic stem cells is known since Virchow [47]. Glioma cells may derive through tumor transformation from immature glia cells [48,49], or primitive neuroepithelial cells or neural stem cells (NSCs) and many experimental demonstrations are available on this matter [50,51]. Glioma-initiating cells (GICs) and GSCs [52,53] share with NSCs some properties, *i.e.* proliferation and self-renewal, and GSCs share with malignant gliomas similar genetic alterations. In contrast to the hypothesis of the transformation of NSCs or neural progenitor cells (NPCs) into GSCs [54], either occurring *in situ* during embryogenesis or during migration and their relationship with GICs, the origin of GSCs has also been referred to dedifferentiation.

Dedifferentiation may refer to two distinct biological processes. The first one is represented by a multi-step process accompanied by genetic alterations that lead to the progressive transformation of normal cells into highly malignant cells. They require self-sufficiency growth signal, insensitivity to anti-growth signals, escape from apoptosis, proliferation potential, angiogenesis and invasion [55]. By combining activation of specific oncogenes and loss of tumor suppressor genes, it is possible to induce GBM from cortical astrocytes [56]. Examples are the combination of p16(INK4a)-p19(ARF) loss with K-Ras and Akt activation [57], p16(INK4a) and p19(ARF) loss with EGFR activation [58] and p53 loss with myr-Akt and c-Myc overexpression in mature astrocytes [59]. Basically, the capacity of transformation inversely correlates with differentiation. It is easier to get transformation from Nestin+ progenitors than from mature astrocytes by Ras and Akt activation [60].

A second meaning of dedifferentiation refers to tumor cells that would acquire stemness properties instead of reflecting the nature of the primitive cells [50,61].

Today, the existence of cell subpopulations, called cancer stem cells (CSCs) or GSCs, with stem cell-like properties such as multipotency, ability to self-renewal or to form neurospheres *in vitro*, is generally accepted, also for gliomas [62].

The origin of gliomas from NSCs has been repeatedly demonstrated by the experimental induction of brain tumors by nitrosourea derivatives [63]. Moreover, NSCs have been accepted as the source of gliomas, also because the signaling that regulates their self-renewal, proliferation and differentiation occurs, altered, in gliomas. Several studies demonstrated that GBM may arise from the subventricular zone (SVZ) [64,65] that is the source of stem cells and progenitors in adults [66,67]. The latter are represented by neuroblasts (type A cells) and oligodendrocyte precursor cells (OPCs), by quiescent type B cells that give origin to highly proliferative cells, and by transit-amplifying progenitor cells (type C cells), that differentiate into two lineage-restricted progenitor cells [68,69]. These cells accumulate mutations up to give rise to gliomas [70], not excluding the intervention of human Cytomegalovirus (HCMV) [71].

GBM is a heterogeneous tumor and its heterogeneity might be explained by either the hierarchical model mechanism [72] or the stochastic mechanism of development [73]. Progenitor cells are at risk of malignant transformation since they show the activation of the adequate cell machinery, represented by telomerase activity, promitotic and antiapoptotic genes [54]. Abnormal developmental patterns are Sonic hedgehog (Shh) pathway, EGFR and phosphatase and tensin homologue (PTEN) signaling. Although their clonal origin is from a small fraction of transformed NSCs, gliomas are heterogeneous as a consequence of an anomalous tumor cell differentiation [74]. The diversity within gliomas is due to changes of the subclones, being all of them generated by multipotent tumor cells, but also through an arrest of the differentiation process.

Recently, other cells have been supposed to give origin to GBM.

4. Origin of GSCs and glioma heterogeneity

The hypothesis of GSCs is based on the concept that a rare subset of cells within GBM may have significant expansion capacity and the ability to generate new tumors [72]. The remainder of tumor cells, which predominantly resemble GBM, may represent partially differentiated cells with limited progenitor capacity or terminally differentiated non-tumorigenic cells. A possible origin of gliomas is also from mature astrocytes by acquiring stemness properties through a dedifferentiation process, as above mentioned [54,75] or from NG2 cells that fit better with tumors arising far from the ventricles or with secondary GBMs [76]. Also reactive astrocytes can be candidate for gliomas [77,78], since they can acquire a stem-like phenotype [79].

In spite of the great similarity between SVZ NSCs or progenitors and GICs, the relationship with GSCs remains unresolved. Are they equivalent, or the latter have nothing to share with the former, if not the stemness properties? An answer can be that over time GICs can acquire sufficient alterations to engender GSCs. GICs are the first genetically aberrant cells that can initiate tumor development and that are responsible for the bulk of tumor cells. OPCs, the major dividing cell population in the adult brain that gives origin to oligodendrocytes, distributed in the SVZ and in the gray and white matter, remain a further unresolved problem. The EGFR and prostaglandin-endoperoxide synthase 2 (PTGS2) inhibition prevents the tumorigenesis of transformed OPCs and GICs for anaplastic oligodendroglioma but not the tumorigenesis of transformed NSCs or GICs for GBM, suggesting that the latter can arise from OPCs or NSCs [80].

In mice models, by using the retrovirus replication-competent avian sarcoma-leukosis virus long terminal repeat with splice acceptor (RCAS) [81], OPCs expressing 2′, 3′-cyclic-nucleotide 3′-phosphodiesterase (CNP) could be targeted later in their development or in the adult. Low grade oligodendrogliomas were obtained by RCAS-platelet-derived growth factor subunit beta (PDGF-β) expressing OPC markers such as sex-determining region Y (SRY)-box2 (SOX2), oligodendrocyte transcription factor 2 (OLIG2), NG2 and PDGF receptor (PDGFR), interpreted as indicating a slight dedifferentiation of tumor cells [82]. OPCs could serve as cells of origin of gliomas [83]. According to the already mentioned experiments by mosaic analysis with double markers (MADM), aberrant growth of precancerous lesions could only be found in cells differentiated along the oligodendrocyte lineage to become OPCs but not in any other lineage or in NSCs [84]. These demonstrations, however, do not exclude that aberrant growth can occur in NSCs, responsible for a direct origin of malignant tumors.

Heterogeneity in gliomas is not due to the occurrence in the same tumor of different non-tumor cells of various species, but to the cellular complexity formed by tumor cells that differ among themselves for a series of phenotypic and molecular characteristics affecting cell proliferation, invasion, *etc.* [85,86]. Cells are at risk of transformation only when demanded to proliferate, such as progenitors, opposite, for example, to B cells of SVZ that are protected [87]. The passage from B cells to amplifying cells implies a chromatin rearrangement from a quiescent to a proliferating status where genetic lesions, if not repaired, pass to the following dividing cells. There are interactions among DNA repair, epigenetics and stem cells. In the niche a homeostatic regulation of stem cells occurs, with a balance between self-renewal and differentiation, and with proliferation starting in response to a stimulating signal. Uncontrolled proliferation would take place when stem cells become independent of growth signal, because of mutations, or they resist anti-growth signals [88]. The homeostatic balance would be regulated by the interaction between Wnt/β-catenin pathway, that promotes cell growth, and bone morphogenetic protein (BMP) signaling that inhibits it. This can be the starting point of heterogeneity, largely dependent on the microenvironment. Gliomas with different genetic signatures may as well originate from different cell subtypes [89].

The same molecular mechanisms of NSCs regulate gliomas [90] that can undergo epigenetic changes and genetic mutations favoring evolution toward malignancy. During their lifespan, they can be exposed to genotoxic stress, to which they respond through repair mechanisms [76]. GBM has many molecular signatures depending on its polyclonality, and the events themselves may have an effect on the clonality. The greater is the potency of stem cells, the more anaplastic is the tumor.

The molecular profile of malignant gliomas has led to the distinction of proneural, proliferative and mesenchymal types associated to NSC profiles [91] or to the distinction of proneural, classic and mesenchymal types, the former expressing genes associated to progenitors and the latter two to stem cells [92]. The stemness would reflect the cell of origin, but it could also be acquired in the niche in adult gliomas [93]. On this basis, the contrasting results obtained on GBM can be explained by the finding of different series of TICs characterized by different phenotypic and molecular profiles [86,94].

5. Migration of NSCs or NPCs toward tumors

NPCs can migrate from the SVZ toward a tumor and target it [95]. Today, this migration may represent a new goal for therapeutic purposes. NSCs exhibit tumor-homing capability. In mice experiments, immortalized murine NSCs, implanted into glioma-bearing rodents, distributed within and around tumors, even migrating to the contralateral hemisphere [96]. Genetically engineered NSCs show a tropism for gliomas, on which may have an adverse effect [97-100], especially if they are also transduced with herpes simplex virus-thymidine kinase (HSVtk) gene and followed by the administration of systemic Ganciclovir [101-103]. Human NSCs implanted in rat brains containing a C6 glioma, migrated in the direction of the expanding tumor [104]. The same properties are shown by mesenchymal stem cells (MSCs) injected either into carotid arteries or intracerebrally [105,106] and by hematopoietic progenitor cells [107]. Endogeneous progenitor cells have been observed to migrate from the SVZ toward a murine experimental GBM [108]. The migrated Nestin+ cells were also actively cycling, as shown by Ki-67/MIB.1 positivity, and 35% of them expressed Musashi-1 [109]. In transgenic mice, virally labeled proliferating cells of the SVZ demonstrated that NPCs accumulate around gliomas, diverted from their physiological migratory pathway to the olfactory bulb [110].

Chemokines, angiogenic cytokines and glioma-produced ECM can play a role in the NSC tropism [111]. It is possible to take advantage of the natural capacity of chemokines to initiate migratory responses and to use this ability to enhance the tumor inhibitory capacity by NPCs to target an intracranially growing glioma [112]. The therapeutic possibilities offered by NSCs are continuously increasing. For example, they can be engineered as sources of secreted therapeutics, exploiting their mobility toward CNS lesions. They could function as minipumps [113].

Rat embryonic progenitor cells, transplanted at distance from a glioma grown in the *striatum*, migrate and co-localize with it. They modify their phenotype, express Vimentin and reduce the tumor volume, demonstrating that a cross-talk exists between them and the tumor [114]. It has been shown that hypoxia is a key factor in determining NSC tropism to glioma by stromal-derived factor 1 (SDF-1) and its receptor (CXCR4), urokinase-type plasminogen activator (uPA) and its receptor (uPAR) and VEGF and its receptor (VEGFR) [115]. It could be interesting to try to enhance motility of adult NSCs toward CNS injury or disease and to take into account that EGFR could play a role, because of its participation to malignant transformation [116]. It has also been recognized that a limitation exists to the possibility of migration of neural precursors from SVZ to an induced cortical GBM in mice. The limitation is caused by the age and the proliferation potential of the SVZ. Adult mice supply fewer cells than younger mice, depending on the expression of D-type Cyclins, because with aging Cyclin D1 is lost and only Cyclin D2 is expressed [110]. Recently, novel treatment strategies using NSCs have been proposed, for example the suicide gene therapy using converting enzymes [117]. New strategies will emerge from further NSC and brain tumor stem cell (BTSC) studies [118]. Is it possible that tumors grow from transplanted NSCs [119]?

6. Perivascular niches (PVN). Relationship between NPCs/GSCs and endothelial cells

GBM is composed of three concentric zones: a central necrotic area, surrounded by an intermediate zone containing large vessels with thrombosis or altered walls; a surrounding proliferation zone that abruptly or progressively flows into the normal tissue and invades it [63]. Neo-angiogenesis takes place in the proliferating zone or in normal surrounding tissue after tumor cell invasion. In the latter, new capillaries are formed from the pre-existing venules. Basically, new capillary formation is due to the endothelial proliferation that mimics angiogenesis in normal embryonic conditions, with buds and new tubule formation. In comparison with normal angiogenesis, tumor angiogenesis is often dysregulated until the formation of *glomeruli* (Figure 3C). In the invasion zone, tumor cells wrap around vessels (co-option). In invaded cortex, the vascular tree coming down from the meningeal vessels is assailed by advancing and invading tumor cells and it progressively deforms through endothelial cell hypertrophy and hyperplasia. It becomes less adequate to perfuse the increased mass of tumor cells coming up from the white matter, because transformed into a lumpy tree with irregular lumina. The generated microvascular proliferations (MVPs) (Figure 3D) are mainly found at the transition from central necrosis to the proliferation zone, where circumscribed necroses with pseudopalisading develop [120]. As a consequence, areas very rich in capillaries and small vessels, produced by an intense angiogenesis, coexist in tumors beside areas poorly vascularized where necroses develop.

Vasculogenesis is a mechanism of tumor neovascularization that has been also attributed to circulating bone marrow (BM)-derived cells known as endothelial progenitor cells (EPCs). Its importance is debated [121,122], but it was shown that mesenchymal progenitors from bone marrow can differentiate into proliferating endothelial cells [123,124]. Also BM-derived TAMs, including TIE-2 expressing monocytes/macrophages (TEMs), circulate in the blood, home at sites of pathological neovascularization and differentiate into endothelial cells or macrophages [125,126].

Another type of vascularization is represented by the "vascular mimicry" due to the capacity of tumor cells to form a functional net of channels coated by themeselves. Two types of vascular mimicry have been described. The patterned matrix type is composed of a basement membrane, lined by tumor cells, forming channels with flowing blood [127]. Vasculogenic mimicry of the tubular type may be morphologically confused with endothelial cell-lined blood vessels. In both types, cells express endothelium-associated genes, as in embryonic vasculogenesis [128,129]. These properties are associated with CSCs [130]. By fluorescent *in situ* hybridization (FISH) and immunophenotyping, these non-endothelial cell-lined vessels have been demonstrated to be primary tumor cells. In *vitro* CD133+ GSCs are vasculogenetic even with vascular smooth muscle-like cell differentiation. The cells do not express CD34 and show EGFR gene amplification [131]. It must be remarked, however, that usually cells of tumor vessels and MVPs never show either isocitrate dehydrogenase 1 and 2 (IDH1/2) mutations or EGFR gene amplification, never exceeding 1 or 2 copies [132]. They do not share with tumor cells genetic alterations and this is in line with the lack of TP53 mutations in MVPs [133].

In tumors transplanted into mice and irradiated, recruitment through hypoxia of BM-derived cells occurs, able to restore circulation through SDF1 and CXCR4 [134]; among these cells, EPCs prevail [121,135-137]. Vasculogenesis can be blocked by pharmacological inhibition or antibodies toward SDF1 and CXCR4 [134].

Interestingly, also a GBM-endothelial cell transdifferentiation is considered to contribute to tumor vascularization, favored by hypoxia [138], independently of VEGF [139]. It has been observed that a quota of GBM CD31+ endothelial cells shares with tumors cells chromosomal aberrations [140] and that a quota of GBM CD105+ endothelial cells harbours the same somatic mutations identified within tumor cells, such as amplification of EGFR and chromosome 7 [141]. In a GBM model, it was demonstrated that the tumor-derived endothelial cells originated from TICs [138]. This finding is of paramount importance because of the possibility to use an anti-VEGF antibody (Bevacizumab) for therapy [142]. Unfortunately, the effects of the drug are only transient [143] and the reason of the failure is the activation of other pro-angiogenic pathways, the recruitment of BM-derived cells and the increase of pericyte protection and tumor invasion [144,145]. The possibility that the tumor becomes more aggressive after therapy has been contemplated [146].

The problem of transdifferentiation and the role that CSCs play in this process are still under discussion [139]. All the observations have been made in animals or from animal models, and *in vivo* experiments of transdifferentiation have been challenged [85]. In human pathology, the contribution of tumor cells to the GBM vasculature has never been demonstrated and vessel cells with typical genetic changes of tumor cells, such as those of EGFR, PDGFR, PTEN, TP53, IDH1/2 have never been found in GBM [132].

By intussusception, pre-existing brain capillaries can be multiplied by transluminal endothelial bridges and by lumen partitioning; it is an early phenomenon [147].

As NPCs or NSCs reside in the normal SVZ niche at close contact with endothelial cells, in GBM, GSCs and/or NPCs are located in PVN. In the latter, a strict similarity exists with what happens in the normal SVZ niche, where the intimate association between normal NSCs and endothelial cells regulates self-renewal and differentiation of the former. In PVN, angiogenesis is activated by VEGF produced by NSCs/GSCs [88,148], whereas their stemness is maintained by Notch produced by endothelial cells through nitric oxide [19,149,150]. Notch is constitutively active in high grade gliomas and conditions their progression [104]. PVNs are strictly correlated with tumor progression. There would be a bidirectional communication between endothelial cells and TICs or GSCs [151].

The PVN composition has been carefully described in GBM, with the inclusion, beside cells of the environment, of ECM, integrins, cell adhesion signaling, cadherin family, *etc.* [152]. In GBMs, strong evidence for the existence of an endothelial mesenchymal transition (EMT) process is still lacking, but this process is increasingly reported as instrumental to tumor growth and diffusion [153,154]. It is defined by the possibility that differentiated epithelial cells establish stable contacts with neighbor cells, assume a mesenchymal cell phenotype with loss of cell-cell interactions, reduce cellular adhesion, active production of ECM proteases, increase cytoskeletal dynamics and changes in transcription factor expression, and acquire a stem cell program, all of them leading to increased migration and invasion ability [155]. The three major groups of transcription factors, the SNAI, Twist-related protein 1 (TWIST1) and Zinc-finger enhancer binding (ZEB) family members, have been reported to be altered in GBM. Their over-expression follows the activation of Wnt/β-catenin pathway and results *in vitro* in an increased cell migration and invasion [156,157]. It is likely that the high expression of mesenchymal genes in the mesenchymal subset of human GBMs [91] can be considered to be reminiscent of the EMT program [92] or that the aberrant activation of EMT factors during gliomagenesis can trigger the mesenchymal shift in GBM [158].

The influence that GSCs can exert on BM-derived endothelial cells has been summarized as follows [159]: to elicit angiogenesis, to home at the tumor the BM-derived EPCs and to promote their differentiation into blood vessels that incorporate into the existing vasculature. Trans-differentiation into endothelial-like cells contributes to the formation of blood vessels [140,160].

The PVN concept was substantiated by the demonstration of Nestin+ and CD133+ cells on capillaries, forming a microvasculature in which the microenvironment that maintains CSCs and their renewal is given by endothelial cells that, in turn, are stimulated by CSCs [149]. A positive correlation was found between the CD133+ niches and CD133+ blood vessels, similar to the correlation between the Nestin+ niches and Nestin+ blood vessels [161]. A good PVN demonstration has been given [2] and beautiful and useful schemes have been provided [159, 162]. It can be added that angiogenesis and self-renewal would represent a resistance to chemo- and radio-therapy.

The location of GSCs in PVN was confirmed by several studies using either CD133 positivity [163] or side population signature genes, such as aspartate beta-hydroxylase domain-containing protein 2 (ASPHD2) or nuclear factor erythroid 2-related factor 2 (NFE2L2) or hypoxia-inducible factor 2 (HIF-2) [164]; they increase with malignancy [161]. By comparing xenografts of C6 glioma with a high or low fraction of GSCs, it was observed that the former exhibit an increased microvessel density and an increased recruitment of BM-derived endothelial progenitors [123]. The relevance of the hypoxia will be discussed later.

6.1. Pericytes

Pericytes, the last PVN component, are perivascular cells that support blood vessels [165], control blood vessel stability, function through paracrine factors and direct cell-cell contacts, and promote vascular maturation (Figure 3E,F). They express different markers including PDGFR-β, α-smooth muscle Actin (α-SMA), Desmin, and NG2. They originate from mesoderm-derived MSCs or from neuroectoderm-derived neural crest cells, depending on their location within the brain. Pericytes are an essential element of the neurovascular unit and contribute to the function of blood-brain-barrier (BBB) [166]. Gliomas can induce the differentiation of MSCs into pericytes [167]. MSCs injected into brain tumors in mouse models have been shown to closely associate with the tumor vasculature and also with up-regulation of the expression of pericyte markers [168].

Pathology observations show that pericytes increase in number in GBM and wrap around vessels with endothelial hyperplasia.

7. PVN neuropathology

The description of the niches must be obviously a survey of the different vascular structures in GBM with their surrounding cell components. The first question to give an answer is: does each vascular structure represent a niche, or are they distributed in the tumor and how? The second question is: is the cell composition of the niches a constant one or does it vary from one another? In the literature, GSCs have been demonstrated in perivascular position [149], as well in perinecrotic niches [164,169] as discussed later. Good schemes of PVN are provided including all the cells that can be encountered in such position [62,159,162]. Such schemes, obviously, are not encounted as real occurrences in the histological examination of GBMs.

By examining the vascular structures in the different tumor zones, in infiltration areas capillaries, arterioles, venules or penetrating vessels from the meninges occur. Around them, there are tumor stem cells/progenitors, often forming cuffings (co-option), or Nestin+ cells adherent to the walls, or reactive GFAP+ astrocytes (Figure 4A–D). Scattered in the tissue, microglia/macrophages occur rather regularly, occasionally distributed in perivascular position (Figure 2). Reactive astrocytes continue to be present also in more intense infiltration, recognizable for their GFAP positivity and for what remains of their long and thick processes; however, they are regularly distributed in the tumor tissue and occasionally they can be found in perivascular position.

In areas of intense tumor cell proliferation, many small vessels can be found either with or without endothelial hyperplasia, sometimes forming a dense net. Around them, tumor cells, mostly Nestin+ and SOX2+, crowded, that can easily be considered as undifferentiated and containing sometimes cells with stemness properties, associated with occasional CD68+ cells. In proliferating areas, larger vessels can be found, with walls thicker than in capillaries, surrounded by a dense cuffing of cells that are Nestin+ in the inner part and GFAP+ outside (Figure 4E,F). In most vessels, pericytes appear wrapping the channel outside the endothelial cell layer; they are well evident in MVPs or in *glomeruli* that, on the other hand, do not appear to be surrounded by other cell types, if not tumor cells.

In intermediate areas or near the central necrosis, many vessels of different size and nature are associated with edema or tissue dissociation and they do not show to be surrounded by any special cell kind. Scattered in the tumor, myeloid cells can be found in variable quantity, associated or not with other types of cells among which macrophages seem to be the most frequent. Microglia/macrophages are distributed in small or large clusters around necroses or around vessels where they can be associated or not with some of the other cell types. The association with myeloid cells is the most striking.

The neuropathological study provides the information that PVN represents a theoretical picture where the different cell types can be represented and where cross-talks occur among the different signalings that support some tumor activities such as invasion, growth, *etc.* Of course, the most important dialogue in these structures occurs between GSCs and endothelial cells, and this is feasible around capillaries and small vessels, even though the thickness of the vessel walls could not in absolute be an insuperable obstacle.

8. Hypoxia and necroses – Perinecrotic niches

In GBM, there are two main types of necrosis: large necroses, usually at the tumor center, of thrombotic origin, and circumscribed necroses, occurring in the proliferative areas and representing a hallmark of the tumor. Hypoxia is, therefore, a tumor characteristic [170], mediated by HIF-1/2 composed of two subunits, an oxygen insensitive HIF-β subunit and an oxygen regulated HIF-α subunit [171]. Under normoxic conditions, HIF-α is rapidly degraded following hydroxylation by the oxygen-dependent prolyl-hydroxylase domain proteins (PHDs), that mark it for ubiquitination and proteasomal degradation [172]. Hypoxia stabilizes HIF-1α by preventing its hydroxylation and degradation; together with HIF-2α, it is critically involved in the regulation of GSCs [164]. Hypoxia directly promotes the GSCs expansion. In human GBM biopsies, GSCs are enriched in perinecrotic regions, where the oxygen tension is reduced and HIF-1α and HIF-2α are activated [164,173]. HIF-2α remains elevated under chronic hypoxia, while HIF-1α is only transiently upregulated [174].

Hypoxia through HIF-1α promotes the expansion of GSCs through the phosphatidylinositol 3-kinase (PI3K)/Akt and ERK1/2 pathways, the inhibition of which reduces the fraction of CD133+ GSCs [175]. In perinecrotic regions hypoxia regulates many properties [159]. In GSCs under hypoxic conditions, it activates Notch by inducing its ligands and the activation of target genes Hes1 and Hey2 [164,176]. Blockade of Notch signaling with γ-secretase inhibitors depletes the GSC population, reduces the expression of GSC markers such as CD133, Nestin, Bmi1 and OLIG2 and inhibits the growth of tumor neurospheres and xenografts [177].

GSCs can be demonstrated to lie around circumscribed necroses or scattered in the tissue by CD133 positivity [169] or other specific antigens [164].

Hypoxia is generally realized when tumor growth exceeds neovascularization, and it would not only regulate tumor cell proliferation, metabolism, differentiation, but also induce key stem cell genes such as Nanog, Oct4 and c-Myc [178].

Necroses are the place where hypoxia occurs, but it must be taken into account that usually its occurrence is histologically deduced from its pathologic effects, *i.e.*, necrosis in the tissue. Hypoxia at its very beginning could not yet be visible as necrosis, but already efficient for other signs. It is possible that tissue features in an area not suspected to be hypoxic, are indeed due to hypoxia. An example is given by apoptosis. Apoptotic nuclei are found in proliferating tumor areas due to an intrinsic or transcriptional pathway *via* mitochondria and focused on TP53 [179], or in hypoxic areas through an extrinsic pathway or TNF [180].

It is, however, possible that isolated apoptotic nuclei in a proliferating area are not due to the first type of apoptosis, *i.e.* the intrinsic one, but to the extrinsic type, consequence of a not yet morphologically evident hypoxia [181]. As a matter of fact, HIF-1α expression can be mainly demonstrated around circumscribed necroses, but also in scattered cells in proliferating areas (Figure 5A,B) [45].

Circumscribed necroses in GBM are the hallmark of the tumor, but their origin and development are still discussed. They have been carefully described and codified [139,182,183] as due to an ischemic process following a vascular occlusion or to a pathology of the endothelium.

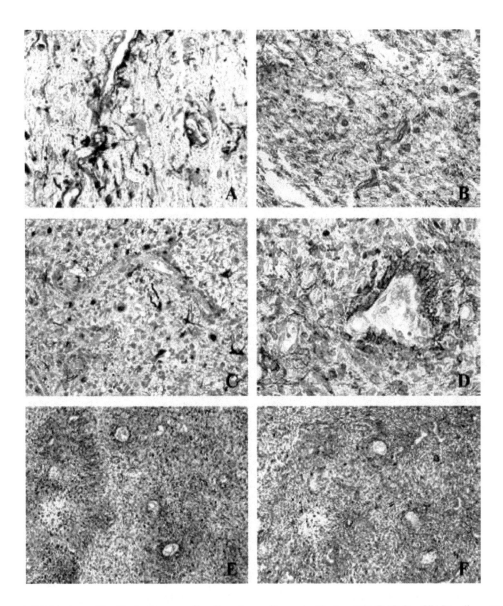

Figure 4. Glioblastoma. D – Nestin+ tumor cells adhere to small vessels; Nestin, x200, DAB. B – GFAP+ cells scattered in the tissue or in relation with vessels directly or by vascular feet: tumor cells or reactive astrocytes; double staining GFAP-CD34, x200, DAB and Alkaline Phosphatase Red, respectively. C – *Id.* with a cuffing of GAFP+ cells in the outer layer; GFAP, x200, DAB. D – Cuffing of Nestin+ cells on a medium size vessel; Nestin, DAB, x200. E – Infiltrative area with Nestin+ cells on small vessels; Nestin, x200, DAB. F – *Id.* Some GFAP+ tumor cells adhere to vessels; GFAP, x200, DAB.

The consequent hypoxia would stimulate angiogenesis, through HIF-1 and VEGF. Another interpretation can be given: necroses develop in hyperproliferating areas, with a high Ki-67/MIB.1 labeling index (LI) and a high Nestin expression in comparison with GFAP, due to the focal insufficiency of angiogenesis to feed a very large number of tumor cells, because of the imbalance between the high tumor cell proliferation capacity and the low one of endothelial cells (Figure 6A–F and Figure 7) [184-186].

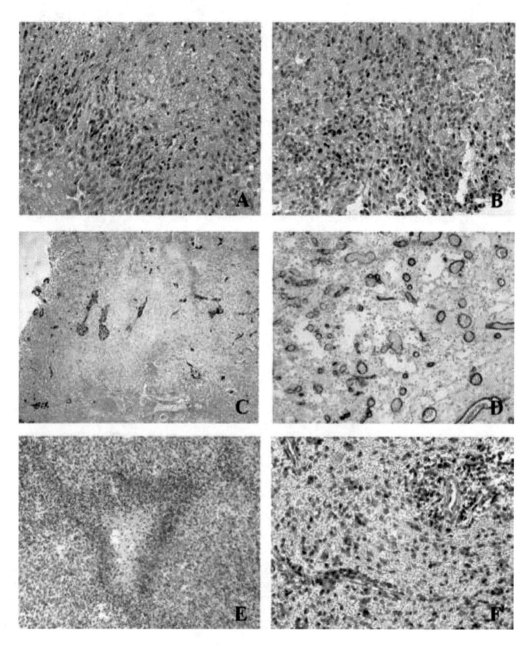

Figure 5. Glioblastoma. A – HIF-1+ cells in perinecrotic position; HIF-1, x200, DAB. B – HIF-1+ cells scattered in a pro-liferative area; HIF-1, x200, DAB. C – A large avascular area; CD34, x25, DAB. D – High vessel density; CD34, x100, DAB. E – Perinecrotic palisade with high density of SOX2+ cells; SOX2, x200, DAB. F – Cuffing of SOX2+ cells around vessels; SOX2, x200, DAB.

This observation does not exclude that inside necroses regressive pathological vessels occur [183]. In GBMs, beside areas with a high vessel density due to an active neoangiogenesis, large avascular areas occur where necroses develop (Figure 5C,D).

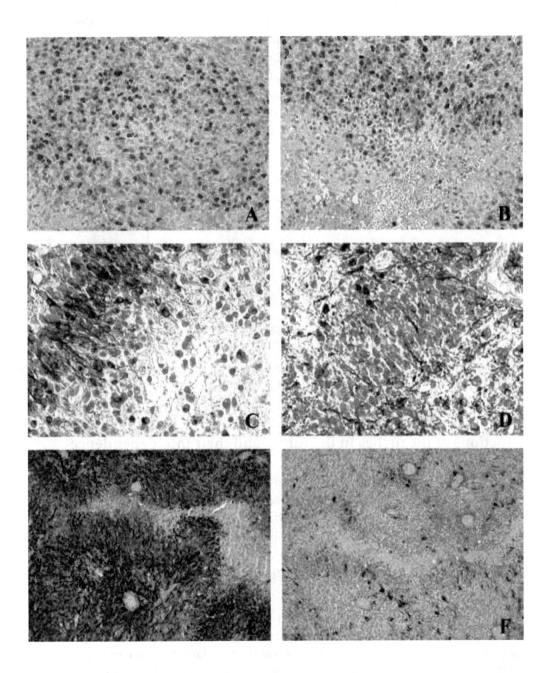

Figure 6. Glioblastoma. A – High Ki-67/MIB.1 labeling index (LI) in a hyperproliferating area; Ki-67/MIB.1, x200, DAB. B – High Ki67/MIB.1 LI in the perinecrotic palisade; Ki-67/MIB.1, x200, DAB. C – Perinecrotic palisade with high density of Nestin+ cells; Nestin, x400, DAB. D – *Id.* with only rare GFAP+ cells; GFAP, x400, DAB. E – A circumscribed necrosis in hyperproliferating Nestin+ area; Nestin, x200, DAB. F – *Id.* only rare GFAP+ tumor cells; GFAP, x200, DAB.

The palisades would be the remnants of the hyperproliferating area after necrosis develop-ment. Both are composed of a high number of cells positive for stemness markers such as CD133, Nestin, SOX2, and RE-1-silencing transcription factor (REST), and have a high proliferation index (Figure 5E,F) [163,187,188]. GSCs can be conceived as deriving from dedifferentiated tumor cells that acquired stemness properties [189]; they would be concen-trated in the above mentioned malignant tumor areas where circumscribed necroses develop because of the vascular insufficiency. It is likely that GSCs around necroses represent the quota of GSCs that populated the hyperproliferating areas and remained unaffected by necrosis development. The palisadings themselves would be the remnants of hyperproliferating areas, spared by necrosis [45,189].

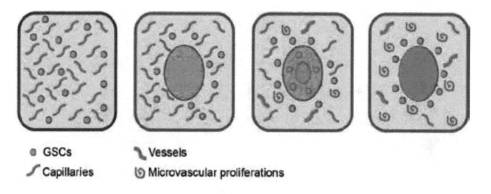

	GSCs		Vessels
	Capillaries		Microvascular proliferations

Figure 7. Progression from hyperproliferating areas with GSCs/progenitors → development of avascular area → ap-pearance of necrosis → necrosis surrounded by GSCs/progenitors.

9. Functions of the niches in the tumor and their interdependence

The GSC maintenance is provided by the signalings that occur in the niches; they can expand and form new ones that, in turn, drive the tumor growth [190]. Signalings involved in the GSC regulation are Oct4, c-Myc, Notch, TGF-β, Wnt/β-catenin pathways. Genes associated with shorter patient survival, as already observed [91], are overexpressed in the side population found by Seidel *et al* [164] and, *viceversa*, downregulated in those associated with longer survival. The overexpression concerns more primary than secondary glioblastomas that show a reduced CSC component [191] that, however, may still support tumor growth.

Perivascular and perinecrotic niches are not separated entities, first of all for temporal reasons. Hypoxia is the main cause of angiogenesis, but this is realized through factors, such as VEGF, Angiopoietin 1 and 2, SDF1 produced by GSCs and, at the same time, the imbalance between the high proliferation rate of tumor cells and the low one of endothelial cells makes angiogen-esis insufficient and causes necrosis development. Moreover, besides tumor areas rich in small neo-formed vessels and capillaries, MVPs due to a dysregulated angiogenesis do not show sufficient exchanges with tumor cells and are responsible for hypoxia [63]. Another important question, widely discussed [172], is how hypoxia and the vasculature regulate macrophages and immune cells through HIFs and nuclear factor kappa-light-chain-enhancer of activated B cells (NF-kB) [192,193] and CXCR4 [194].

It cannot be established whether GSCs of perivascular and perinecrotic niches belong to the same population, because, although showing the same stemness antigens, they still represent progenitors that can be in different state of differentiation. The significance conferred to GSCs in perinecrotic position as dedifferentiated tumor cells which reached stemness beyond a certain point of dedifferentiation, cannot be recognized to GSCs in perivascular niches [45,189]. Letting aside the transdifferentiation of tumor cells into endothelial cells, which did not received sufficient support, another point of link between the two microenvironments is represented by cell migration through EMT that is promoted by hypoxia and bound to GSCs [155]. GSCs can migrate along newly formed vessels and favor tumor diffusion.

The most important question in this topic is the occurrence of circumscribed necroses in the tumor areas with the highest malignant phenotype including both avascular districts and districts with a high vessel density, so that perinecrotic niches appear to be associated with perivascular niches to characterize these malignant areas [45,189,195].

10. Conclusions

The origin of gliomas has been outlined as traceable back to the transformation of primitive neuroepithelial cells or NSCs, capable of self-renewal and proliferation, *i.e.* endowed with stemness properties, or to the dedifferentiation of adult glia to reach stemness properties. The CSC responsibility for tumor proliferation, recurrence and resistance to therapies falls today into the most credited hypothesis. Many experiments have shown that GSCs derive by transformation of NSCs or they represent a simple functional stemness status. Some aspects of the problem remain unresolved, for example, the relationship between TICs and CSCs or the CSCs location in the tumor, as well as the existence in the tumor of NSCs that continuously renew the CSCs quota.

Recently, a new concept arose to indicate everything in the tumor, outside cancer cells, that regulates tumor proliferation, invasion, differentiation, resistance to therapies as the microenvironment, with its innumerable molecular pathways and numberless signalings and crosstalks. Major expressions of the microenvironment are in GBM the perivascular and the perinecrotic niches. The former are important for the endothelial cell/CSC relationship that, on one side, maintains the stemness status of CSCs and, on the other side, gives origin to angiogenesis. The latter are important for the occurrence of hypoxia through HIF-1/2 that can induce CSC formation.

The neuropathological study of GBMs with the final goal to find a concrete expression to the perinecrotic niche concept, provides an alternative interpretation to that considering perinecrotic CSCs as induced by hypoxia. They can be the remnants of CSCs that crowded the hyperproliferating and malignant areas of the tumor in which necrosis developed for insufficient vascularization. Perivascular niches are usually very well depicted as schemes that contemplate all the cells that can be in contact with vessels/endothelial cells. This event, however, is not observed to be realized with all the identified cells in all the vessels, going from capillaries or small vessels to larger vessels, MVPs or *glomeruli* in the different tumor areas. The cells described in the schemes never occur concurrently in one or all the vessels, so that the schemes themselves remain as a theoretical indication of possible relationships that can be established between tumor cells and vessels as a consequence of a general molecular regulation that is realized in the microenvironment.

Acknowledgements

This work was supported by Grant n. 4011 SD/cv 2011-0438 from Compagnia di San Paolo, Turin, Italy.

Author details

Davide Schiffer[1*], Marta Mellai[1], Laura Annovazzi[1], Cristina Casalone[2] and Paola Cassoni[3]

*Address all correspondence to: davide.schiffer@unito.it

1 Neuro-Bio-Oncology Research Center / Policlinico di Monza Foundation, Consorzio di Neuroscienze, University of Pavia, Vercelli, Italy

2 Istituto Zooprofilattico, Turin, Italy

3 Dpt. Medical Sciences, University of Turin, Turin, Italy

References

[1] Swartz MA, Iida N, Roberts EW, Sangaletti S, Wong MH, et al. Tumor microenvironment complexity: emerging roles in cancer therapy. Cancer Res. 2012; 72(10): 2473–2480.

[2] Lorger M. Tumor microenvironment in the brain. Cancers (Basel). 2012; 4(1): 218–243.

[3] Graeber MB, Streit WJ. Microglia: immune network in the CNS. Brain Pathol. 1990; 1(1): 2–5.

[4] Hao C, Parney IF, Roa WH, Turner J, Petruk KC, et al. Cytokine and cytokine receptor mRNA expression in human glioblastomas: evidence of Th1, Th2 and Th3 cytokine dysregulation. Acta Neuropathol. 2002; 103(2): 171–178.

[5] Frei K, Nohava K, Malipiero UV, Schwerdel C, Fontana A. Production of macrophage colony-stimulating factor by astrocytes and brain macrophages. J Neuroimmunol. 1992; 40(2-3): 189–195.

[6] Deininger MH, Seid K, Engel S, Meyermann R, Schluesener HJ. Allograft inflammatory factor–1 defines a distinct subset of infiltrating macrophages/microglialcells in rat and human gliomas. Acta Neuropathol. 2000; 100(6): 673–680.

[7] Mizutani M, Pino PA, Saederup N, Charo IF, Ransohoff RM, et al. The fractalkine receptor but not CCR2 is present on microglia from embryonic development throughout adulthood. J Immunol. 2012; 188(1): 29–36.

[8] Gomez Perdiguero E, Schulz C, Geissmann F. Development and homeostasis of "resident" myeloid cells: the case of the microglia. Glia. 2013; 61(1): 112–120.

[9] Roggendorf W, Strupp S, Paulus W. Distribution and characterization of microglia/macrophages in human brain tumors. Acta Neuropathol. 1996; 92(3): 288–293.

[10] Morimura T, Neuchrist C, Kitz K, Budka H, Scheiner O, et al. Monocyte subpopulations in human gliomas: expression of Fc and complement receptors and correlation with tumor proliferation. Acta Neuropathol. 1990; 80(3): 287–294.

[11] Sutter A, Hekmat A, Luckenbach GA. Antibody-mediated tumor cytotoxicity of microglia. Pathobiology. 1991; 59(4): 254–258.

[12] Flügel A, Bradl M, Kreutzberg GW, Graeber MB. Transformation of donor-derived bone marrow precursors into host microglia during autoimmune CNS inflammation and during the retrograde response to axotomy. J Neurosci Res. 2001; 66(1): 74–82.

[13] Huettner C, Czub S, Kerkau S, Roggendorf W, Tonn JC. Interleukin 10 is expressed in human gliomas in vivo and increases glioma cell proliferation and motility in vitro. Anticancer Res. 1997; 17(5A): 3217–3224.

[14] Graeber MB, Streit WJ. Microglia: biology and pathology. Acta Neuropathol. 2010; 119(1): 89–105.

[15] Abou-Ghazal M, Yang DS, Qiao W, Reina–Ortiz C, Wei J, et al. The incidence, correlation with tumor–infiltrating inflammation, and prognosis of phosphorylated STAT3 expression in human gliomas. Clin Cancer Res. 2008; 14(24): 8228–8235.

[16] Kanamori M, Kawaguchi T, Berger MS, Pieper RO. Intracranial microenvironment reveals independent opposing functions of host alphaVbeta3expression on glioma growth and angiogenesis. J Biol Chem. 2006; 281(48): 37256–37264.

[17] Somasundaram R, Herlyn D. Chemokines and the microenvironment in neuroectodermal tumor-host interaction. Semin Cancer Biol. 2009; 19(2): 92–96.

[18] Yi L, Xiao H, Xu M, Ye X, Hu J, et al. Glioma-initiating cells: a predominant role in microglia/macrophages tropism to glioma. J Neuroimmunol. 2011; 232(1-2): 75–82.

[19] Charles N, Ozawa T, Squatrito M, Bleau AM, Brennan CW, et al. Perivascular nitric oxide activates notch signaling and promotes stem-like character in PDGF-induced glioma cells. Cell Stem Cell. 2010; 6(2): 141–152.

[20] Markovic DS, Glass R, Synowitz M, Rooijen Nv, Kettenmann H. Microglia stimulate the invasiveness of glioma cells by increasing the activity of metalloprotease-2. Neuropathol Exp Neurol. 2005; 64(9): 754–762.

[21] Markovic DS, Vinnakota K, Chirasani S, Synowitz M, Raguet H, et al. Gliomas induce and exploit microglial MT1-MMP expression for tumor expansion. Proc Natl Acad Sci U S A. 2009; 106(30): 1230–1235.

[22] Held-Feindt J, Hattermann K, Müerköster SS, Wedderkopp H, Knerlich-Lukoschus F, et al. CX3CR1 promotes recruitment of human glioma-infiltrating microglia/macrophages (GIMs). Exp Cell Res. 2010; 316(9): 1553–1566.

[23] Zhai H, Heppner FL, Tsirka SE. Microglia/macrophages promote glioma progression. Glia. 2011; 59(3): 472–485.

[24] Burke B, Sumner S, Maitland N, Lewis CE. Macrophages in gene therapy: cellular delivery vehicles and in vivo targets. J Leukoc Biol. 2002; 72(3): 417–428.

[25] Bingle L, Brown NJ, Lewis CE. The role of tumor-associated macrophages in tumor progression: implications for new anticancer therapies. J Pathol. 2002; 196(3): 254–265.

[26] Lejeune F, Liénard D, Eggermont A. Regional administration of recombinant tumor necrosis factor-alpha in cancer, with special reference to melanoma. BioDrugs. 1998; 9(3): 211–218.

[27] Orosz P, Echtenacher B, Falk W, Rüschoff J, Weber D, et al. Enhancement of experimental metastasis by tumor necrosis factor. J Exp Med. 1993; 177(5): 1391–1398.

[28] Villeneuve J, Tremblay P, Vallières L. Tumor necrosis factor reduces brain tumor growth by enhancing macrophage recruitment and microcyst formation. Cancer Res. 2005; 65(9): 3928–3936.

[29] Pollard JW. Tumor-educated macrophages promote tumor progression and metastasis. Nat Rev Cancer. 2004; 4(1): 71–78.

[30] Naganuma H, Sasaki A, Satoh E, Nagasaka M, Nakano S, et al. Transforming growth factor-beta inhibits interferon-gamma secretion by lymphokine-activated killer cells stimulated with tumor cells. Neurol Med Chir (Tokyo). 1996; 36(11): 789–795.

[31] Watters JJ, Schartner JM, Badie B. Microglia function in brain tumors. Neurosci Res. 2005; 81(3): 447–455.

[32] Sielska M, Przanowski P, Wylot B, Gabrusiewicz K, Maleszewska M, et al. Distinct roles of CSF family cytokines in macrophage infiltration and activation in glioma progression and injury response. J Pathol. 2013; 230(3): 310–321.

[33] Tran CT, Wolz P, Egensperger R, Kösel S, Imai Y, et al. Differential expression of MHC class II molecules by microglia and neoplastic astroglia: relevance for the escape of astrocytoma cells from immune surveillance. Neuropathol Appl Neurobiol. 1998; 24(4): 293–301.

[34] Komohara Y, Ohnishi K, Kuratsu J, Takeya M. Possible involvement of the M2 anti–inflammatory macrophage phenotype in growth of humangliomas. J Pathol. 2008; 216(1): 15–24.

[35] Zhou W, Bao S. Reciprocal Supportive Interplay between Glioblastoma and Tumor-Associated Macrophages. Cancers (Basel). 2014; 6(2): 723–740.

[36] Bao S, Ouyang G, Bai X, Huang Z, Ma C, et al. Periostin potently promotes metastatic growth of colon cancer by augmenting cell survival viathe Akt/PKB pathway. Cancer Cell. 2004; 5(4): 329–339.

[37] Zhou W, Ke SQ, Huang Z, Flavahan W, Fang X, et al. Periostin secreted by glioblastoma stem cells recruits M2 tumour–associated macrophages and promotes malignant growth. Nat Cell Biol. 2015; 17(2): 170–182.

[38] Mikheev AM, Mikheeva SA, Trister AD, Tokita MJ, Emerson SN, et al. Periostin is a novel therapeutic target that predicts and regulates glioma malignancy. Neuro Oncol. 2014. pii: nou161.

[39] Squadrito ML, De Palma M. A niche role for periostin and macrophages in glioblastoma. Nat Cell Biol. 2015; 17(2): 107–109.

[40] Bushong EA, Martone ME, Ellisman MH. Maturation of astrocyte morphology and the establishment of astrocyte domains during postnatal hippocampal development. Int J Dev Neurosci. 2004; 22(2): 73–86.

[41] Clarke SR, Shetty AK, Bradley JL, Turner DA. Reactive astrocytes express the embryonic intermediate neurofilament nestin. Neuroreport. 1994; 5(15): 1885–1888.

[42] Eliasson C, Sahlgren C, Berthold CH, Stakeberg J, Celis JE, et al. Intermediate filament protein partnership in astrocytes. J Biol Chem. 1999; 274(34): 23996–24006.

[43] Mandonnet E, Capelle L, Duffau H. Extension of paralimbic low grade gliomas: toward an anatomical classification based on white matter invasion patterns. J Neurooncol. 2006; 78(2): 179–185.

[44] Ellingson BM, LaViolette PS, Rand SD, Malkin MG, Connelly JM, et al. Spatially quantifying microscopic tumor invasion and proliferation using a voxel-wise solution to a glioma growth model and serial diffusion MRI. Magn Reson Med. 2011; 65(4): 1131–1143.

[45] Schiffer D, Mellai M, Annovazzi L, Caldera V, Piazzi A, et al. Stem cell niches in glioblastoma: a neuropathological view. Biomed Res Int. 2014; 2014: 725921.

[46] Tamagno I, Schiffer D. Nestin expression in reactive astrocytes of human pathology. J Neurooncol. 2006; 80(3): 227–233.

[47] Virchow R. Die krankhaften Geschwülste. Berlin: Hirschwald; 1863-1865.

[48] Reynolds BA, Weiss S. Generation of neurons and astrocytes from isolated cells of the adult mammalian central nervous system. Science. 1992; 255(5052): 1707–1710.

[49] Doetsch F, Caillé I, Lim DA, García-Verdugo JM, Alvarez-Buylla A. Subventricular zone astrocytes are neural stem cells in the adult mammalian brain. Cell. 1999; 97(6): 703–716.

[50] Visvader JE, Lindeman GJ. Cancer stem cells in solid tumors: accumulating evidence and unresolved questions. Nat Rev Cancer. 2008; 8(10): 755–768.

[51] De Filippis L, Binda E. Concise review: self-renewal in the central nervous system: neural stem cells from embryo to adult. Stem Cells Transl Med. 2012; 1(4): 298–308.

[52] Singh SK, Clarke ID, Terasaki M, Bonn VE, Hawkins C, et al. Identification of a cancer stem cell in human brain tumors. Cancer Res. 2003; 63(18): 5821–5828.

[53] Singh SK, Clarke ID, Hide T, Dirks PB. Cancer stem cells in nervous system tumors. Oncogene. 2004; 23(43): 7267–7273.

[54] Sanai N, Alvarez-Buylla A, Berger MS. Neural stem cells and the origin of gliomas. N Engl J Med. 2005; 353(8): 811–822.

[55] Hanahan D, Weinberg RA. The hallmarks of cancer. Cell. 2000; 100(1): 57–70.

[56] Stiles CD, Rowitch DH. Glioma stem cells: a midterm exam. Neuron. 2008; 58(6): 832–846.

[57] Uhrbom L, Dai C, Celestino JC, Rosenblum MK, Fuller GN, et al. Ink4a-Arf loss cooperates with KRas activation in astrocytes and neural progenitors to generate glioblastomas of various morphologies depending on activated Akt. Cancer Res. 2002; 62(19): 5551–5558.

[58] Bachoo RM, Maher EA, Ligon KL, Sharpless NE, Chan SS, et al. Epidermal growth factor receptor and Ink4a/Arf: convergent mechanisms governing terminal differentiation and transformation along the neural stem cell to astrocyte axis. Cancer Cell. 2002; 1(3): 269–277.

[59] Radke J, Bortolussi G, Pagenstecher A. Akt and c-Myc induce stem-cell markers in mature primary p53$^{-/-}$ astrocytes and render these cells gliomagenic in the brain of immunocompetent mice. PLoS One. 2013; 8(2): e56691.

[60] Holland EC, Celestino J, Dai C, Schaefer L, Sawaya RE, et al. Combined activation of Ras and Akt in neural progenitors induces glioblastoma formation in mice. Nat Genet. 2000; 25(1): 55–57.

[61] Schiffer D, Mellai M, Annovazzi L, Piazzi A, Monzeglio O, et al. Glioblastoma cancer stem cells: basis for a functional hypothesis. Stem Cell Discovery 2012; 2(3): 122–131.

[62] Goffart N, Kroonen J, Rogister B. Glioblastoma-initiating cells: relationship with neural stem cells and the micro-environment. Cancers (Basel). 2013; 5(3): 1049-1071.

[63] Schiffer D. Brain tumors: biology, pathology and clinical references. Berlin, Heidelberg, New York: Springer; 1997.

[64] Lim DA, Cha S, Mayo MC, Chen MH, Keles E, et al. Relationship of glioblastoma multiforme to neural stem cell regions predicts invasive and multifocal tumor phenotype. Neuro Oncol. 2007; 9(4): 424–429.

[65] Alcantara Llaguno S, Chen J, Kwon CH, Jackson EL, Li Y, et al. Malignant astrocytomas originate from neural stem/progenitor cells in a somatic tumor suppressor mouse model. Cancer Cell. 2009; 15(1): 45–56.

[66] Luskin MB. Restricted proliferation and migration of postnatally generated neurons derived from the forebrain subventricular zone. Neuron. 1993; 11(1): 173–189.

[67] Lois C, Alvarez-Buylla A. Long-distance neuronal migration in the adult mammalian brain. Science. 1994; 264(5162): 1145–1148.

[68] Hack MA, Saghatelyan A, de Chevigny A, Pfeifer A, Ashery-Padan R, et al. Neuronal fate determinants of adult olfactory bulb neurogenesis. Nat Neurosci. 2005; 8(7): 865–872.

[69] Menn B, Garcia-Verdugo JM, Yaschine C, Gonzalez-Perez O, Rowitch D, et al. Origin of oligodendrocytes in the subventricular zone of the adult brain. J Neurosci. 2006; 26(30): 7907–7918.

[70] Jackson EL, Garcia-Verdugo JM, Gil-Perotin S, Roy M, Quinones-Hinojosa A, et al. PDGFR alpha-positive B cells are neural stem cells in the adult SVZ that form glioma-like growths in response to increased PDGF signaling. Neuron. 2006; 51(2): 187–199.

[71] Price RL, Song J, Bingmer K, Kim TH, Yi JY, et al. Cytomegalovirus contributes to glioblastoma in the context of tumor suppressor mutations. Cancer Res. 2013; 73(11): 3441–3450.

[72] Holland EC. Progenitor cells and glioma formation. Curr Opin Neurol. 2001; 14(6): 683–688.

[73] Adams JM, Strasser A. Is tumor growth sustained by rare cancer stem cells or dominant clones? Cancer Res. 2008; 68(11): 4018–4021.

[74] Reya T, Morrison SJ, Clarke MF, Weissman IL. Stem cells, cancer, and cancer stem cells. Nature. 2001; 414(6859): 105–111.

[75] Assanah M, Lochhead R, Ogden A, Bruce J, Goldman J, et al. Glial progenitors in adult white matter are driven to form malignant gliomas by platelet-derived growth factor-expressing retroviruses. J Neurosci. 2006; 26(25): 6781–6790.

[76] Siebzehnrubl FA, Reynolds BA, Vescovi A, Steindler DA, Deleyrolle LP. The origins of glioma: E Pluribus Unum? Glia. 2011; 59(8): 1135–1147.

[77] Dufour C, Cadusseau J, Varlet P, Surena AL, de Faria GP, et al. Astrocytes reverted to a neural progenitor-like state with transforming growth factor alpha are sensitized to cancerous transformation. Stem Cells. 2009; 27(10): 2373–2382.

[78] Silver DJ, Steindler DA. Common astrocytic programs during brain development, injury and cancer. Trends Neurosci. 2009; 32(6): 303–311.

[79] Buffo A, Rite I, Tripathi P, Lepier A, Colak D, et al. Origin and progeny of reactive gliosis: A source of multipotent cells in the injured brain. Proc Natl Acad Sci U S A. 2008; 105(9): 3581–3586.

[80] Hide T, Takezaki T, Nakatani Y, Nakamura H, Kuratsu J, et al. Combination of a ptgs2 inhibitor and an epidermal growth factor receptor-signaling inhibitor prevents tumorigenesis of oligodendrocyte lineage-derived glioma-initiating cells. Stem Cells. 2011; 29(4): 590–599.

[81] Moore LM, Holmes KM, Fuller GN, Zhang W. Oncogene interactions are required for glioma development and progression as revealed by a tissue specific transgenic mouse model. Chin J Cancer. 2011; 30(3): 163–172.

[82] Persson AI, Petritsch C, Swartling FJ, Itsara M, Sim FJ, et al. Non-stem cell origin for oligodendroglioma. Cancer Cell. 2010; 18(6): 669–682.

[83] Lindberg N, Kastemar M, Olofsson T, Smits A, Uhrbom L. Oligodendrocyte progenitor cells can act as cell of origin for experimental glioma. Oncogene. 2009; 28(23): 2266–2275.

[84] Jiang Y, Uhrbom L. On the origin of glioma. Ups J Med Sci. 2012; 117(2): 113–121.

[85] Lathia JD, Gallagher J, Myers JT, Li M, Vasanji A, et al. Direct in vivo evidence for tumor propagation by glioblastoma cancer stem cells. PLoS One. 2011; 6(9): e24807.

[86] Mazzoleni S, Galli R. Gliomagenesis: a game played by few players or a team effort? Front Biosci (Elite Ed). 2012; 4: 205–213.

[87] Foroni C, Galli R, Cipelletti B, Caumo A, Alberti S, et al. Resilience to transformation and inherent genetic and functional stability of adult neural stem cells ex vivo. Cancer Res. 2007; 67(8): 3725–3733.

[88] Li L, Neaves WB. Normal stem cells and cancer stem cells: the niche matters. Cancer Res. 2006; 66(9): 4553–4557.

[89] Furnari FB, Fenton T, Bachoo RM, Mukasa A, Stommel JM, et al. Malignant astrocytic glioma: genetics, biology, and paths to treatment. Genes Dev. 2007; 21(21): 2683–2710.

[90] Zheng H, Ying H, Yan H, Kimmelman AC, Hiller DJ, et al. p53 and Pten control neural and glioma stem/progenitor cell renewal and differentiation. Nature. 2008; 455(7216): 1129–1133.

[91] Phillips HS, Kharbanda S, Chen R, Forrest WF, Soriano RH, et al. Molecular subclasses of high-grade glioma predict prognosis, delineate a pattern of disease progression, and resemble stages in neurogenesis. Cancer Cell. 2006; 9(3): 157–173.

[92] Verhaak RG, Hoadley KA, Purdom E, Wang V, Qi Y, et al. Integrated genomic analysis identifies clinically relevant subtypes of glioblastoma characterized by abnormalities in PDGFRA, IDH1, EGFR, and NF1. Cancer Cell. 2010; 17(1): 98–110.

[93] Swartling FJ, Hede SM, Weiss WA. What underlies the diversity of brain tumors? Cancer Metastasis Rev. 2013; 32(1-2): 5–24.

[94] Chen R, Nishimura MC, Bumbaca SM, Kharbanda S, Forrest WF, et al. A hierarchy of self-renewing tumor-initiating cell types in glioblastoma. Cancer Cell. 2010; 17(4): 362–375.

[95] Shah K, Bureau E, Kim DE, Yang K, Tang Y, et al. Glioma therapy and real-time imaging of neural precursor cell migration and tumor regression. Ann Neurol. 2005; 57(1): 34–41.

[96] Aboody KS, Brown A, Rainov NG, Bower KA, Liu S, et al. Neural stem cells display extensive tropism for pathology in adult brain: evidence from intracranial gliomas. Proc Natl Acad Sci U S A. 2000; 97(23): 12846–12851.

[97] Ehtesham M, Kabos P, Kabosova A, Neuman T, Black KL, et al. The use of interleukin 12-secreting neural stem cells for the treatment of intracranial glioma. Cancer Res. 2002; 62(20): 5657–5663.

[98] Shah AC, Benos D, Gillespie GY, Markert JM. Oncolytic viruses: clinical applications as vectors for the treatment of malignant gliomas. J Neurooncol. 2003; 65(3): 203–226.

[99] Kim SK, Cargioli TG, Machluf M, Yang W, Sun Y, et al. PEX-producing human neural stem cells inhibit tumor growth in a mouse glioma model. Clin Cancer Res. 2005; 11(16): 5965–5970.

[100] Uhl M, Weiler M, Wick W, Jacobs AH, Weller M, et al. Migratory neural stem cells for improved thymidine kinase-based gene therapy of malignant gliomas. Biochem Biophys Res Commun. 2005; 328(1): 125–129.

[101] Li ZB, Zeng ZJ, Chen Q, Luo SQ, Hu WX. Recombinant AAV-mediated HSVtk gene transfer with direct intratumoral injections and Tet-On regulation for implanted human breast cancer. BMC Cancer. 2006; 6: 66.

[102] Rath P, Shi H, Maruniak JA, Litofsky NS, Maria BL, et al. Stem cells as vectors to deliver HSV/tk gene therapy for malignant gliomas. Curr Stem Cell Res Ther. 2009; 4(1): 44–49.

[103] Tyler MA, Ulasov IV, Sonabend AM, Nandi S, Han Y, et al. Neural stem cells target intracranial glioma to deliver an oncolytic adenovirus in vivo. Gene Ther. 2009; 16(2): 262–278.

[104] Jeon JY, An JH, Kim SU, Park HG, Lee MA. Migration of human neural stem cells toward an intracranial glioma. Exp Mol Med. 2008; 40(1): 84–91.

[105] Nakamura K, Ito Y, Kawano Y, Kurozumi K, Kobune M, et al. Antitumor effect of genetically engineered mesenchymal stem cells in a rat glioma model. Gene Ther. 2004; 11(14): 1155–1164.

[106] Nakamizo A, Marini F, Amano T, Khan A, Studeny M, et al. Human bone marrow-derived mesenchymal stem cells in the treatment of gliomas. Cancer Res. 2005; 65(8): 3307–3318.

[107] Tabatabai G, Bähr O, Möhle R, Eyüpoglu IY, Boehmler AM, et al. Lessons from the bone marrow: how malignant glioma cells attract adult haematopoietic progenitor cells. Brain. 2005; 128(Pt 9): 2200–2211.

[108] Glass R, Synowitz M, Kronenberg G, Walzlein JH, Markovic DS, et al. Glioblastoma-induced attraction of endogenous neural precursor cells is associated with improved survival. J Neurosci. 2005; 25(10): 2637–2646.

[109] Pirzkall A, Nelson SJ, McKnight TR, Takahashi MM, Li X, et al. Metabolic imaging of low-grade gliomas with three-dimensional magnetic resonance spectroscopy. Int J Radiat Oncol Biol Phys. 2002; 53(5): 1254–1264.

[110] Walzlein JH, Synowitz M, Engels B, Markovic DS, Gabrusiewicz K, et al. The antitumorigenic response of neural precursors depends on subventricular proliferation and age. Stem Cells. 2008; 26(11): 2945–2954.

[111] Xu F, Zhu JH. Stem cells tropism for malignant gliomas.Neurosci Bull. 2007; 23(6): 363–369.

[112] Honeth G, Staflin K, Kalliomäki S, Lindvall M, Kjellman C. Chemokine-directed migration of tumor-inhibitory neural progenitor cells towards an intracranially growing glioma. Exp Cell Res. 2006; 312(8): 1265–1276.

[113] Chen HI, Bakshi A, Royo NC, Magge SN, Watson DJ. Neural stem cells as biological minipumps: a faster route to cell therapy for the CNS? Curr Stem Cell Res Ther. 2007; 2(1): 13–22.

[114] Staflin K, Lindvall M, Zuchner T, Lundberg C. Instructive cross-talk between neural progenitor cells and gliomas. J Neurosci Res. 2007; 85(10): 2147–2159.

[115] Zhao D, Najbauer J, Garcia E, Metz MZ, Gutova M, et al. Neural stem cell tropism to glioma: critical role of tumor hypoxia. Mol Cancer Res. 2008; 6(12): 1819–1829.

[116] Ayuso-Sacido A, Graham C, Greenfield JP, Boockvar JA. The duality of epidermal growth factor receptor (EGFR) signaling and neural stem cell phenotype: cell enhancer or cell transformer? Curr Stem Cell Res Ther. 2006; 1(3): 387–394.

[117] Barresi V, Belluardo N, Sipione S, Mudò G, Cattaneo E, et al. Transplantation of pro-drug-converting neural progenitor cells for brain tumor therapy. Cancer Gene Ther. 2003; 10(5): 396–402.

[118] Oh MC, Lim DA. Novel treatment strategies for malignant gliomas using neural stem cells. Neurotherapeutics. 2009; 6(3): 458–464.

[119] Amariglio N, Hirshberg A, Scheithauer BW, Cohen Y, Loewenthal R, et al. Donor-derived brain tumor following neural stem cell transplantation in an ataxia telangiectasia patient. PLoS Med. 2009; 6(2): e1000029.

[120] Schiffer D, Chiò A, Giordana MT, Mauro A, Migheli A, et al. Vascular response to irradiation in malignant gliomas. J Neurooncol. 1990; 8(1): 73–84.

[121] Lyden D, Hattori K, Dias S, Costa C, Blaikie P, et al. Impaired recruitment of bone-marrow-derived endothelial and hematopoietic precursor cells blocks tumor angiogenesis and growth. Nat Med. 2001; 7(11): 1194–1201.

[122] Machein MR, Renninger S, de Lima-Hahn E, Plate KH. Minor contribution of bone marrow-derived endothelial progenitors to the vascularization of murine gliomas. Brain Pathol. 2003; 13(4): 582–597.

[123] Folkins C, Shaked Y, Man S, Tang T, Lee CR, et al. Glioma tumor stem-like cells promote tumor angiogenesis and vasculogenesis via vascular endothelial growth factor and stromal-derived factor 1. Cancer Res. 2009; 69(18): 7243–7251.

[124] Burrel K, Zadeh G. Molecular mechanism of Tumor angiogenesis. In: Lichtor T. (ed.) Tumor angiogenesis. Rijeka: InTech; 2012. p275–296.

[125] Lewis CE, De Palma M, Naldini L. Tie2-expressing monocytes and tumor angiogenesis: regulation by hypoxia and angiopoietin-2. Cancer Res. 2007; 67(18): 8429–8432.

[126] Venneri MA, De Palma M, Ponzoni M, Pucci F, Scielzo C, et al. Identification of proangiogenic TIE2-expressing monocytes (TEMs) in human peripheral blood and cancer. Blood. 2007; 109(12): 5276–5285.

[127] Maniotis AJ, Folberg R, Hess A, Seftor EA, Gardner LM, et al. Vascular channel formation by human melanoma cells in vivo and in vitro: vasculogenic mimicry. Am J Pathol. 1999; 155(3): 739–752.

[128] Seftor EA, Meltzer PS, Schatteman GC, Gruman LM, Hess AR, et al. Expression of multiple molecular phenotypes by aggressive melanoma tumor cells: role in vasculogenic mimicry. Crit Rev Oncol Hematol. 2002; 44(1): 17–27.

[129] Liu C, Huang H, Doñate F, Dickinson C, Santucci R, et al. Prostate-specific membrane antigen directed selective thrombotic infarction of tumors. Cancer Res. 2002; 62(19): 5470–5475.

[130] Bonnet D, Dick JE. Human acute myeloid leukemia is organized as a hierarchy that originates from a primitive hematopoietic cell. Nat Med. 1997; 3(7): 730–737.

[131] El Hallani S, Boisselier B, Peglion F, Rousseau A, Colin C, et al. A new alternative mechanism in glioblastoma vascularization: tubular vasculogenic mimicry. Brain. 2010; 133(Pt 4): 973–982.

[132] Rodriguez FJ, Orr BA, Ligon KL, Eberhart CG. Neoplastic cells are a rare component in human glioblastoma microvasculature. Oncotarget. 2012; 3(1): 98–106.

[133] Kulla A, Burkhardt K, Meyer-Puttlitz B, Teesalu T, Asser T, et al. Analysis of the TP53 gene in laser-microdissected glioblastoma vasculature. Acta Neuropathol. 2003; 105(4): 328–332.

[134] Kioi M, Vogel H, Schultz G, Hoffman RM, Harsh GR, et al. Inhibition of vasculogenesis, but not angiogenesis, prevents the recurrence of glioblastoma after irradiation in mice. J Clin Invest. 2010; 120(3): 694–705.

[135] Takahashi T, Kalka C, Masuda H, Chen D, Silver M, et al. Ischemia- and cytokine-induced mobilization of bone marrow-derived endothelial progenitor cells for neovascularization. Nat Med. 1999; 5(4): 434–438.

[136] Orlic D, Kajstura J, Chimenti S, Bodine DM, Leri A, et al. Bone marrow stem cells regenerate infarcted myocardium. Pediatr Transplant. 2003; 7 (S3): 86–88.

[137] Greenfield JP, Cobb WS, Lyden D. Resisting arrest: a switch from angiogenesis to vasculogenesis in recurrent malignant gliomas. J Clin Invest. 2010; 120(3): 663–667.

[138] Soda Y, Marumoto T, Friedmann-Morvinski D, Soda M, Liu F, et al. Transdifferentiation of glioblastoma cells into vascular endothelial cells. Proc Natl Acad Sci U S A. 2011; 108(11): 4274–4280.

[139] Hardee ME, Zagzag D. Mechanisms of glioma-associated neovascularization. Am J Pathol. 2012; 181(4): 1126–1141.

[140] Ricci-Vitiani L, Pallini R, Biffoni M, Todaro M, Invernici G, et al. Tumor vascularization via endothelial differentiation of glioblastoma stem-like cells. Nature. 2010; 468(7325): 824–828.

[141] Wang Y, Zhu M, Zhang R, Yang H, Wang Y, et al. Whole genome amplification of the rust Puccinia striiformis f. sp. tritici from single spores. J Microbiol Methods. 2009; 77(2): 229–234.

[142] Jain RK, di Tomaso E, Duda DG, Loeffler JS, Sorensen AG, et al. Angiogenesis in brain tumors. Nat Rev Neurosci. 2007; 8(8): 610–622.

[143]   Vredenburgh JJ, Desjardins A, Herndon JE 2nd, Dowell JM, Reardon DA, et al. Phase II trial of bevacizumab and irinotecan in recurrent malignant glioma. Clin Cancer Res. 2007; 13(4): 1253–1259.

[144]   Bergers G, Hanahan D. Modes of resistance to anti-angiogenic therapy. Nat Rev Cancer. 2008; 8(8): 592–603.

[145]   Shojaei F, Ferrara N. Refractoriness to antivascular endothelial growth factor treatment: role of myeloid cells. Cancer Res. 2008; 68(14): 5501–5504.

[146]   Pàez-Ribes M, Allen E, Hudock J, Takeda T, Okuyama H, et al. Antiangiogenic therapy elicits malignant progression of tumors to increased local invasion and distant metastasis. Cancer Cell. 2009; 15(3): 220–231.

[147]   Winkler F, Kienast Y, Fuhrmann M, Von Baumgarten L, Burgold S, et al. Imaging glioma cell invasion in vivo reveals mechanisms of dissemination and peritumoral angiogenesis. Glia. 2009; 57(12): 1306–1315.

[148]   Bao S, Wu Q, Sathornsumetee S, Hao Y, Li Z, et al. Stem cell-like glioma cells promote tumor angiogenesis through vascular endothelial growth factor. Cancer Res. 2006; 66(16): 7843–7848.

[149]   Calabrese C, Poppleton H, Kocak M, Hogg TL, Fuller C, et al. A perivascular niche for brain tumor stem cells. Cancer Cell. 2007; 11(1): 69–82.

[150]   Hambardzumyan D, Becher OJ, Rosenblum MK, Pandolfi PP, Manova-Todorova K, et al. PI3K pathway regulates survival of cancer stem cells residing in the perivascular niche following radiation in medulloblastoma in vivo. Genes Dev. 2008; 22(4): 436–348.

[151]   Gilbertson RJ, Rich JN. Making a tumor's bed: glioblastoma stem cells and the vascular niche. Nat Rev Cancer. 2007; 7(10): 733–736.

[152]   Brooks MD, Sengupta R, Snyder SC, Rubin JB. Hitting them where they live: targeting the glioblastoma perivascular stem cell niche. Curr Pathobiol Rep. 2013; 1(2): 101–110.

[153]   Pala A, Karpel-Massler G, Wirtz CR, Halatsch ME. Epithelial to mesenchymal transition and progression of Glioblastoma. In: Lichtor T. (ed.) Clinical menagment and evolving novel therapeutic strategies for patients with brain Tumors. Rijeka: InTech; 2013. p277–289.

[154]   Ortensi B, Setti M, Osti D, Pelicci G. Cancer stem cell contribution to glioblastoma invasiveness. Stem Cell Res Ther. 2013; 4(1): 18.

[155]   Mani SA, Guo W, Liao MJ, Eaton EN, Ayyanan A, et al. The epithelial-mesenchymal transition generates cells with properties of stem cells. Cell. 2008; 133(4): 704–715.

[156] Jin X, Jeon HY, Joo KM, Kim JK, Jin J, et al. Frizzled 4 regulates stemness and invasiveness of migrating glioma cells established by serial intracranial transplantation.
Cancer Res. 2011; 71(8): 3066–3075.

[157] Kahlert UD, Maciaczyk D, Doostkam S, Orr BA, Simons B, et al. Activation of canoni-
cal WNT/β-catenin signaling enhances in vitro motility of glioblastoma cells by activation of ZEB1 and other activators of epithelial-to-mesenchymal transition. Cancer
Lett. 2012; 325(1): 42–53.

[158] Bhat KP, Salazar KL, Balasubramaniyan V, Wani K, Heathcock L, et al. The transcriptional coactivator TAZ regulates mesenchymal differentiation in malignant glioma.
Genes Dev. 2011; 25(24): 2594–2609.

[159] Filatova A, Acker T, Garvalov BK. The cancer stem cell niche(s): the crosstalk between glioma stem cells and their microenvironment. Biochim Biophys Acta. 2013;
1830(2): 2496–2508.

[160] Wang R, Chadalavada K, Wilshire J, Kowalik U, Hovinga KE, et al. Glioblastoma
stem-like cells give rise to tumor endothelium. Nature. 2010; 468(7325): 829–833.

[161] He H, Li MW, Niu CS. The pathological characteristics of glioma stem cell niches. J
Clin Neurosci. 2012; 19(1): 121–127.

[162] Charles NA, Holland EC, Gilbertson R, Glass R, Kettenmann H. The brain tumor microenvironment. Glia. 2012; 60(3): 502–514.

[163] Christensen K, Schrøder HD, Kristensen BW. CD133 identifies perivascular niches in
grade II-IV astrocytomas. J Neurooncol. 2008; 90(2): 157–170.

[164] Seidel S, Garvalov BK, Wirta V, von Stechow L, Schänzer A, et al. A hypoxic niche
regulates glioblastoma stem cells through hypoxia inducible factor 2 alpha. Brain.
2010; 133(Pt 4): 983–995.

[165] Bergers G, Song S. The role of pericytes in blood-vessel formation and maintenance.
Neuro Oncol. 2005; 7(4): 452–464.

[166] Armulik A, Genové G, Mäe M, Nisancioglu MH, Wallgard E, et al. Pericytes regulate
the blood-brain barrier. Nature. 2010; 468(7323): 557–561.

[167] Birnbaum T, Hildebrandt J, Nuebling G, Sostak P, Straube A. Glioblastoma-depend-
ent differentiation and angiogenic potential of human mesenchymal stem cells in vitro. J Neurooncol. 2011; 105(1): 57–65.

[168] Bexell D, Gunnarsson S, Tormin A, Darabi A, Gisselsson D, et al. Bone marrow multipotent mesenchymal stroma cells act as pericyte-like migratory vehicles in experimental gliomas. Mol Ther. 2009; 17(1): 183–190.

[169] Christensen K, Schrøder HD, Kristensen BW. CD133+ niches and single cells in glioblastoma have different phenotypes. J Neurooncol. 2011; 104(1): 129–143.

[170] Evans SM, Judy KD, Dunphy I, Jenkins WT, Hwang WT, et al. Hypoxia is important in the biology and aggression of human glial brain tumors. Clin Cancer Res. 2004; 10(24): 8177–8184.

[171] Keith B, Johnson RS, Simon MC. HIF1α and HIF2α: sibling rivalry in hypoxic tumor growth and progression. Nat Rev Cancer. 2011; 12(1): 9–22.

[172] Wang GL, Jiang BH, Rue EA, Semenza GL. Hypoxia-inducible factor 1 is a basic-helix-loop-helix-PAS heterodimer regulated by cellular O2 tension. Proc Natl Acad Sci U S A. 1995; 92(12): 5510–5514.

[173] Rankin EB, Giaccia AJ. The role of hypoxia-inducible factors in tumorigenesis. Cell Death Differ. 2008; 15(4): 678–685.

[174] Holmquist-Mengelbier L, Fredlund E, Löfstedt T, Noguera R, Navarro S, et al. Recruitment of HIF-1alpha and HIF-2alpha to common target genes is differentially regulated in neuroblastoma: HIF-2alpha promotes an aggressive phenotype. Cancer Cell. 2006; 10(5): 413–423.

[175] Soeda A, Park M, Lee D, Mintz A, Androutsellis-Theotokis A, et al. Hypoxia promotes expansion of the CD133-positive glioma stem cells through activation of HIF-1alpha. Oncogene. 2009; 28(45): 3949–3959.

[176] Bar EE, Lin A, Mahairaki V, Matsui W, Eberhart CG. Hypoxia increases the expression of stem-cell markers and promotes clonogenicity in glioblastoma neurospheres. Am J Pathol. 2010; 177(3): 1491–1502.

[177] Fan X, Khaki L, Zhu TS, Soules ME, Talsma CE, et al. NOTCH pathway blockade depletes CD133-positive glioblastoma cells and inhibits growth of tumor neurospheres and xenografts. Stem Cells. 2010; 28(1): 5–16.

[178] Heddleston JM, Li Z, McLendon RE, Hjelmeland AB, Rich JN. The hypoxic microenvironment maintains glioblastoma stem cells and promotes reprogramming towards a cancer stem cell phenotype. Cell Cycle. 2009; 8(20): 3274–3284.

[179] Green DR, Reed JC. Mitochondria and apoptosis. Science. 1998; 281(5381): 1309–1312.

[180] Ashkenazi A, Dixit VM. Apoptosis control by death and decoy receptors. Curr Opin Cell Biol. 1999; 11(2): 255–260.

[181] Mellai M, Schiffer D. Apoptosis in brain tumors: prognostic and therapeutic considerations. Anticancer Res. 2007 Jan; 27(1A): 437–448.

[182] Fischer I, Gagner JP, Law M, Newcomb EW, Zagzag D. Angiogenesis in gliomas: biology and molecular pathophysiology. Brain Pathol. 2005; 15(4): 297–310.

[183] Rong Y, Durden DL, Van Meir EG, Brat DJ. 'Pseudopalisading' necrosis in glioblastoma: a familiar morphologic feature that links vascular pathology, hypoxia, and angiogenesis. J Neuropathol Exp Neurol. 2006; 65(6): 529–539.

[184] Schiffer D, Chiò A, Giordana MT, Mauro A, Migheli A, Vigliani MC. The vascular response to tumor infiltration in malignant gliomas. Morphometric and reconstruction study. Acta Neuropathol. 1989; 77(4): 369–378.

[185] Kargiotis O, Rao JS, Kyritsis AP. Mechanisms of angiogenesis in gliomas. J Neurooncol. 2006; 78(3): 281–293.

[186] Schiffer D, Manazza A, Tamagno I. Nestin expression in neuroepithelial tumors. Neurosci Lett. 2006; 400(1-2): 80–85.

[187] Annovazzi L, Mellai M, Caldera V, Valente G, Schiffer D. SOX2 expression and amplification in gliomas and glioma cell lines. Cancer Genomics Proteomics. 2011; 8(3): 139–147.

[188] Conti L, Crisafulli L, Caldera V, Tortoreto M, Brilli E, et al. REST controls self-renewal and tumorigenic competence of human glioblastoma cells. PLoS One. 2012; 7(6): e38486.

[189] Caldera V, Mellai M, Annovazzi L, Piazzi A, Lanotte M, et al. Antigenic and genotypic similarity between primary glioblastomas and their derived neurospheres. J Oncol. 2011; 2011: 314962.

[190] Clarke MF, Fuller M. Stem cells and cancer: two faces of eve. Cell. 2006; 124(6): 1111–1115.

[191] Beier D, Hau P, Proescholdt M, Lohmeier A, Wischhusen J, et al. CD133(+) and CD133(-) glioblastoma-derived cancer stem cells show differential growth characteristics and molecular profiles. Cancer Res. 2007; 67(9): 4010–4015.

[192] Cummins EP, Berra E, Comerford KM, Ginouves A, Fitzgerald KT. Prolyl hydroxylase-1 negatively regulates IkappaB kinase-beta, giving insight into hypoxia-induced NFkappaB activity. Proc Natl Acad Sci U S A. 2006; 103(48): 18154–18159.

[193] Taylor CT, Cummins EP. The role of NF-kappaB in hypoxia-induced gene expression. Ann N Y Acad Sci. 2009; 1177: 178–184.

[194] Tafani M, Di Vito M, Frati A, Pellegrini L, De Santis E, et al. Pro-inflammatory gene expression in solid glioblastoma microenvironment and in hypoxic stem cells from human glioblastoma. J Neuroinflammation. 2011; 8: 32.

[195] Bar EE. Glioblastoma, cancer stem cells and hypoxia. Brain Pathol. 2011; 21(2): 119–129.

10

Minimally Invasive but Maximally Effective Treatment of Anterior Skull Based Tumors — The Combination of Advanced Neuroendoscopy and Intraoperative Imaging with iMRI and O-Arm

Kaveh Asadi-Moghaddam, Joseph C. Taylor and
Todd W. Vitaz

1. Introduction

The use of endoscopic techniques for the treatment of anterior skull based tumors has seen and exponential rise over the past 15 years. As a result of this rapid growth newer more powerful endoscopic systems with better surgical instruments have been developed which has increased the armamentarium and further broadened the scope of potentially treatable lesions [1,2]. However, even with these newer systems as well as angled surgical telescopes; visual lines of sight and normal anatomical structures can still hinder visualization. In addition, the steep learning curve associated with this type of procedure as well as the loss of the normal surgical feedback such as direct 3d visualization and tactile feedback also increase the challenges associated with such procedures. Therefore, in many cases it may be difficult to determine when the surgical goals of complete resection or safest maximal debulking have been obtained. The addition of advanced intraoperative imaging with intraoperative MRI or O-Arm (Medtronic, Minneapolis, MN) technology to some of these cases enables surgeons to obtain radiographic feedback during the procedure and thus further assess their work and adds another factor into surgical decision making [3].

2. Surgical corridors and types of lesion approaches treatable with extended endonasal approach

The treatment of both benign and malignant lesions of the anterior skull base can be performed with this approach. This technique requires a team approach with an ENT and neurosurgeon who both must be experienced in endoscopic principles, skull base anatomy and have a vast understanding of all potential treatment options[1,2,4-6]. An enormous learning curve exists not only for performing the surgical approach but also for dissection and removal of the lesion and subsequent reconstruction of the surgical defect and complication avoidance. Most authors have reported this learning curve with much higher complication rates in the earlier portions of their series[1,6-8]. We like most other teams have modified and fine-tuned our technique as we have continued to gain experience. Most authors recommend starting with straight forward midline lesions (figure 1.) and then broadening their technique to more challenging and invasive para-midline lesions as their comfort level and experience grows. In addition, the inclusion of frameless navigation systems and even more modern advanced imaging techniques such as O-Arm and intraoperative MRI also improve the safety and broaden the scope of lesions that may be amenable to such treatment approaches.

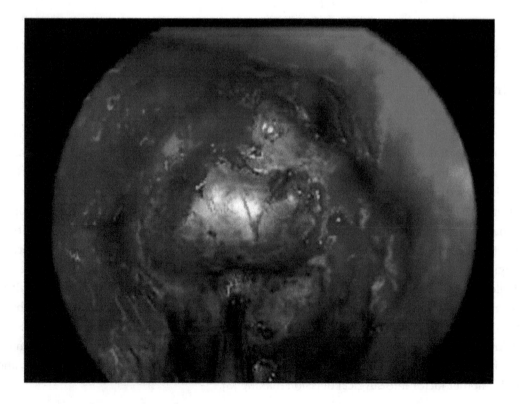

Figure 1. Intraoperative photograph from endoscopic endonasal approach to a small midline pituitary tumor, after straightforward midline approach and bone removal illustrating exposed sellar dura.

Lesions from the crista galli all the way down to the body of C2 can be treated with different variations of this approach[1,2,6,8-11]. Superiorly the medial orbits serve as a lateral limit on exposure [6]; however, more advanced techniques utilizing an oculoplastic surgeon and a small conjunctival incision can even expand this border (figure 2.). Traditionally the carotid arteries served as the lateral extent at the level of the sella [6,10]; however more advanced techniques now allow lateral exposure all the way to the infratemporal fossa [2,5].

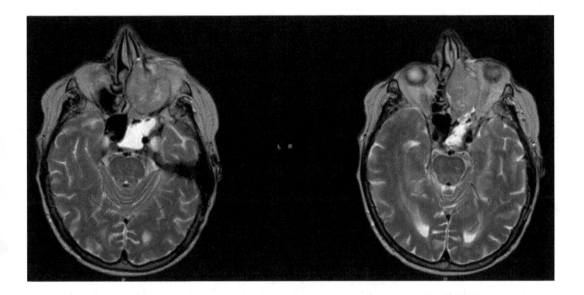

Figure 2. Preoperative axial T2-wieghted preoperative MRI showing primary sinus melanoma with left orbital compression in an 86 year old gentleman. Patient underwent endoscopic removal with aide of a small subconjunctival incision for palliative debulking of the lesion without globe removal.

Studies comparing endoscopic techniques with more traditional transcranial procedures have found either equivalent or superior results with endoscopic approaches[7,8]. However, limitations with endoscopic techniques continue to exist. These include anatomical constraints that may place major neural or vascular structures ventral to the pathology and thus increase the surgical risks and minimize utility. Limitations in visualization have been overcome with newer endoscopic lighting and camera systems. The 2 dimensional view with endoscopic techniques may create some challenges; however, experienced surgeons have learned to accommodate to these limitations. Newer 3D systems will soon become readily commercially available and as these systems evolve will likely overcome this limitation all together. Hemostasis and repair of postoperative CSF leaks have been the two most challenging aspects of these procedures [1,2,6,8,10,12]. Various commercially available products and surgical nuances can be used to overcome many of the challenges with hemostasis. In addition, vascular lesions are approached from the ventral side of dural involvement thus allowing devascularization of the lesion prior to any tumor manipulation or debulking. Control of postoperative CSF leaks deserves special mention and will be discussed below. Finally, the method of tumor removal must be modified to safely perform these techniques. While en bloc resection may be possible for small midline lesions this is not safely feasible for the majority of tumors. This becomes especially important in the realm of malignant tumor management where the historical standard has always been en bloc resection with negative margins. Even though this may be the goal, studies have shown that this in actually only obtained in 70% of cases of "open" resections for these lesions [13,14]. There is no convincing evidence to prove that a less invasive piecemeal resection portends to a worse prognosis and studies in this area are lacking [8].

3. Complications associated with EEA

Major neurological complications following this type of procedure are rare. They are typically related to either damage to major vascular structures or perforating vessels, optic nerve and chiasm or cranial nerves [1,2,4-8]. New or worsening visual symptoms are rare and their occurrence varies considerably based on pathology. Intraoperative monitoring of cranial nerve 3, 4, 6 may minimize the risk of damage to these structures.

Unlike transcranial approaches there is no skin incision or autologous bone flap, thus the risk of wound infection is almost entirely eliminated [7]. During the early experience with this exposure the concern for operating through a contaminated nasal corridor and the associated risk of meningitis or intracranial abscess was an enormous concern; however, experience has shown that this risk is minimal and usually limited to the setting of postoperative CSF leakage. In fact most authors recommend standard perioperative gram positive antibiotic coverage (cefazolin, clindamycin, vancomycin) for 24-48 hours [1,2,4,7]. In addition, because the pathological process is approached from the ventral bone interface, brain retraction and manipulation is minimal in these procedures. Therefore the risk of postoperative seizures, cognitive or other detrimental neurological changes from brain retraction and manipulation are almost entirely eliminated.

3.1. Postoperative CSF leaks

The creation of postoperative CSF fistulas has been one of the most challenging limitations to overcome with these techniques. Direct repair with suturing is not possible because of the deep surgical corridor and limited lateral exposure. Rates of postoperative CSF leakage vary between (0%-30%)[15-19]; and most surgeons have shown a direct relationship to experience with higher rates early on in their series despite progressing to more complex and invasive modifications of this procedure as their experience grew [1,2,4,6-8].

To try to prevent the occurrence of these events numerous reconstructive procedures have been attempted. These include the use of various autologous, allogenic and synthetic sub-strates from abdominal fat, fascia lata, nasal mucosa or turbinates, temporalis muscle, peri-cardium, and synthetic dural substitutes. In addition, bone reconstruction has been attempted with various autologous and synthetic commercial substances. These implants may be inserted as inlay or onlay grafts as well as the "gasket seal" techniques [20]. The addition of biological sealants such as Tisseal (Baxter Bioscience, Deerfield, IL) and DuraSeal (Integra, Plainsboro, NJ) are often commonly used as well.

A recent advancement has been the use of vascularized nasoseptal flaps [1,2,6,7,10,12]. These flaps which are typically developed at the beginning of the procedure prior to bone removal to reduce the risk of damage to the vascularity, have significantly decreased the risk of postoperative CSF leaks in cases where opening of the dura and arachnoid is anticipated [6]. A complete understanding of the vascular anatomy of this region is required to ensure that adequate vascularized tissue is available for reconstruction at the end of the procedure. Harvesting of such grafts lengthens surgical times only slightly but does increase postoperative nasal crusting and discomfort. Typically the septum is remucosalized by 3 months [6].

4. Combination of endoscopic techniques with advanced imaging technology

Despite the fact that endoscopic techniques may actually improve illumination and visualization over conventional microsurgical techniques there are many instances where it may be difficult to determine whether or not the surgical goals have been obtained. The use of angled (30, 45, 70 degree) telescopes can help surgeons evaluate around corners but not through objects. The surgical goals vary from case to case and depend on patient age, comorbidities, preoperative neurological status and pathology. While gross total resection may be the goal for most procedures in some lesion debulking for symptom control followed by stereotactic radiosurgery to the capsule may be the safest approach to minimize surgical morbidity (figure 3).

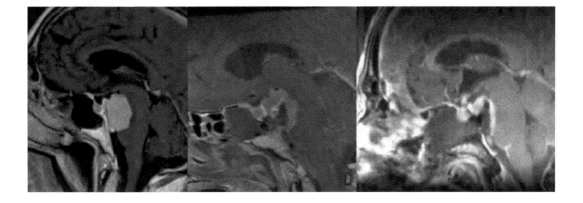

Figure 3. Sagittal T1-weighted post contrast preoperative, first intraoperative and second intraoperative MRI in 78 year old myelopathic gentleman with clival meningioma with significant brainstem compression. The surgical goal was to debulk the lesion leaving a small capsule however endoscopically it was difficult to determine how much residual tumor persisted behind the pituitary gland which is clearly seen on the middle image. On the final image the capsule can be seen falling away from the diencephalon and chiasmatic region.

O-Arm (Medtronic, Minneapolis, MN) and similar technologies may be useful in defining bone anatomy during some very complex procedures. The lack of tissue differentiation makes this technology very limiting for determining the extent of tumor removal for most cases. We have found this extremely useful in verifying adequate surgical results in cases of basilar invagination treated with the EEA. Following what is felt to be complete resection of the compressive pathology imaging can be obtained to verify the actual surgical results (figure 4). In addition, this technology can also be used in cases where more lateral temporal bone removal is required to verify actual bone removal prior to dural opening and tumor resection.

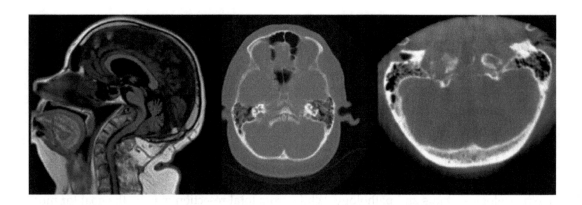

Figure 4. Preoperative Sagittal T1-weighted MRI and axial CT scan; and axial post midline decompression O-Arm image (sagittal reformatted images show complete decompression from clivus to C2/3 level) in 44 year old myelopathic female with platybasia and basilar invagination with brainstem compression, treated via endoscopic approach with O-Arm assisted navigation.

Another more common technology is the use of Intraoperative MRI. This technology has been extensively utilized for endoscopic removal of pituitary tumors for more than ten years [3,21]. We have found this exceptionally helpful in cases of giant pituitary tumors (figure 5) and other skull base cases such as meningiomas and craniopharyngiomas (figure 6). Following completion of resection imaging can be performed and then additional tumor resection can occur if significant residual is appreciated on these scans. Extreme care must be used in interpreting these results as surgical induced changes on peritumoral structures or capsule can mimic significant residual tumor in some instances.

We have found intraoperative imaging helpful in cases of large pituitary macroademonas where the capsule/diaphragm fails to prolapse into the field (figure 7). Imaging can be performed to determine the degree of residual tumor and decide whether opening the capsule and proceeding with extracapsular dissection is warranted. Finally, in cases where surgical debulking may be the primary goal intraoperative imaging can be performed to ensure that adequate results are obtained.

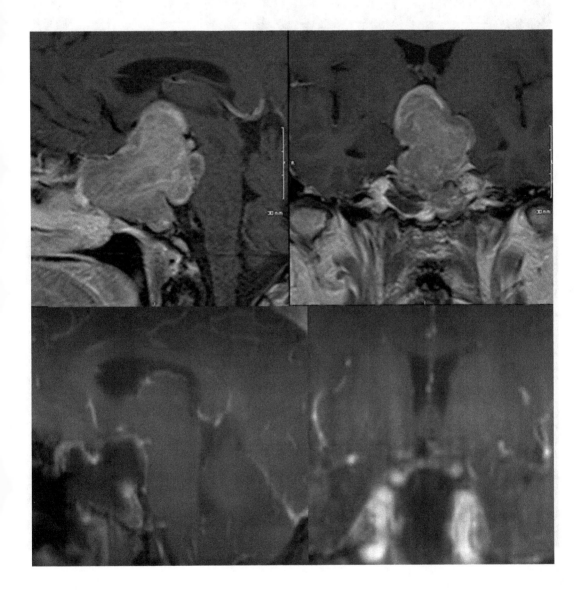

Figure 5. Post contrast T1-weighted sagittal and coronal preoperative (upper) and intraoperative (lower) images from a patient with a giant pituitary macroadenoma.

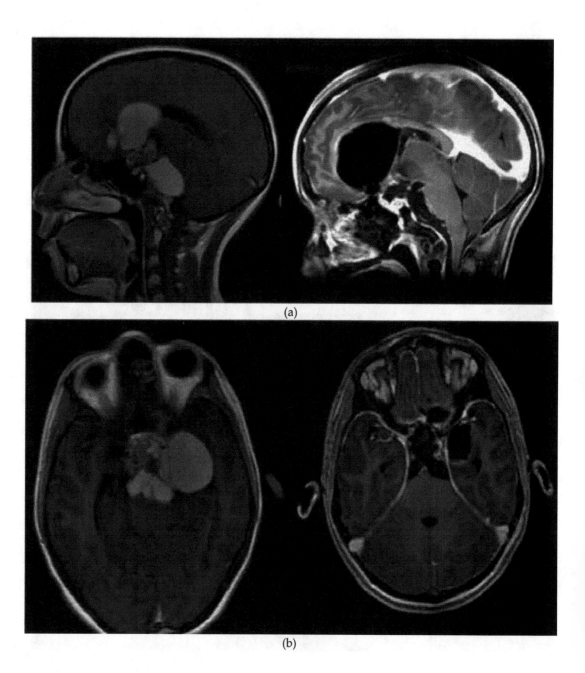

(a)

(b)

Figure 6. Post contrast T1-weighted preoperative and intraoperative Sagittal (a.) and axial (b.) images in 12 year old female with giant polycystic Craniopharyngioma with 2 cm enhancing nodule. iMRI was helpful in determining complete removal of enhancing nodule and drainage of all major cyst compartments following endoscopic midline approach from posterior ethmoids to clivus, working above and below pituitary gland, air visualized on intraoperative images was irrigated out of ventricles prior to closure.

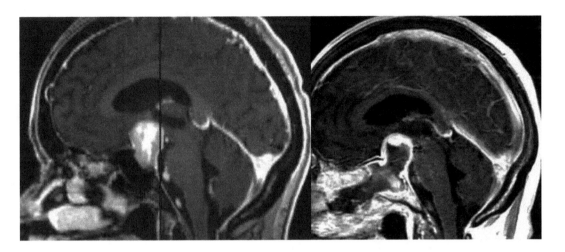

Figure 7. Post contrast sagittal preoperative and intraoperative sagittal MRI scans for a 76 year old female with a large pituitary macroadenoma, tumor capsule failed to prolapse into field during resection, visual inspection following imaging showed mostly blood products with a small amount of residual tumor along the superior aspect, given the patients age and preoperative visual status it was decided that a more aggressive resection was not in the patients best interest.

Author details

Kaveh Asadi-Moghaddam[1], Joseph C. Taylor[2] and Todd W. Vitaz[1*]

*Address all correspondence to: todd.vitaz@spectrumhealth.org

1 Department of Clinical Neurosciences Spectrum Health Medical Group, and College of Human Medicine Michigan State University, Grand Rapids, MI, USA

2 Grand Rapids Ear Nose and Throat, Grand Rapids, MI, USA

References

[1] Kassam AB, Snyderman CH, Mintz A, Gardner P, Carrau RL. Expanded endonasal approach: the rostrocaudal axis. Part I. Crista Galli to the sella turcica. Neurosurgical Focus 2005;19(E3): 1-12.

[2] Kassam AB, Gardner P, Snyderman C, Mintz A, Carrau R. Expanded endonasal approach: fully endoscopic, completely transnasal approach to the middle third of the clivus, petrous bone, middle cranial fossa, and infratemporal fossa. Neurosurgical Focus 2005;19(E3): 1-10.

[3] Anand VK, Schwartz TH, Hiltzik DH, Kacker A. Endoscopic transphenoidal pituitary surgery with real-time intraoperative magnetic resonance imaging. American Journal of Rhinology 2006;20: 401-405.

[4] Ensenat J, de Notaris M, Sanchez M, Fernandez C, Ferrer E, Bernal-Sprekelsen M, Alobid I. Endoscopic Endonasal surgery for skull base tumours: technique and preliminary results in a consecutive case series report. Rhinology 2013;51: 37-46.

[5] Ceylan S, Koc K, Anik I. endoscopic endonasal transsphenoidal approach for pituitary adenomas invading the cavernous sinus. Journal of Neurosurgery 2010;112: 99-107.

[6] Verillaud B, Bresson D, Sauvaget E, Mandonnet E, Georges B, Kania R, Herman P. Endoscopic endonasal skull base surgery. European Annals of Otorhinolaryngology, Head and Neck Diseases 2012;129: 190-196.

[7] Komotar RJ, Starke RM, Raper DM, Anand VK, Schwartz TH. Endoscopic endonasal compared with microscopic transcranial resection of craniopharyngiomas. World Neurosurgery 2012;77(2): 329-341.

[8] Greenfield JP, Anand VK, Kacker A, Seibert MJ, Singh A, Brown SM, Schwartz TH. Endoscopic endonasal transethmoidal transcribriform transfoveal ethmoidalis approach to the anterior cranial fossa skull base. Neurosurgery 2010;66: 883-892.

[9] Visocchi M, Doglietto F, Della Pepa GM, Esposito G, La Rocca G, Di Rocca C, Maira G, Fernandez E. Endoscope-assisted microsurgical transoral approach to the anterior craniovertebral junction compressive pathologies. European Spine Journal 2011;20: 1518-1525.

[10] Abuzayed B, Tanriover N, Gazioglu N, Sanus G, Ozlen F,Biceroglu H et al. Endoscopic endonasal anatomy and approaches to the anterior skull base: a neurosurgeon's perspective. The Journal of Craniofacial Surgery 2010;21(2): 529-537.

[11] Catapano D, Sloffer C, Frank G, Pasquini E, D'Angelo V, Lanzino G. Comparison between the microscope and endoscope in direct endonasal extended transsphenoidal approach: anatomical study. Journal of Neurosurgery 2006;104: 419-425.

[12] Cavallo LM, Messina A, Esposito F, De Vivitiis O, Dal Fabbro M, De Divittiis E, Cappabianca P. Skull base reconstruction in the extended endoscopic transsphenoidal approach for suprasellar lesions. Journal of Neurosurgery 2007;107: 713-720.

[13] Patel SG, Singh B, Polluri A, Bridger PG, Cantu G, Cheesman AD, et al. Craniofacial surgery for malignant skull base tumours: report of an international collaborative study. Cancer 2003;98: 1179-1187.

[14] Ganly I, Patel SG, Singh B, Kraus DH, Bridger PG, Cantu G, et al. Craniofacial resection for malignant paranasal sinus tumours: report of an international collaborative study. Head and Neck 2005;27: 575-584.

[15] de Vivitiis E, Cappabianca P, Cavallo LM, Esposito F, de Divitiis O, Messina A. Extended endoscopic transsphenoidal approach for extrasellar craniopharyngiomas. Neurosurgery 2007; 61: 219-228.

[16] Frank G, Pasquini E, Doglietto F, Mazzatenta D, Sciarretta V, Farneti G, Calbucci F. The endoscopic extended transsphenoidal approach for craniopharyngiomas. Neurosurgery 2006;59: 75-83.

[17] Jane Jr JA, Kiehna E, Payne SC, Early SV, Laws Jr ER. Early outcomes of endoscopic transsphenoidal surgery for adult craniopharyngiomas. Neurosurgical Focus 2010;28: E9.

[18] Leng LZ, Greenfield JP, Souweidane MM, Anand VK, Schwartz TH. Endoscopic resection of craniopharyngiomas: analysis of outcome including extent of resection, cerebrospinal fluid leak, return to preoperative productivity, and body mass index. Neurosurgery 2012;70: 110-123.

[19] Stamm AC, Vellutin E, Harvey RJ, Nogeir Jr JF, Herman DR. Endoscopic transnasal craniotomy and the resection of Craniopharyngioma. Laryngoscope 2008;118: 1142-1148.

[20] Leng LZ, Brown S, Anand K, Schwartz TH. "Gasket-seal" watertight closure in minimal-access endoscopic cranial base surgery. Neurosurgery 2008;62: 342-342.

[21] Vitaz TW, Inkabi KE, Carruba CJ. Intraoperative MRI for transphenoidal procedures: short-term outcome for 100 consecutive cases. Clinical Neurology and Neurosurgery 2011;113: 731-735.

11

Brain Tumor Metabolism — Unraveling its Role in Finding New Therapeutic Targets

Vera Miranda Gonçalves, Fátima Baltazar and
Rui Manuel Reis

1. Introduction

Primary tumors of brain account for approximately 2-3% of all cancers, with annual incidence approximately 15 patients per 100,000 people and the prevalence has been estimated in 69 patients per 100,000 people. Several brain tumor types evolve from glial or neuronal precursors, being the tumors of glial cells the most common and denominated gliomas [1, 2]. Gliomas are histologically classified according to the World Health Organization (WHO) classification into four malignancy grades[3, 4]. Pilocytic astrocytomas (WHO grade I) are benign tumors that can usually be cured after surgical resection. Diffuse astrocytomas (WHO grade II) exhibit a slow growth, but have an inevitable tendency to progress to higher grade lesions, such as anaplastic gliomas (WHO grade III) and glioblastomas (WHO grade IV). Anaplastic gliomas are rapidly growing malignant tumors that, in addition to surgery, require aggressive adjuvant therapy. Glioblastomas (GBMs) are the most malignant and frequent type of gliomas, which are preferentially manifested in aged adults with a peak of incidence between 50-60 years old [4]. Glioblastomas may evolve from lower grade tumors as described and are mentioned secondary glioblastomas, although most of GBMs arise rapidly without the evidence of less malignant lesion, and are denominated *de novo* or primary glioblastomas [2, 4].

The current standard therapy for GBM includes tumor resection followed by radiation and concomitant chemotherapy, with temozolomide being the only approved drug that shows some efficacy in this disease [5]. In the last decade, specific inhibitors of oncogenic signaling pathways such as EGFR, PI3K/Akt, and VEGF have made progress with some of them currently tested in clinical trials. Nowadays, bevacizumab (avastin®), a humanized monoclonal antibody against VEGF is approved as a second line of treatment for recurrent GBMs and is currently in phase III clinical trials for the treatment of initial GBMs [6]. Antiangiogenic therapy with avastin improved radiographic response and 6 month of progression free survival, however with modest or little effect on overall survival, when in combination with TMZ during and after radiotherapy [7, 8]. Besides, its role in promoting vascular normalization, the effect on tumor cell invasion is still controversial. Avastin treatment induces infiltration in U87 xenograft model and also was associated with diffusing invasive recurrence in some GBM patients [9, 10]. Additionally, it was observed that vasculature normalization with bevacizumab treatment leads to increased hypoxia and consequently acquisition of resistance [11]. Despite progress in new molecular-based therapies, the prognosis of glioblastomas patients is still very dismal [12, 13]. Thus, exploitation of new molecular targets becomes crucial in neuro-oncology.

In recent years, understanding the regulation of tumor metabolism has significantly improved. Accumulating evidence showed that tumor cells reprogram their metabolism to meet high energy demands, coordinate markedly elevated biosynthetic processes and energy production, which in turn promote rapid growth and division of tumor cells [14-17]. Thus, targeting metabolism has become a novel promising strategy for treating cancers, particularly glioblastomas.

2. Tumor metabolism

During cancer progression, molecular changes are associated to metabolic reprogramming [18, 19], which is nowadays defined as a new hallmark of cancer [20]. In mammalian cells, namely quiescent cells or differentiated tissues, glycolysis is reduced in the presence of oxygen and energy production arises from mitochondrial oxidative phosphorylation which oxidizes pyruvate to CO_2 and H_2O, known as "Pasteur effect" (Figure 1) [21]. However, in tumor cells, like proliferating tissues, there is high glycolytic activity even in the presence of oxygen, being glycolysis the major source of energy. This phenomenon is known as "Warburg effect". As a result, tumor cells convert most of the incoming glucose into lactate (around 85 %) rather than metabolizing pyruvate in the mitochondria through oxidative phosphorylation (around 5%) (Figure 1) [16, 21, 22].

2.1. Glycolytic metabolism in brain tumors

As above mentioned, in tumor cells, even in the presence of oxygen, glucose is converted into lactate instead of being oxidized in mitochondria, being glycolysis the major source of energy [16]. It has been described that glioblastomas present metabolic remodeling, increasing glycolytic activity about 3-fold when compared to normal brain tissue [23, 24]. Thus, an increase in several glycolytic enzymes was observed, such as hexokinase II (HKII), pyruvate kinase (PKM), as well as the glucose transporters (GLUTs). Importantly, several studies reported these molecules as important mediators in glycolytic metabolism, constituting attractive molecular targets (Figure 2).

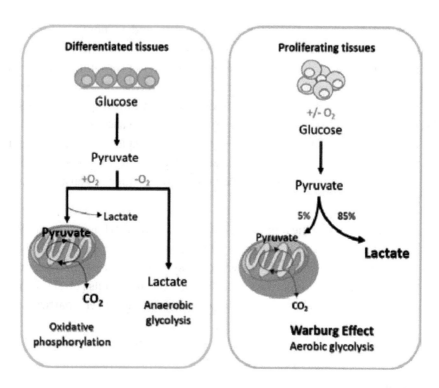

Figure 1. Schematic representation of the metabolic differences between differentiated tissues and proliferating tissues. In the presence of oxygen, non-proliferating tissues metabolize glucose to pyruvate and oxidize it in mitochondria through oxidative phosphorylation. On the other hand, glucose is metabolized to lactate when in the absence of oxygen. In proliferative tissues, like tumor cells, glucose is metabolized to pyruvate and even in the presence of oxygen pryruvate is converted into lactate,a phenomenon denominated aerobic glycolysis or Warburg effect.

2.1.1. Glucose Transporters (GLUTs)

Glucose is the main source of energy in most tissues, including brain. GLUTs are transmembrane transporters that perform the uptake of glucose into the cell. The GLUT family is composed by 12 isoforms, however only GLUT1, GLUT3, and GLUT12 have been described as transporters of glucose [25]. GLUT1 is ubiquitously expressed and it is responsible for providing basal glucose to different tissues and cells. In brain, GLUT1 is expressed in astrocytes, whereas GLUT3 is observed in neurons [26].

In the tumoral context, overexpression of specific isoforms of GLUTs has been reported [27, 28]. Most frequently, an increase in GLUT1 expression has been observed in several solid tumors compared with the corresponding normal tissue [27, 28]. However, it has been verified that their expression is tissue specific and some tumors overexpressed other isoforms, such as GLUT12 in prostate cancer [29]. Concerning brain tumors, few studies have evaluated GLUT expression, where it is described that glioblastomas have an increased expression of GLUT1 and GLUT3 when compared with low grade gliomas and normal brain [30, 31]. In fact, both the isoforms are downstream targets of hypoxia-inducible factor 1α (HIF-1α), a transcription factor that is frequently present in glioblastomas. GLUT1 expression is observed in vessels of the normal brain tissues and presents a focal expression in the perinecrotic regions of GBMs, suggesting that their expression is associated with hypoxic regions in glioblastomas (Miranda-

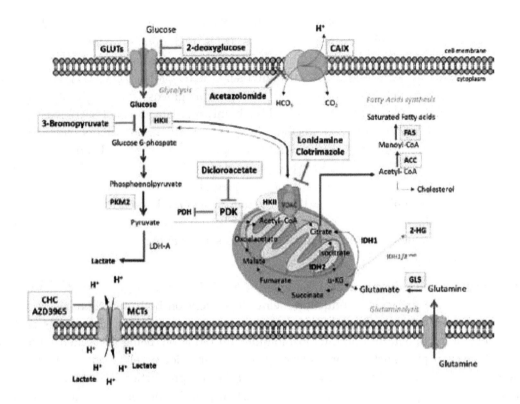

Figure 2. Potential molecular targets in metabolic remodeling of glioblastomas. The green boxes represent the potential metabolic molecular targets in glioblastomas: enzymes involved in glycolytic metabolism, glutamine metabolism, lipid metabolism; different transporters and also the oncometabolite 2-hydroxyglutarate. Yellow boxes represent the different inhibitors of the specific molecular targets described. Abbreviations: GLUTs, glucose transporters; MCTs, monocarboxylate transporters; CAIX, carbonic anhydrase IX; HKII, hexokinase II, PKM2, pyruvate kinase M2; LDH-A, lactate dehydrogenase A; PDH, pyruvate dehydrogenase; PDK, pyruvate dehydrogenase kinase; IDH1/2, isocitrate dehydrogenase 1/2; IDH1/2 [mut], isocitrate dehydrogenase ½ mutation; 2-HG, 2-hydroxyglutarate; GLS, glutaminase; ACC, acetyl-CoA carboxylase; FAS, fatty acid synthase; α-KG, α-ketoglutarate; VDAC, voltage-dependent anion channel; CHC, α-cyanohydroxycinnamic acid.

Gonçalves V. *et al*, submitted). Several *in vitro* studies also reported overexpression of GLUT1 expression in GBMs cells when compared with normal astrocytes [32].

These findings raise the importance of GLUT inhibition in tumor therapy, however, at the moment, a glucose transporter inhibitor is not available at the clinical level. Nevertheless, *in vitro* studies have been using 2-deoxy-D-glucose has an inhibitor of glucose uptake promoting a decrease on tumor cell proliferation [33] (Figure 2). These studies reported the high dependence of brain tumors on glucose as source of energy and also for catabolic processes.

2.1.2. Hexokinase II

HK is one of the most important enzymes of the glycolytic pathway, which is responsible for the phosphorylation of glucose to glucose-6-phosphate (G6P), thereby preventing the efflux of glucose from the cell [34]. This enzyme has four isoforms (I-IV) identified in different mammalian tissues [35].

In most solid tumors, hexokinases type I and II are the most frequently upregulated [36]. In glioblastomas, HKII is highly expressed, whereas HKI is predominantly expressed in normal brain and low grade gliomas [37]. Additionally, HKII is expressed at low levels in neuronal tissue, but is highly expressed in mesenchymal subtype of glioblastomas [37]. As the first enzyme involved in the glycolytic pathway, HK controls glucose flux in glycolysis or the pentose phosphate pathway (PPP) [38]. HKII is a highly regulated form of hexokinase, being regulated by HIF-1α, glucose, p53, insulin, glucagon, cAMP, among others [36]. The four hexokinase types are normally expressed in the cytoplasm, however type I and II can bind to the outer membrane of the mitochondria *via* voltage-dependent anion channel (VDAC) (Figure 2) [39]. The translocation of HKII to mitochondria is regulated by growth factors and signaling pathways, such as EGFR and PI3K/AKT activation, which are known to be upregulated in glioblastomas [40]. Moreover, the association of HKII with mitochondria in gliomas, besides maintaining high glucose influx, also renders cells resistant to apoptosis, due to the prevention of cytochrome c release [41].

Several studies have described that the expression of HKII in gliomas promotes proliferation and increase in lactate production, being dependent on both mitochondrial localization and kinase activity [42]. Additionally, HKII overexpression in glioblastomas confers resistance to treatment with both temozolomide and radiation, being associated with poor overall survival [43]. Furthermore, silencing of HKII in glioma cells leads to decrease in glycolytic metabolism, observed by a decrease in lactate production and increase expression of OXPHOS proteins and oxygen consumption [43]. Finally, it was also demonstrated that reduction of HKII expression impaired tumor growth *in vivo* both on subcutaneous and intracranial xenograft models [37, 43].

Some drugs have been proposed for chemical inhibition of HKII (Figure 2). 3-bromopyruvate (3-BrPA), a pyruvate analogue, is an alkylating agent and also an inhibitor of glycolysis that decreases tumor growth, without apparent toxicity in subcutaneous hepatocellular carcinoma [44]. However, it is effective only at high concentrations (mM) and to the best our knowledge is not under clinical trials. Other known inhibitor is lonidamine, an inhibitor of HKII binding to the mitochondria, which is currently in clinical trials. *In vitro* studies showed a decrease in lactate production in high grade gliomas but not in low grade [33]. Despite that lonidamine treatment leads to a decrease in tumor growth in different solid tumors without adverse effects, the results of a phase I/II efficacy trial was disappointing in gliomas [45, 46]. Clotrimazole is another inhibitor of HKII localization that demonstrated promising results *in vivo*. In gliomas, clotrimazole increased the sensitivity to radiotherapy and also leads to decrease in tumor growth [47, 48].

2.1.3. Pyruvate Kinase (PK)

PK is an enzyme involved in the last irreversible step of the glycolytic pathway, converting phosphoenolpyruvate (PEP) to pyruvate [49, 50]. It is also regulated allosterically by the phosphotyrosine binding or phosphorylation and its expression is regulated by isoform selection [50]. Thus, PKM1 is mostly present in adult tissues, such as adult brain and muscle, whereas PKM2 is more frequent in proliferating tissues and embryonic tissues, namely in fetal brain and tumor cancer cells [49]. PKM1 and PKM2 presented different properties, which results in different activities. PKM1 is constitutively active, but PKM2 is regulated by fructose-1,6-biphosphate, presenting reduced activity, which allows the accumulation of glycolytic intermediates and promotes the entry of G6P into the oxidative metabolism of PPP for the production of energy and biosynthesis of proteins, lipids and nucleotides (macromolecules) [50-53]. In cancer cells, like glioblastomas, there is upregulation of PKM2 that favors aerobic glycolysis, increasing lactate production [51, 54, 55]. On the other hand, PKM2 favors the biosynthetic pathway, leading to increased biomass. This dual function potentiates tumor proliferation and aggressiveness. The dimeric form of PKM2 delays pyruvate formation and allows the accumulation of upstream glycolytic intermediates for biosynthetic pathways, whereas the tetrameric form favors aerobic glycolysis, increasing lactate production [56].

In lung cancer cell lines, replacing PKM2 by PKM1 decreases lactate production and increases oxygen consumption (reverse Warburg effect) and also decreases the proliferative capacity of cancer cells in nude mice [54]. It was demonstrated in glioblastomas that knockdown of PKM2 decreased cell proliferation and survival but this did not favor the switch from aerobic glycolysis to oxidative phosphorylation, unlike HKII knockdown [43]. Interestingly, PKM2 was identified as essential for survival of glioma stem cells [57].

Another important function of PKM2 has been associated to epigenetic regulation, being a regulator of histone phosphorylation and acetylation of EGFR-driven glioblastomas [58, 59]. Additionally, in glioblastomas, it was demonstrated that PKM2 is involved in the EGFR signaling pathway that induces its phosphorylation and translocation into the nucleus, which in turn promotes activation of the transcription factor *c-Myc* with consequent activation of downstream targets, namely genes involved in glycolytic metabolism [60]. Taken together, inhibition of PKM2, in order to deplete the dimer and tetramer formation, can be a new therapeutic strategy, since it can lead to inhibition of glycolysis, decreasing energy production and at the same time blocking the anabolic process in tumor cells (Figure 2).

2.2. Mitochondrial metabolism in brain tumors

In addition to glycolytic dependence, most tumors present abnormalities in the number and function of mitochondria, as the case of glioblastomas [61]. Otto Warburg hypothesized that the increase on glycolytic metabolism in cancer was due to mitochondrial dysfunction, however nowadays we know that most tumors maintain functional mitochondria [22, 62-64]. Moreover, increased glycolytic metabolism can be a consequence of mitochondrial metabolism impairment, due to abnormalities in components of the tricarboxylic acid (TCA) cycle, alterations in electron transport chain or deficiencies in oxidative phosphorylation [65, 66]. Concerning the selection theory in cancer cells, the dependence on glycolysis occurs gradually in order to compensate the respiratory failure. In contrast to normal brain cells, in which glycolysis and respiration are tightly coupled, tumor cells are defective in their ability to connect glycolysis and respiration [66].

Two mitochondrial enzymes are important in glioblastomas, such as pyruvate dehydrogenase kinase (PDK) and isocitrate dehydrogenases 1 and 2 (IDH1 and IDH2). The presence of mutations in IDH1 and IDH2 has been recently associated with gliomagenesis.

2.2.1. Pyruvate Dehydrogenase Kinase (PDK)

Pyruvate dehydrogenase (PDH) is a mitochondrial enzyme that controls the entry of pyruvate into mitochondria, promoting its oxidative decarboxylation into acetyl-CoA [67, 68]. The activity of PDH is inhibited by phosphorylation through PDK, resulting in its accumulation in the cytosol and consequent conversion into lactate [67, 68]. PDK is an important mitochondrial matrix protein comprising four isoforms (PDK1 to PDK4), being PDK2 highly expressed in glioblastomas compared to normal adjacent brain tissue [69].

Tumor cells present high levels of glycolysis as a consequence of increased hypoxic microenvironment, which leads to activation of HIF-1α and consequent upregulation of downstream target genes involved in glycolytic metabolism, such as PDK [67]. This enzyme is responsible for the uncoupling between glycolysis and mitochondrial oxidation of glucose, preventing the entry of pyruvate into the mitochondria with consequent increase in glycolytic rates, which confers resistance to apoptosis [67, 68]. Thus, PDK became an important target for glycolytic tumors (Figure 2). Dichloroacetate (DCA), a chemical PDK inhibitor, has been studied in several *in vitro* and *in vivo* models [68]. DCA promotes dephosphorylation of PDH, leading to entry of pyruvate into the mitochondria, decreasing glycolytic rates and lactate production [68, 70]. This leads to activation of oxidative phosphorylation, depolarization of mitochondria and consequent increase in production of reactive oxygen species (ROS), which promotes apoptosis of cancer cells, decreasing tumor cell proliferation [68, 70]. DCA treatment has demonstrated promising results in some tumors, particularly in non-small cell lung, breast and endometrial cancer, either experimentally using *in vitro* and *in vivo* models, as well as in clinical trials [70-73]. In glioblastomas, inhibition of PDK with DCA was evaluated pre-clinically. In C6 glioma cells, it was observed a decrease in lactate production, increase in ROS production, as well as depolarization of mitochondria, which results in a decrease on cell proliferation and induction of apoptosis [74]. *In vivo* it was verified that DCA decreased not only tumor growth but also the angiogenic capacity of glioma cells [74]. The effect of DCA was also tested in a series of glioblastoma patients with congenital acidosis, with a reduction in lactate levels, decrease in HKII localization in the mitochondria, as well as a decrease in mitochondrial polarization, which rendered tumor cells more sensitive to apoptosis [69]. Despite these encouraging results, no exact conclusions can yet be made regarding the efficacy and toxicity of DCA in glioblastoma patients. Thus, a large and randomized clinical study would be important to define the efficacy and toxicity of DCA. Additionally, whether DCA can sensitize GBM cells to temozolomide and radiotherapy remains undetermined.

2.2.2. Isocitrate Dehydrogenase (IDH)

IDH is an enzyme that catalyzes the oxidative decarboxylation of isocitrate to α-ketoglutarate, generating NADH in the mitochondria or NADPH in the cytoplasm [75]. It is composed by 5 genes, being the *IDH1* and *IDH2* the most explored and important in gliomas. IDH1 is presented in the cytoplasm and peroxisome, whereas IDH2 is presented in the mitochondria [76].

In 2008, recurrent somatic hotspot mutations of *IDH1* and *IDH2* were found in low grade gliomas and secondary glioblastomas [77, 78]. These mutations cause amino acid single change in one of the two alleles of the gene (arginine 132 for *IDH1* and arginine 172 for *IDH2*), being classified has a dominant mutation [79]. It is described that the arginine mutation occurs in the binding site of the substrate isocitrate [42]. *IDH1* mutations are reported in more than 80% secondary glioblastomas, but only 5% in primary glioblastomas [76, 80, 81]. Additionally, it occurs in 80% of diffuse astrocytomas (WHO grade II). These mutations are more frequent in younger patient secondary glioblastomas, associated with a proneural subtype and also with increased survival [82]. It was reported that the presence of IDH mutations leads to a decrease in α-ketoglutarate that is required for prolyl hydroxylase (PHD) activity that promote degradation of HIF-1α (ref). Thus, downregulation of intracellular α-ketoglutarate contributes to stabilization of HIF-1α, leading to pseudohypoxia [83]. Nevertheless, subsequent studies did not verify an alteration in α-ketoglutarate on mutant IDH1/2, instead, a gain of function activity it was found, which converts α-ketoglutarate to 2-hydroxyglutarate (Figure 2) [84, 85]. The latter has been recognized as an oncometabolite, which inhibits enzymes involved in the α-ketoglutarate pathway. Additionally, it was described that 2-hydroxyglutarate is involved in epigenetic regulation, promoting a hypermethylator phenotype in gliomas [86] and also keep cells in an undifferentiated *status*, or stem cell-like, which can be more permissive to transformation [17]. The presence of pseudohypoxia, due to the constitutive stabilization of HIF-1α, indicates that *IDH1/2* mutations are involved in HIF-1α signaling pathway, which promotes glucose metabolism, angiogenesis and invasion [83]. These results suggest the paramount role of IDH mutations on the metabolic remodeling of glioblastomas, contributing to the "Warburg effect". Therefore, study the involvement of *IDH1/2* mutations in metabolic remodelling and in aerobic glycolysis opens a new window for investigation. Overall, IDH1 is an attractive target for therapy (Figure 2) since they are early events in the progression from low grade to high grade gliomas.

2.3. Glutamine metabolism and lipid synthesis in brain tumors

Like glucose, glutamine is a source of energy for tumor cells, functioning as a nitrogen donor [87, 88]. Glutamine metabolism has been reported to be upregulated in some tumors, being crucial for the biosynthetic processes, namely synthesis of cholesterol and fatty acids [14, 89, 90]. The shift to glutamine metabolism to produce the precursor acetyl-CoA for lipid biosynthesis is a mechanism of adaptation to glycolytic metabolism that prevents the entry of pyruvate into mitochondria, due to upregulation of PDK [91]. In fact, it has been observed an increased expression of glutaminase (GLS) enzyme in tumor cells. GLS is located in the mitochondria and catalyzes the conversion of glutamine to glutamate being transcriptionally regulated by the oncogenes *c-Myc* and *NFκB*. [92-94], An increased concentration of glutamine in glioblastomas compared to normal brain tissue was demonstrated by nuclear magnetic resonance (NMR) [95]. Additionally, there is a low expression of glutamine synthase that correlates with a better prognosis in glioblastomas [96].

Beyond the altered glycolytic and glutamine metabolism in tumor cells, the alteration in lipid metabolism is also recognized as a component of the metabolic reprogramming. It has been observed that tumor cells present reactivation of *de novo* fatty acid synthesis, important for the biogenesis of cellular membranes [97, 98]. Glioblastomas contain higher levels of unsaturated fatty acids compared to normal brain, indicating the presence of exacerbated lipogenesis, which is regulated by several key genes, such as SREBP-1 and its down-stream-targeted genes acetyl-CoA carboxylase (ACC), fatty acid synthase (FAS) and low-density lipoprotein receptor (LDLR), which are upregulated in these tumors [99]. Importantly, the EGFR/PI3K/AkT signaling pathway regulates the metabolic reprogramming in glioblastomas [100]. Cholesterol is also an important component of cell membranes and cholesterol esters have been found to be abundantly present in high grade gliomas, but undetectable in normal tissues by NMR techniques [101, 102]. Recently, low density lipoprotein receptor (LDLR) has been described to be upregulated in GBM patients, xenografts and cell lines, and this upregulation was correlated with high levels of cholesterol esters in GBM cells [103]. Interestingly, LDLR is also be upregulated by EGFR/PI3K/Akt signaling, which was been shown to be mediated by SREBP-1 in GBMs [100]. However, little is known about the altered lipid metabolism in cancer cells, namely glioblastomas, and their role in the tumor context, being possible that lipogenesis in cancer cells could support the cell growth located within nutrient-limited areas, thereby contributing to symbiotic relationships within tumors. Once more, lipid metabolism, as well as glutamine metabolism, and their key enzymes are interesting targets in glioblastomas (Figure 2)

3. Lactate transport and pH regulation in brain tumors

A constitutive increase in the glycolytic phenotype of cancer cells leads to acute and chronic acidification of tumor microenvironment. Important proteins involved in acidification of the extracellular space are monocarboxylate transporters (MCTs) that co-transport H+and lactate, and carbonic anhydrases (CAIXs), which are activated by growth factors, oncogenic transformation, hypoxia, and low intracellular pH [21]. As it is known, tumor acidity is associated with cancer cell invasion behavior, i.e. increased migration, invasion and metastasis [104]. Further, tumor acidosis and lactate contributes to several features of tumor progression and malignancy, like immune escape, angiogenesis, and radioresistance, making lactate a key player in cancer aggressiveness. [105]. Still in line with a potential involvement of lactate in the invasion behavior, it has been shown that lactate up-regulates the expression of transforming growth factor (TGF-β2), which is associated with increased migration in glioblastomas [106].

3.1. Monocarboxylate transporters

The MCT family comprises 14 members with similar topology; however, only 4 isoforms (MCT1–MCT4) are proton-linked monocarboxylate transporters, performing the transmembrane transport of monocarboxylates, such as lactate, coupled with a proton, in an equimolar manner [107, 108].

In the last years, several studies reported up-regulation of MCTs in different human solid tumors, showing the importance of MCTs in cancer biology [109]. In brain tumors, the scare studies point to the importance of MCT expression, especially MCT1. Strong expression of MCT1 in the plasma membrane was found in high grade gliomas compared with low-grade lesions and normal adjacent tissues, which exhibited negative or weak MCT1 staining [110, 111],. A study in neuroblastomas showed, by mRNA quantification, that MCT1 was differently expressed and that its activity was highly associated with MYCN amplification, leading to the hypothesis that expression of MCT1 could be associated with higher malignancy [112]. Further, expression analysis revealed that SLC16A1 transcript, encoding MCT1, was elevated in 90% of the medulloblastomas analyzed [113]. It was also reported that inhibition of MCT activity, particularly MCT1, decreased the glycolytic phenotype (low glucose consumption and lactate production), cell proliferation and invasion, promoting increase in cell death [111, 114, 115]. This elucidates the importance of MCT1 activity in intracellular pH homeostasis and tumor aggressiveness of glioblastomas.

Although MCTs are not the major H^+ transporters, the data available in the literature support the hypothesis of a major contribution of MCTs to the hyper-glycolytic and acid-resistant phenotype, as major adaptation to the hypoxic microenvironment [116]. Thus, MCT inhibition may be a useful therapeutic approach in brain tumors (Figure 2). Actually, it was demonstrated that *in vitro* MCT1 inhibition decreases intracellular pH, leads to cell death and, importantly, enhances cancer cell radiosensivity in gliomas [114, 115]. Importantly, promising results using *in vivo* models have also been reported, where treatment with the chemical inhibitor CHC retarded tumor growth, rendered tumor cells sensitive to radiation and decreased invasion [114, 117]. However, CHC is not a specific MCT inhibitor, having also other targets. Recently, novel MCT1 inhibitors have been designed and may constitute an effective strategy to block MCT1 activity in cancer [118]. A orally administered related compound, AZD3965 (AstraZeneca), is currently in Phase I/II clinical trials for advanced solid tumors [119].

3.2. Carbonic anhydrases

Carbonic anhydrase catalyzes the conversion of extracellular bicarbonate to CO_2 and protons (H^+), thereby contributing to extracellular acidification [120]. This family is composed by 15 isoforms described in mammals, which differ in cellular localization, catalytic activity and susceptibility to different class of inhibitors. Two carbonic anhydrases are overexpressed in many solid tumors, namely CAIX and CAXII, being associated with tumor progression and response to therapy [121]. It is verified that CAIX is mostly negative in normal tissues but increase in the corresponding tumor tissues, whereas CAXII present a diffuse distribution in healthy tissues [122, 123]. Glioblastomas present high levels of intratumoral hypoxia, with consequent HIF-1α activation which contributes to increased expression of glycolysis-related genes [124], including CAIX [125]. CAIX is overexpressed in these tumors with focal plasma membrane expression close to peri-necrotic regions (hypoxic) [126], being negative in normal adjacent tissues, making it a feasible treatment target [127]. Furthermore, it has been described that CAIX is associated to poor overall survival, because it confers resistance to chemotherapy, radiotherapy and anti-angiogenic therapy [128]. Increased expression of CAIX in advanced stages/grades of many tumor types also suggests its association with dedifferentiation [129].

In vitro and *in vivo* approaches have demonstrated the potential of CAIX inhibition (Figure 2). Knockdown of CAIX decreased tumor cell ATP levels under hypoxic and glycolytic

conditions [126]. In addition, the susceptibility of U251 glioblastoma cells to chemotherapy and radiation treatment was strongly enhanced after CAIX downregulation, which is
supported by a recent *in vivo* study [126]. Similarly, CAIX inhibition enhanced the effect of
anti-angiogenic therapy with the anti-VEGF antibody bevacizumab [130]. Some inhibitors
have been developed to inhibit CA activity, particularly CAIX and CAXII. Acetazolo-
mide, enhances the apoptotic response of glioma cells to temozolomide [131] and an *in vivo*
study using derivatives of acetazolamide showed retardation of mice carcinoma xenograft
growth after 1 month of treatment [131]. Other studies have identified coumarins as CA
inhibitors, however they were not tested yet in the cancer context [132, 133]. Furthermore, specific monoclonal antibodies for the mostly expressed isoforms in tumors, namely
CAIX, have been developed, *i.e*, the M75 and WX-G250 for colorectal cancer and renal cell
carcinoma, respectively [134, 135].

4. Future perspectives and conclusions

Metabolic transformation plays a major role in gliomas development, tumor progression and
adaptation to tumor microenvironment. The interplay between tumor angiogenesis, hypoxia,
pH regulation and energy metabolism, glycolysis related enzymes and transporters, as well
as pH regulator transporters, may provide promising molecular targets for drug development.
In addition to glycolysis, glutaminolysis and fatty acid synthesis represent key metabolic
events with potentially interesting drug targets. Furthermore, mutations in *IDH1/2*, detected
in a genome wide screen on GBMs, point to new specific transforming events in gliomas. These
metabolic pathways are tightly linked and also controlled by signaling events often deregu-
lated in gliomas, underlying the flexibility of glioma cells to develop adaptive mechanisms
when exposed to oxygen or nutrient deprivation. This highlights the need of targeting several
pathways simultaneously and linking the metabolic targets to the genetic makeup of GBM
tumors.

Author details

Vera Miranda Gonçalves[1,2], Fátima Baltazar[1,2] and Rui Manuel Reis[1,2,3*]

*Address all correspondence to: ruireis.hcb@gmail.com

1 Life and Health Sciences Research Institute (ICVS), School of Health Sciences, University
of Minho, Braga, Portugal

2 ICVS/3B's-PT Government Associate Laboratory, Braga/Guimarães, Portugal

3 Molecular Oncology Research Center, Barretos Cancer Hospital, Barretos, São Paulo, Brazil

References

[1] Ohgaki, H. and P. Kleihues, *Epidemiology and etiology of gliomas.* Acta Neuropathol, 2005. 109(1): p. 93-108.

[2] Huse, J.T. and E.C. Holland, *Targeting brain cancer: advances in the molecular pathology of malignant glioma and medulloblastoma.* Nat Rev Cancer, 2010. 10(5): p. 319-31.

[3] Louis, D.N., et al., *The 2007 WHO classification of tumours of the central nervous system.* Acta Neuropathol, 2007. 114(2): p. 97-109.

[4] Riemenschneider, M.J. and G. Reifenberger, *Molecular neuropathology of gliomas.* Int J Mol Sci, 2009. 10(1): p. 184-212.

[5] Stupp, R., et al., *Radiotherapy plus concomitant and adjuvant temozolomide for glioblastoma.* N Engl J Med, 2005. 352(10): p. 987-96.

[6] Lai, A., et al., *Phase II study of bevacizumab plus temozolomide during and after radiation therapy for patients with newly diagnosed glioblastoma multiforme.* J Clin Oncol, 2011. 29(2): p. 142-8.

[7] Chinot, O.L., et al., *Bevacizumab plus radiotherapy-temozolomide for newly diagnosed glioblastoma.* N Engl J Med, 2014. 370(8): p. 709-22.

[8] Weathers, S.P. and M.R. Gilbert, *Advances in treating glioblastoma.* F1000Prime Rep, 2014. 6: p. 46.

[9] de Groot, J.F., et al., *Tumor invasion after treatment of glioblastoma with bevacizumab: radiographic and pathologic correlation in humans and mice.* Neuro Oncol, 2010. 12(3): p. 233-42.

[10] Narayana, A., et al., *Bevacizumab in recurrent high-grade pediatric gliomas.* Neuro Oncol, 2010. 12(9): p. 985-90.

[11] Mesti, T., et al., *Metabolic impact of anti-angiogenic agents on U87 glioma cells.* PLoS One, 2014. 9(6): p. e99198.

[12] Gaspar, N., et al., *MGMT-independent temozolomide resistance in pediatric glioblastoma cells associated with a PI3-kinase-mediated HOX/stem cell gene signature.* Cancer Res, 2010. 70(22): p. 9243-52.

[13] Costa, B.M., et al., *Prognostic value of MGMT promoter methylation in glioblastoma patients treated with temozolomide-based chemoradiation: a Portuguese multicentre study.* Oncol Rep, 2010. 23(6): p. 1655-62.

[14] DeBerardinis, R.J., et al., *The biology of cancer: metabolic reprogramming fuels cell growth and proliferation.* Cell Metab, 2008. 7(1): p. 11-20.

[15] DeBerardinis, R.J. and C.B. Thompson, *Cellular metabolism and disease: what do metabolic outliers teach us?* Cell, 2012. 148(6): p. 1132-44.

[16] Vander Heiden, M.G., L.C. Cantley, and C.B. Thompson, *Understanding the Warburg effect: the metabolic requirements of cell proliferation*. Science, 2009. 324(5930): p. 1029-33.

[17] Schulze, A. and A.L. Harris, *How cancer metabolism is tuned for proliferation and vulnerable to disruption*. Nature, 2012. 491(7424): p. 364-73.

[18] Dang, C.V. and G.L. Semenza, *Oncogenic alterations of metabolism*. Trends Biochem Sci, 1999. 24(2): p. 68-72.

[19] Gatenby, R.A. and R.J. Gillies, *A microenvironmental model of carcinogenesis*. Nat Rev Cancer, 2008. 8(1): p. 56-61.

[20] Hanahan, D. and R.A. Weinberg, *Hallmarks of cancer: the next generation*. Cell, 2011. 144(5): p. 646-74.

[21] Gatenby, R.A. and R.J. Gillies, *Why do cancers have high aerobic glycolysis?* Nat Rev Cancer, 2004. 4(11): p. 891-9.

[22] Warburg, O., *On respiratory impairment in cancer cells*. Science, 1956. 124(3215): p. 269-70.

[23] Oudard, S., et al., *High glycolysis in gliomas despite low hexokinase transcription and activity correlated to chromosome 10 loss*. Br J Cancer, 1996. 74(6): p. 839-45.

[24] Tabatabaei, P., et al., *Glucose metabolites, glutamate and glycerol in malignant glioma tumours during radiotherapy*. J Neurooncol, 2008. 90(1): p. 35-9.

[25] Zhao, F.Q. and A.F. Keating, *Functional properties and genomics of glucose transporters*. Curr Genomics, 2007. 8(2): p. 113-28.

[26] Leybaert, L., *Neurobarrier coupling in the brain: a partner of neurovascular and neurometabolic coupling?* J Cereb Blood Flow Metab, 2005. 25(1): p. 2-16.

[27] Medina, R.A. and G.I. Owen, *Glucose transporters: expression, regulation and cancer*. Biol Res, 2002. 35(1): p. 9-26.

[28] Macheda, M.L., S. Rogers, and J.D. Best, *Molecular and cellular regulation of glucose transporter (GLUT) proteins in cancer*. J Cell Physiol, 2005. 202(3): p. 654-62.

[29] Chandler, J.D., et al., *Expression and localization of GLUT1 and GLUT12 in prostate carcinoma*. Cancer, 2003. 97(8): p. 2035-42.

[30] Boado, R.J., K.L. Black, and W.M. Pardridge, *Gene expression of GLUT3 and GLUT1 glucose transporters in human brain tumors*. Brain Res Mol Brain Res, 1994. 27(1): p. 51-7.

[31] Flynn, J.R., et al., *Hypoxia-regulated protein expression, patient characteristics, and preoperative imaging as predictors of survival in adults with glioblastoma multiforme*. Cancer, 2008. 113(5): p. 1032-42.

[32]   Jensen, R.L., *Brain tumor hypoxia: tumorigenesis, angiogenesis, imaging, pseudoprogression, and as a therapeutic target.* J Neurooncol, 2009. 92(3): p. 317-35.

[33]   Stieber, D., S.A. Abdul Rahim, and S.P. Niclou, *Novel ways to target brain tumour metabolism.* Expert Opin Ther Targets, 2011. 15(10): p. 1227-39.

[34]   Smith, T.A., *Mammalian hexokinases and their abnormal expression in cancer.* Br J Biomed Sci, 2000. 57(2): p. 170-8.

[35]   Wilson, J.E., *Isozymes of mammalian hexokinase: structure, subcellular localization and metabolic function.* J Exp Biol, 2003. 206(Pt 12): p. 2049-57.

[36]   Pedersen, P.L., et al., *Mitochondrial bound type II hexokinase: a key player in the growth and survival of many cancers and an ideal prospect for therapeutic intervention.* Biochim Biophys Acta, 2002. 1555(1-3): p. 14-20.

[37]   Wolf, A., et al., *Hexokinase 2 is a key mediator of aerobic glycolysis and promotes tumor growth in human glioblastoma multiforme.* J Exp Med, 2011. 208(2): p. 313-26.

[38]   Agnihotri, S., et al., *A GATA4-regulated tumor suppressor network represses formation of malignant human astrocytomas.* J Exp Med, 2011. 208(4): p. 689-702.

[39]   Mathupala, S.P., Y.H. Ko, and P.L. Pedersen, *Hexokinase-2 bound to mitochondria: cancer's stygian link to the "Warburg Effect" and a pivotal target for effective therapy.* Semin Cancer Biol, 2009. 19(1): p. 17-24.

[40]   Mellinghoff, I.K., et al., *Molecular determinants of the response of glioblastomas to EGFR kinase inhibitors.* N Engl J Med, 2005. 353(19): p. 2012-24.

[41]   Pastorino, J.G., N. Shulga, and J.B. Hoek, *Mitochondrial binding of hexokinase II inhibits Bax-induced cytochrome c release and apoptosis.* J Biol Chem, 2002. 277(9): p. 7610-8.

[42]   Wolf, A., S. Agnihotri, and A. Guha, *Targeting metabolic remodeling in glioblastoma multiforme.* Oncotarget, 2010. 1(7): p. 552-62.

[43]   Wolf, A., et al., *Developmental profile and regulation of the glycolytic enzyme hexokinase 2 in normal brain and glioblastoma multiforme.* Neurobiol Dis, 2011. 44(1): p. 84-91.

[44]   Ko, Y.H., et al., *Advanced cancers: eradication in all cases using 3-bromopyruvate therapy to deplete ATP.* Biochem Biophys Res Commun, 2004. 324(1): p. 269-75.

[45]   Oudard, S., et al., *Phase II study of lonidamine and diazepam in the treatment of recurrent glioblastoma multiforme.* J Neurooncol, 2003. 63(1): p. 81-6.

[46]   Carapella, C.M., et al., *The potential role of lonidamine (LND) in the treatment of malignant glioma. Phase II study.* J Neurooncol, 1989. 7(1): p. 103-8.

[47]   Liu, H., Y. Li, and K.P. Raisch, *Clotrimazole induces a late G1 cell cycle arrest and sensitizes glioblastoma cells to radiation in vitro.* Anticancer Drugs, 2010. 21(9): p. 841-9.

[48] Khalid, M.H., et al., *Inhibition of tumor growth and prolonged survival of rats with intracranial gliomas following administration of clotrimazole.* J Neurosurg, 2005. 103(1): p. 79-86.

[49] Altenberg, B. and K.O. Greulich, *Genes of glycolysis are ubiquitously overexpressed in 24 cancer classes.* Genomics, 2004. 84(6): p. 1014-20.

[50] Mazurek, S., et al., *Pyruvate kinase type M2 and its role in tumor growth and spreading.* Semin Cancer Biol, 2005. 15(4): p. 300-8.

[51] Mazurek, S., et al., *Pyruvate kinase type M2: a crossroad in the tumor metabolome.* Br J Nutr, 2002. 87 Suppl 1: p. S23-9.

[52] Christofk, H.R., et al., *Pyruvate kinase M2 is a phosphotyrosine-binding protein.* Nature, 2008. 452(7184): p. 181-6.

[53] Eigenbrodt, E., et al., *Double role for pyruvate kinase type M2 in the expansion of phosphometabolite pools found in tumor cells.* Crit Rev Oncog, 1992. 3(1-2): p. 91-115.

[54] Christofk, H.R., et al., *The M2 splice isoform of pyruvate kinase is important for cancer metabolism and tumour growth.* Nature, 2008. 452(7184): p. 230-3.

[55] Kefas, B., et al., *Pyruvate kinase M2 is a target of the tumor-suppressive microRNA-326 and regulates the survival of glioma cells.* Neuro Oncol, 2010. 12(11): p. 1102-12.

[56] Soga, T., *Cancer metabolism: key players in metabolic reprogramming.* Cancer Sci, 2013. 104(3): p. 275-81.

[57] Goidts, V., et al., *RNAi screening in glioma stem-like cells identifies PFKFB4 as a key molecule important for cancer cell survival.* Oncogene, 2012. 31(27): p. 3235-43.

[58] Yang, W., et al., *PKM2 phosphorylates histone H3 and promotes gene transcription and tumorigenesis.* Cell, 2012. 150(4): p. 685-96.

[59] Yang, W., et al., *EGFR-induced and PKCepsilon monoubiquitylation-dependent NF-kappaB activation upregulates PKM2 expression and promotes tumorigenesis.* Mol Cell, 2012. 48(5): p. 771-84.

[60] Yang, W., et al., *ERK1/2-dependent phosphorylation and nuclear translocation of PKM2 promotes the Warburg effect.* Nat Cell Biol, 2012. 14(12): p. 1295-304.

[61] Katsetos, C.D., H. Anni, and P. Draber, *Mitochondrial dysfunction in gliomas.* Semin Pediatr Neurol, 2013. 20(3): p. 216-27.

[62] Warburg, O., *On the origin of cancer cells.* Science, 1956. 123(3191): p. 309-14.

[63] Pedersen, P.L., *Tumor mitochondria and the bioenergetics of cancer cells.* Prog Exp Tumor Res, 1978. 22: p. 190-274.

[64] Meixensberger, J., et al., *Metabolic patterns in malignant gliomas.* J Neurooncol, 1995. 24(2): p. 153-61.

[65] Seyfried, T.N. and P. Mukherjee, *Targeting energy metabolism in brain cancer: review and hypothesis.* Nutr Metab (Lond), 2005. 2: p. 30.

[66] Seyfried, T.N., et al., *Metabolic management of brain cancer.* Biochim Biophys Acta, 2011. 1807(6): p. 577-94.

[67] Kim, J.W., et al., *HIF-1-mediated expression of pyruvate dehydrogenase kinase: a metabolic switch required for cellular adaptation to hypoxia.* Cell Metab, 2006. 3(3): p. 177-85.

[68] Michelakis, E.D., L. Webster, and J.R. Mackey, *Dichloroacetate (DCA) as a potential metabolic-targeting therapy for cancer.* Br J Cancer, 2008. 99(7): p. 989-94.

[69] Michelakis, E.D., et al., *Metabolic modulation of glioblastoma with dichloroacetate.* Sci Transl Med, 2010. 2(31): p. 31ra34.

[70] Bonnet, S., et al., *A mitochondria-K+channel axis is suppressed in cancer and its normalization promotes apoptosis and inhibits cancer growth.* Cancer Cell, 2007. 11(1): p. 37-51.

[71] Cairns, R.A., et al., *Metabolic targeting of hypoxia and HIF1 in solid tumors can enhance cytotoxic chemotherapy.* Proc Natl Acad Sci U S A, 2007. 104(22): p. 9445-50.

[72] Cao, W., et al., *Dichloroacetate (DCA) sensitizes both wild-type and over expressing Bcl-2 prostate cancer cells in vitro to radiation.* Prostate, 2008. 68(11): p. 1223-31.

[73] Wong, J.Y., et al., *Dichloroacetate induces apoptosis in endometrial cancer cells.* Gynecol Oncol, 2008. 109(3): p. 394-402.

[74] Duan, Y., et al., *Antitumor activity of dichloroacetate on C6 glioma cell: in vitro and in vivo evaluation.* Onco Targets Ther, 2013. 6: p. 189-98.

[75] Reitman, Z.J. and H. Yan, *Isocitrate dehydrogenase 1 and 2 mutations in cancer: alterations at a crossroads of cellular metabolism.* J Natl Cancer Inst, 2010. 102(13): p. 932-41.

[76] Kim, W. and L.M. Liau, *IDH mutations in human glioma.* Neurosurg Clin N Am, 2012. 23(3): p. 471-80.

[77] Parsons, D.W., et al., *An integrated genomic analysis of human glioblastoma multiforme.* Science, 2008. 321(5897): p. 1807-12.

[78] Yan, H., et al., *IDH1 and IDH2 mutations in gliomas.* N Engl J Med, 2009. 360(8): p. 765-73.

[79] Fu, Y., et al., *Glioma-derived mutations in IDH: from mechanism to potential therapy.* Biochem Biophys Res Commun, 2010. 397(2): p. 127-30.

[80] DeAngelis, L.M. and I.K. Mellinghoff, *Virchow 2011 or how to ID(H) human glioblastoma.* J Clin Oncol, 2011. 29(34): p. 4473-4.

[81] Watanabe, T., et al., *IDH1 mutations are early events in the development of astrocytomas and oligodendrogliomas.* Am J Pathol, 2009. 174(4): p. 1149-53.

[82] Verhaak, R.G., et al., *Integrated genomic analysis identifies clinically relevant subtypes of glioblastoma characterized by abnormalities in PDGFRA, IDH1, EGFR, and NF1.* Cancer Cell, 2010. 17(1): p. 98-110.

[83] Zhao, S., et al., *Glioma-derived mutations in IDH1 dominantly inhibit IDH1 catalytic activity and induce HIF-1alpha.* Science, 2009. 324(5924): p. 261-5.

[84] Ward, P.S., et al., *The common feature of leukemia-associated IDH1 and IDH2 mutations is a neomorphic enzyme activity converting alpha-ketoglutarate to 2-hydroxyglutarate.* Cancer Cell, 2010. 17(3): p. 225-34.

[85] Dang, L., et al., *Cancer-associated IDH1 mutations produce 2-hydroxyglutarate.* Nature, 2009. 462(7274): p. 739-44.

[86] Lu, C. and C.B. Thompson, *Metabolic regulation of epigenetics.* Cell Metab, 2012. 16(1): p. 9-17.

[87] Zielke, H.R., C.L. Zielke, and P.T. Ozand, *Glutamine: a major energy source for cultured mammalian cells.* Fed Proc, 1984. 43(1): p. 121-5.

[88] Reitzer, L.J., B.M. Wice, and D. Kennell, *Evidence that glutamine, not sugar, is the major energy source for cultured HeLa cells.* J Biol Chem, 1979. 254(8): p. 2669-76.

[89] DeBerardinis, R.J., et al., *Beyond aerobic glycolysis: transformed cells can engage in glutamine metabolism that exceeds the requirement for protein and nucleotide synthesis.* Proc Natl Acad Sci U S A, 2007. 104(49): p. 19345-50.

[90] Rajagopalan, K.N. and R.J. DeBerardinis, *Role of glutamine in cancer: therapeutic and imaging implications.* J Nucl Med, 2011. 52(7): p. 1005-8.

[91] Daye, D. and K.E. Wellen, *Metabolic reprogramming in cancer: unraveling the role of glutamine in tumorigenesis.* Semin Cell Dev Biol, 2012. 23(4): p. 362-9.

[92] Dang, C.V., A. Le, and P. Gao, *MYC-induced cancer cell energy metabolism and therapeutic opportunities.* Clin Cancer Res, 2009. 15(21): p. 6479-83.

[93] Rathore, M.G., et al., *The NF-kappaB member p65 controls glutamine metabolism through miR-23a.* Int J Biochem Cell Biol, 2012. 44(9): p. 1448-56.

[94] Wang, J.B., et al., *Targeting mitochondrial glutaminase activity inhibits oncogenic transformation.* Cancer Cell, 2010. 18(3): p. 207-19.

[95] Kallenberg, K., et al., *Untreated glioblastoma multiforme: increased myo-inositol and glutamine levels in the contralateral cerebral hemisphere at proton MR spectroscopy.* Radiology, 2009. 253(3): p. 805-12.

[96] Rosati, A., et al., *Epilepsy in glioblastoma multiforme: correlation with glutamine synthetase levels.* J Neurooncol, 2009. 93(3): p. 319-24.

[97] Menendez, J.A. and R. Lupu, *Fatty acid synthase and the lipogenic phenotype in cancer pathogenesis.* Nat Rev Cancer, 2007. 7(10): p. 763-77.

[98]   Abramson, H.N., *The lipogenesis pathway as a cancer target.* J Med Chem, 2011. 54(16): p. 5615-38.

[99]   Gopal, K., et al., *Lipid Composition of Human Intracranial Tumors: A Biochemical Study.* Acta Neurochir (Wien), 1963. 11: p. 333-47.

[100] Guo, D., et al., *EGFR signaling through an Akt-SREBP-1-dependent, rapamycin-resistant pathway sensitizes glioblastomas to antilipogenic therapy.* Sci Signal, 2009. 2(101): p. ra82.

[101] Tugnoli, V., et al., *Characterization of lipids from human brain tissues by multinuclear magnetic resonance spectroscopy.* Biopolymers, 2001. 62(6): p. 297-306.

[102] Yates, A.J., et al., *Lipid composition of human neural tumors.* J Lipid Res, 1979. 20(4): p. 428-36.

[103] Rudling, M.J., et al., *Low density lipoprotein receptor activity in human intracranial tumors and its relation to the cholesterol requirement.* Cancer Res, 1990. 50(3): p. 483-7.

[104] Dhup, S., et al., *Multiple biological activities of lactic acid in cancer: influences on tumor growth, angiogenesis and metastasis.* Curr Pharm Des, 2012. 18(10): p. 1319-30.

[105] Hirschhaeuser, F., U.G. Sattler, and W. Mueller-Klieser, *Lactate: a metabolic key player in cancer.* Cancer Res, 2011. 71(22): p. 6921-5.

[106] Baumann, F., et al., *Lactate promotes glioma migration by TGF-beta2-dependent regulation of matrix metalloproteinase-2.* Neuro Oncol, 2009. 11(4): p. 368-80.

[107] Halestrap, A.P. and N.T. Price, *The proton-linked monocarboxylate transporter (MCT) family: structure, function and regulation.* Biochem J, 1999. 343 Pt 2: p. 281-99.

[108] Enerson, B.E. and L.R. Drewes, *Molecular features, regulation, and function of monocarboxylate transporters: implications for drug delivery.* J Pharm Sci, 2003. 92(8): p. 1531-44.

[109] Pinheiro, C., et al., *Role of monocarboxylate transporters in human cancers: state of the art.* J Bioenerg Biomembr, 2012. 44(1): p. 127-39.

[110] Froberg, M.K., et al., *Expression of monocarboxylate transporter MCT1 in normal and neoplastic human CNS tissues.* Neuroreport, 2001. 12(4): p. 761-5.

[111] Miranda-Goncalves, V., et al., *Monocarboxylate transporters (MCTs) in gliomas: expression and exploitation as therapeutic targets.* Neuro Oncol, 2013. 15(2): p. 172-88.

[112] Fang, J., et al., *The H+-linked monocarboxylate transporter (MCT1/SLC16A1): a potential therapeutic target for high-risk neuroblastoma.* Mol Pharmacol, 2006. 70(6): p. 2108-15.

[113] Li, K.K., et al., *miR-124 is frequently down-regulated in medulloblastoma and is a negative regulator of SLC16A1.* Hum Pathol, 2009. 40(9): p. 1234-43.

[114] Colen, C.B., et al., *Metabolic targeting of lactate efflux by malignant glioma inhibits invasiveness and induces necrosis: an in vivo study.* Neoplasia, 2011. 13(7): p. 620-32.

[115] Colen, C.B., et al., *Metabolic remodeling of malignant gliomas for enhanced sensitization during radiotherapy: an in vitro study.* Neurosurgery, 2006. 59(6): p. 1313-23; discussion 1323-4.

[116] Pouyssegur, J., F. Dayan, and N.M. Mazure, *Hypoxia signalling in cancer and approaches to enforce tumour regression.* Nature, 2006. 441(7092): p. 437-43.

[117] Sonveaux, P., et al., *Targeting lactate-fueled respiration selectively kills hypoxic tumor cells in mice.* J Clin Invest, 2008. 118(12): p. 3930-42.

[118] Bueno, V., et al., *The specific monocarboxylate transporter (MCT1) inhibitor, AR-C117977, a novel immunosuppressant, prolongs allograft survival in the mouse.* Transplantation, 2007. 84(9): p. 1204-7.

[119] Porporato, P.E., et al., *Anticancer targets in the glycolytic metabolism of tumors: a comprehensive review.* Front Pharmacol, 2011. 2: p. 49.

[120] Damaghi, M., J.W. Wojtkowiak, and R.J. Gillies, *pH sensing and regulation in cancer.* Front Physiol, 2013. 4: p. 370.

[121] Supuran, C.T., *Carbonic anhydrases: novel therapeutic applications for inhibitors and activators.* Nat Rev Drug Discov, 2008. 7(2): p. 168-81.

[122] Tureci, O., et al., *Human carbonic anhydrase XII: cDNA cloning, expression, and chromosomal localization of a carbonic anhydrase gene that is overexpressed in some renal cell cancers.* Proc Natl Acad Sci U S A, 1998. 95(13): p. 7608-13.

[123] Hilvo, M., et al., *Biochemical characterization of CA IX, one of the most active carbonic anhydrase isozymes.* J Biol Chem, 2008. 283(41): p. 27799-809.

[124] Brahimi-Horn, M.C., G. Bellot, and J. Pouyssegur, *Hypoxia and energetic tumour metabolism.* Curr Opin Genet Dev, 2011. 21(1): p. 67-72.

[125] Chiche, J., M.C. Brahimi-Horn, and J. Pouyssegur, *Tumour hypoxia induces a metabolic shift causing acidosis: a common feature in cancer.* J Cell Mol Med, 2010. 14(4): p. 771-94.

[126] Proescholdt, M.A., et al., *Function of carbonic anhydrase IX in glioblastoma multiforme.* Neuro Oncol, 2012. 14(11): p. 1357-66.

[127] Zatovicova, M., et al., *Carbonic anhydrase IX as an anticancer therapy target: preclinical evaluation of internalizing monoclonal antibody directed to catalytic domain.* Curr Pharm Des, 2010. 16(29): p. 3255-63.

[128] Sedlakova, O., et al., *Carbonic anhydrase IX, a hypoxia-induced catalytic component of the pH regulating machinery in tumors.* Front Physiol, 2014. 4: p. 400.

[129] Currie, M.J., et al., *Immunohistochemical analysis of cancer stem cell markers in invasive breast carcinoma and associated ductal carcinoma in situ: relationships with markers of tumor hypoxia and microvascularity.* Hum Pathol, 2013. 44(3): p. 402-11.

[130] McIntyre, A., et al., *Carbonic anhydrase IX promotes tumor growth and necrosis in vivo and inhibition enhances anti-VEGF therapy.* Clin Cancer Res, 2012. 18(11): p. 3100-11.

[131] De Simone, G., et al., *Carbonic anhydrase inhibitors: Hypoxia-activatable sulfonamides incorporating disulfide bonds that target the tumor-associated isoform IX.* J Med Chem, 2006. 49(18): p. 5544-51.

[132] Maresca, A., et al., *Non-zinc mediated inhibition of carbonic anhydrases: coumarins are a new class of suicide inhibitors.* J Am Chem Soc, 2009. 131(8): p. 3057-62.

[133] Maresca, A., et al., *Deciphering the mechanism of carbonic anhydrase inhibition with coumarins and thiocoumarins.* J Med Chem, 2010. 53(1): p. 335-44.

[134] Chrastina, A., S. Pastorekova, and J. Pastorek, *Immunotargeting of human cervical carcinoma xenograft expressing CA IX tumor-associated antigen by 125I-labeled M75 monoclonal antibody.* Neoplasma, 2003. 50(1): p. 13-21.

[135] Siebels, M., et al., A clinical phase I/II trial with the monoclonal antibody cG250 (RENCAREX(R)) and interferon-alpha-2a in metastatic renal cell carcinoma patients. World J Urol, 2011. 29(1): p. 121-6.

Permissions

All chapters in this book were first published by InTech Open; hereby published with permission under the Creative Commons Attribution License or equivalent. Every chapter published in this book has been scrutinized by our experts. Their significance has been extensively debated. The topics covered herein carry significant findings which will fuel the growth of the discipline. They may even be implemented as practical applications or may be referred to as a beginning point for another development.

The contributors of this book come from diverse backgrounds, making this book a truly international effort. This book will bring forth new frontiers with its revolutionizing research information and detailed analysis of the nascent developments around the world.

We would like to thank all the contributing authors for lending their expertise to make the book truly unique. They have played a crucial role in the development of this book. Without their invaluable contributions this book wouldn't have been possible. They have made vital efforts to compile up to date information on the varied aspects of this subject to make this book a valuable addition to the collection of many professionals and students.

This book was conceptualized with the vision of imparting up-to-date information and advanced data in this field. To ensure the same, a matchless editorial board was set up. Every individual on the board went through rigorous rounds of assessment to prove their worth. After which they invested a large part of their time researching and compiling the most relevant data for our readers.

The editorial board has been involved in producing this book since its inception. They have spent rigorous hours researching and exploring the diverse topics which have resulted in the successful publishing of this book. They have passed on their knowledge of decades through this book. To expedite this challenging task, the publisher supported the team at every step. A small team of assistant editors was also appointed to further simplify the editing procedure and attain best results for the readers.

Apart from the editorial board, the designing team has also invested a significant amount of their time in understanding the subject and creating the most relevant covers. They scrutinized every image to scout for the most suitable representation of the subject and create an appropriate cover for the book.

The publishing team has been an ardent support to the editorial, designing and production team. Their endless efforts to recruit the best for this project, has resulted in the accomplishment of this book. They are a veteran in the field of academics and their pool of knowledge is as vast as their experience in printing. Their expertise and guidance has proved useful at every step. Their uncompromising quality standards have made this book an exceptional effort. Their encouragement from time to time has been an inspiration for everyone.

The publisher and the editorial board hope that this book will prove to be a valuable piece of knowledge for researchers, students, practitioners and scholars across the globe.

List of Contributors

Caroline Agha, Hannah C. Machemehl and Hassan M. Fathallah-Shaykh
The University of Alabama at Birmingham, Department of Neurology, USA

Zhihua Yang
Department of Neurology, the First Affiliated Hospital, Guangzhou Medical University, Guangdong, China

Shoumin Bai
Department of Oncology, Sun Yat-Sen Memorial Hospital, Sun Yat-Sen University, Guangdong, China

Beibei Gu and Shuling Peng
Department of Anesthesiology, Sun Yat-Sen Memorial Hospital, Sun Yat-Sen University, Guangdong, China

Wang Liao and Jun Liu
Department of Neurology, Sun Yat-Sen Memorial Hospital, Sun Yat-Sen University, Guangdong, China

Mohammad M. Hossain and Mehdi H. Shahi
Interdisciplinary Brain Research Centre, Faculty of Medicine, Aligarh Muslim University, Aligarh, India

Bárbara Meléndez
Molecular Pathology Research Unit, Virgen de la Salud Hospital, Toledo, Spain

Juan A. Rey
IdiPaz Research Unit, La Paz University Hospital, Madrid, Spain

Javier S. Castresana
Department of Biochemistry and Genetics, University of Navarra School of Sciences, Pamplona, Spain

Krzysztof Siemianowicz
Department of Biochemistry, School of Medicine in Katowice, Medical University of Silesia, Poland

Wirginia Likus
Department of Human Anatomy, School of Medicine in Katowice, Medical University of Silesia, Poland

Jarosław Markowski
Department of Laryngology, School of Medicine in Katowice, Medical University of Silesia, Poland

Abdul Aziz Mohamed Yusoff, Farizan Ahmad and Zamzuri Idris
Department of Neurosciences, School of Medical Sciences, Universiti Sains Malaysia, Health Campus, Kubang Kerian, Kelantan, Malaysia

Hasnan Jaafar
Department of Pathology, School of Medical Sciences, Universiti Sains Malaysia, Health Campus, Kubang Kerian, Kelantan, Malaysia

Jafri Malin Abdullah
Department of Neurosciences, School of Medical Sciences, Universiti Sains Malaysia, Health Campus, Kubang Kerian, Kelantan, Malaysia
Center for Neuroscience Services and Research, Universiti Sains Malaysia, Health Campus, Kubang Kerian, Kelantan, Malaysia

Adrianna Ranger
Department of Clinical Neurological Sciences, Division of Neurosurgery, Children's Hospital-London Health Sciences Center, Western University, London, Ontario, Canada

David Diosy
Department of Clinical Neurological Sciences, Division of Neurology, London Health Sciences Center, Western University, London, Ontario, Canada

Ryuya Yamanaka and Azusa Hayano
Graduate School for Health Care Science, Kyoto Prefectural University of Medicine, Kyoto, Japan

Davide Schiffer, Marta Mellai and Laura Annovazzi
Neuro-Bio-Oncology Research Center / Policlinico di Monza Foundation, Consorzio di Neuroscienze, University of Pavia, Vercelli, Italy

Cristina Casalone
Istituto Zooprofilattico, Turin, Italy

Paola Cassoni
Dpt. Medical Sciences, University of Turin, Turin, Italy

Kaveh Asadi-Moghaddam and Todd W. Vitaz
Department of Clinical Neurosciences Spectrum Health Medical Group, and College of Human Medicine, Michigan State University, Grand Rapids, Michigan, USA

Vera Miranda Gonçalves and Fátima Baltazar
Life and Health Sciences Research Institute (ICVS), School of Health Sciences, University of Minho, Braga, Portugal
ICVS/3B's-PT Government Associate Laboratory, Braga/Guimarães, Portugal

Rui Manuel Reis
Life and Health Sciences Research Institute (ICVS), School of Health Sciences, University of Minho, Braga, Portugal
ICVS/3B's-PT Government Associate Laboratory, Braga/Guimarães, Portugal
Molecular Oncology Research Center, Barretos Cancer Hospital, Barretos, São Paulo, Brazil

Index

Printed in the USA
CPSIA information can be obtained
at www.ICGtesting.com
JSHW051349091023
49903JS00006B/83